T

A

P
mu
rea

Chemical Endocrinology

Chemical Endocrinology

EDWARD H. FRIEDEN

Department of Chemistry
Kent State University
Kent, Ohio

ACADEMIC PRESS New York San Francisco London 1976
A Subsidiary of Harcourt Brace Jovanovich, Publishers

ACADEMIC PRESS, INC.
111 Fifth Avenue, New York, New York 10003

United Kingdom Edition published by
ACADEMIC PRESS, INC. (LONDON) LTD.
24/28 Oval Road, London NW1

Library of Congress Cataloging in Publication Data

Frieden, Edward H
Chemical endocrinology.

Bibliography: p.
Includes index.
1. Hormones. 2. Endocrinology. I. Title.
[DNLM: 1. Hormones–Physiology. WK102 F911c]
QP571.F74 596'.01'927 75-13103
ISBN 0–12–268150–9

PRINTED IN THE UNITED STATES OF AMERICA

Contents

Preface

Although the biochemical and endocrinological disciplines have maintained a close working relationship for more than half a century, the particularly fruitful collaboration which has developed between these two during the past two or three decades has resulted in a rapid expansion of knowledge in several areas. One such area is chemical endocrinology, which is concerned with the chemical nature of the naturally occurring hormones, their chemical structures, and their biological activities. A related topic concerns the effect of evolutionary change on hormone structure. Although this aspect is still in its formative stages, it is nevertheless already possible to propose reasonable schemes for the evolution of several important groups of hormones.

Much of the considerable accumulated information concerning these topics has found its way into permanent summaries to be found on library shelves. With a few notable exceptions, however, the available texts are specialized, either in content or in terms of the audience to which they are directed. The impetus for this book arose from the conviction that a reasonably compact source of information would be welcomed not only by endocrinologists but by students and investigators in other fields as well.

The text begins with a brief description of the biological functions of the products of the endocrine glands. The main body of the work is organized around detailed descriptions of the chemistry of the several hormones. In addition, because of the importance I attach to the relationship between structure and function, a separate chapter on the principles of hormone bioassay is included, and bioassay procedures for most of the hormones are described in considerable detail.

Preparation of the manuscript was made possible in part by a research time grant from the Research Committee of Kent State University. I would also like to acknowledge my indebtedness to Dr. Felix Bronner for his patient and constructive editorial advice and to my colleagues Dr. Walter Adams and Dr. Allen Rawitch for reading parts of the text. Most of all I am indebted to my wife Betty, not only for her help in final manuscript preparation but also for her constant support and encouragement. To her this volume is affectionately dedicated.

Edward H. Frieden

List of Abbreviations

ACTH	Adrenocorticotropic hormone; corticotropin
cAMP	3′,5′-Adenosine monophosphate; cyclic AMP
CBG	Corticosteroid-binding globulin
CCK–PZ	Cholecystokinin–pancreozymin
CG	Chorionic gonadotropin
CG-α,β; FSH-α,β; LH-α,β; TSH-α,β	Dissociable glycopeptide subunits of the glycoprotein hormones
CRH	Corticotropin-releasing hormone
CS	Chorionic somatomammotropin; placental lactogen
CT	Calcitonin
DOC	11-Deoxycorticosterone
f/f_0	Asymmetry ratio
FSH	Follicle-stimulating hormone
FSH-RH	Follicle-stimulating hormone-releasing hormone
GH	Growth hormone; somatotropin
GH-RH	Growth hormone-releasing hormone
GH-RIH	Growth hormone-release-inhibiting hormone
Gon-RH	Gonadotropin (FSH and LH)-releasing hormone
Hgb	Hemoglobin
HMG	Human menopausal gonadotropin
K_m	Michaelis constant
LGH	"Large" growth hormone
LH	Luteinizing hormone
LH-RH	Luteinizing hormone-releasing hormone
LtH	Luteotropic hormone, prolactin
MRH	MSH-releasing hormone
MRIH	MSH release-inhibiting hormone
MSH	Melanocyte-stimulating hormone
NEFA	Nonesterified fatty acids
NIH-FSH-S1, NIH-LH, etc.	Hormone reference standards made available by the National Institutes of Health; NIH-FSH-S1 refers to the first of several FSH standards which have been used
NLe	Norleucine

PL	Placental lactogen; chorionic somatomammotropin
Pr	Prolactin; luteotropic hormone
Pr-RH	Prolactin-releasing hormone
Pr-RIH	Prolactin release-inhibiting hormone
PRS	Pregnant rabbit serum
PTH	Parathyroid hormone
s	Sedimentation coefficient
SDS	Sodium dodecyl sulfate
SHBG	Sex hormone-binding globulin
STH	Somatotropin; growth hormone
TBG	Thyroxine-binding globulin
TP	Testosterone propionate
TRH	Thyrotropin-releasing hormone
v, V	Observed and maximum velocities, respectively, of enzyme-catalyzed reactions

Protein hormones from particular species are identified by single letter prefixes: b, bovine; c, canine; h, human; m, monkey; o, ovine; p, porcine; r, rat; etc.

1

Biological Actions of the Hormones

I. Biological Actions of the Thyroid Hormones

In warm-blooded vertebrates, few organs or tissues are free of the influence of the thyroid hormones thyroxine and triiodothyronine. In a very profound way, growth, development, maturation, and reproduction all depend upon a functional thyroid gland. Thyroid deficiency in early life results in the retention of infantile characteristics and dwarfism. If the gland is absent or inactive during a critical period in early life (10–24 days in the rat; 0–1 year in man) normal mental development is irreversibly inhibited and the condition known as *cretinism* results. Subsequently, the continued absence of thyroid secretion results in delay of skeletal maturation and deposition of bone mineral. In many species, gonadal impairment occurs as a result of thyroid hormone deficiency.

One of the best-known indices of thyroid function is its effect upon energy production and oxygen consumption. Heat production and oxygen consumption in homeothermic (warm-blooded) animals are invariably decreased in thyroidectomized animals and increased in hyperthyroid animals. The metabolic effects of iodinated thyronines upon the whole animal are paralleled by effects upon oxygen consumption of various tissues *in vitro;* tissues from thyroidectomized animals displayed lower Q_{O_2}'s than normally observed and those from thyroid-treated animals higher Q_{O_2}'s than normally observed. Liver, heart, and skeletal muscle are most prominently affected, while kidney and brain show reduced responses.

In cold-blooded animals, thyroid effects upon oxygen consumption are difficult to observe and may depend upon the environmental temperature. In some lizards, for example, neither thyroidectomy nor the administration of thyroid extracts affects oxygen consumption if the animals are maintained at 25°; if the temperature is raised to 30°, however, typical effects of thyroid depletion or replacement are observed.

One of the most spectacular expressions of the action of thyroid hormone—indeed, of any hormone—is the induction of metamorphosis in lower vertebrates. The relationship between the thyroid and amphibian metamorphosis was one of the seminal observations of endocrinology, Gudernatsch, in 1912, having observed that feeding thyroid tissue would accelerate the metamorphosis of tadpoles and salamanders. In sensitive species (e.g., *Rana*) thyroidectomy (or hypophysectomy) results in indefinite delay of metamorphosis; the larvae, meanwhile, continue to grow and may reach truly enormous size. In contrast, midget-sized adults may be produced by premature treatment of young tadpoles with thyroid extracts or thyroxine. Both anuran (frogs, toads) and urodele (salamanders, newts) larval metamorphosis are controlled by thyroid secretion.

The multifarious effects of the thyroid hormones appear to have a common basis in their effects upon nucleic acid and protein metabolism. Their growth-promoting effects, as well as their calorigenic and differentiating effects, are blocked by agents (such as actinomycin D and puromycin) which inhibit RNA and protein synthesis. The earliest biochemical event which can be recognized in livers of thyroidectomized rats following a single injection of thyroxine, for example, is initiation of the synthesis of rapidly labeled nuclear RNA; this is followed by the synthesis of nuclear RNA polymerase, of mitochondrial and microsomal proteins, and subsequently, of oxidative enzymes (Frieden and Lipner, 1971). In tadpoles, the initiation of metamorphosis is preceded by the initiation of synthesis of a constellation of new proteins, including hemoglobin, hydrolases, and urea cycle enzymes.

II. Biological Actions of the Adrenal Hormones

The adrenal gland is composed of two kinds of tissue of separate embryonic origin which, in mammals, are organized into medullary (internal) and cortical (external) regions. In other vertebrates this convenient anatomical arrangement does not exist; however, the cytological and functional differentiation of the two kinds of tissue persist in nonmammalian species as well.

Adrenal medullary tissue characteristically secretes two physiologically active substances—epinephrine and norepinephrine—often referred to as catecholamines. Their relative proportions vary with the species; for instance, whale adrenals contain approximately four times as much norepinephrine as epinephrine. In contrast, the adrenals of baboons, rabbits, and guinea pigs contain little or no norepinephrine.

The characteristic effects of epinephrine are exerted in two directions—upon the cardiovascular system and upon carbohydrate metabolism. Epinephrine increases the force, amplitude, and frequency of the heartbeat; at the same time, the peripheral circulatory resistance decreases because skeletal blood vessels are dilated. The result is therefore an increase of systolic blood pressure and a considerable increase in cardiac output. Norepinephrine, on the other hand, constricts the blood vessels of the muscles, viscera, and skin, thus *increasing* total peripheral resistance. In response, both systolic and diastolic blood pressures increase. Thus, both hormones increase blood pressure, but for different reasons.

Epinephrine, acting via adenyl cyclase is glycogenolytic, stimulating the conversion of liver and muscle glycogen, first to glucose 1-phosphate, and subsequently, in the liver, to glucose. Hyperglycemia may therefore result. In fasted animals, with depleted stores of liver glycogen, the principal effect is upon muscle glycogen—glycogenolysis followed by glycolysis to lactic acid. The lactate thus produced is reconverted to glycogen in the liver. The overall result may, therefore, be an increase in liver glycogen at the expense of muscle glycogen.

Epinephrine also increases oxygen consumption and basal metabolic rate, although massive doses may depress both. Norepinephrine, however, is calorigenic only in cold-adapted animals. The principal cardiovascular and metabolic effects of the catecholamines are summarized in Figs. 1.1 and 1.2.

In addition to their cardiovascular, glycogenolytic, and calorigenic effects, the adrenal catecholamines exert a number of peripheral metabolic effects. Epinephrine stimulates the release of ACTH from the anterior pituitary; this hormone, in turn, evokes the release of other hormones from the adrenal cortex. The latter hormones are gluconeogenic—promoting the conversion of amino acids and protein to glucose. In addition, both catecholamines cause a rise in the concentration of free fatty acids in plasma, probably as a result of lipolysis.

As far as is known, the adrenal medullary hormones, while important agents of homeostasis, are not essential for life. It is quite the contrary with the group of compounds secreted by the adrenal cortex. Unless carefully

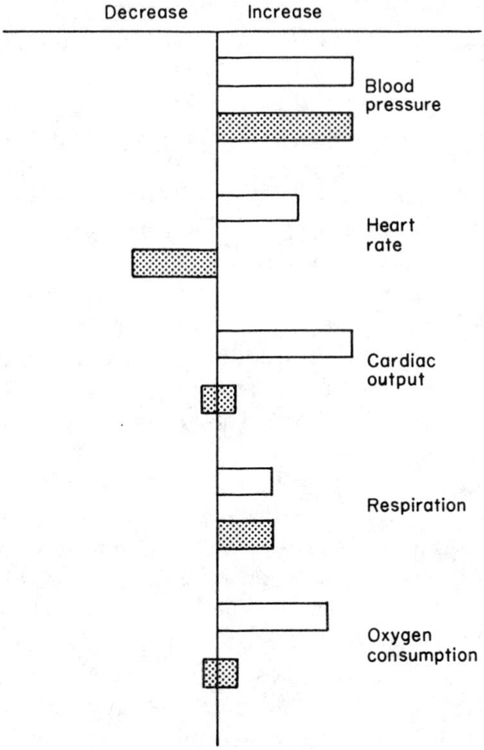

Fig. 1.1 *Comparison of the effects of epinephrine (open bars) and norepinephrine (shaded bars) upon some cardiovascular parameters in man. Bar lengths indicate relative magnitudes when the drugs were infused intravenously.*

maintained, adrenalectomized laboratory animals frequently die within a few days. The death sentence may, however, be stayed indefinitely by the administration of adrenal cortical extracts or salt solutions.

A convenient, though not entirely precise, generalization divides the metabolically active corticoids into two main groups—the *mineralocorticoids* and the *glucocorticoids*. The mineralocorticoids, which are also the most potent in terms of their ability to maintain life in adrenalectomized animals, exert their predominant effects upon body electrolytes and body water. Examples of naturally occurring mineralocorticoids include 11-deoxycorticosterone (DOC) and 18-oxocorticosterone (aldosterone). In mammals an absolute or relative mineralocorticoid insufficiency results in excessive loss of sodium and chloride ions and excessive retention of potassium ions. In consequences of the loss of sodium ions a diuresis also occurs; a metabolic

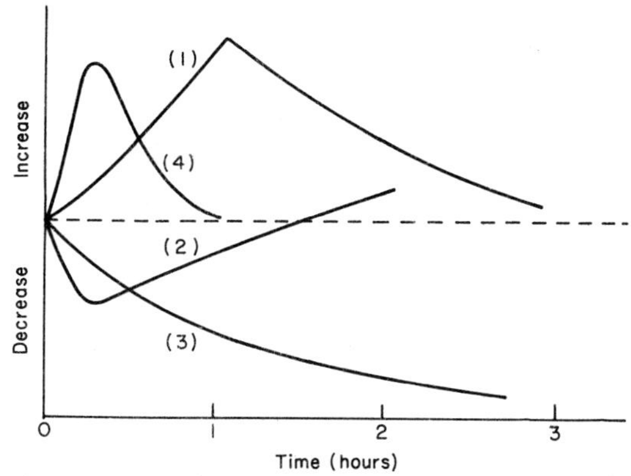

Fig. 1.2 *Time course of metabolic events following a single injection of epinephrine in rats.* (1) *Blood glucose;* (2) *liver glycogen;* (3) *muscle glycogen;* (4) *plasma free fatty acids.*

acidosis may also ensue. All of these symptoms are readily reversed when mineralocorticoids are supplied. Their primary action is to increase tubular reabsorption of sodium chloride and sodium bicarbonate and to promote the exchange of intracellular potassium for sodium.

Electrolyte metabolism is also under adrenal cortical control in other vertebrates, including birds and fishes. The nasal gland of marine birds (for example, albatrosses) secretes a fluid of very high salt content (this enables the albatross to drink seawater), and nasal gland function is under adrenal cortical control. In euryhaline fishes sodium influx through the gills and sodium loss via the kidneys are both regulated by mineralocorticoid hormones.

Besides disturbances in electrolyte metabolism, adrenalectomized animals suffer from a number of other metabolic disturbances. All available metabolic indices (including carbohydrate tolerance, respiratory quotient, and nitrogen excretion) indicate that the conversion of protein to carbohydrate is decreased, the conversion of carbohydrate to fat is increased, and that, overall, the utilization of carbohydrate is increased. In fasted adrenalectomized rats liver glycogen is reduced to very low levels (0.1–0.2%, as compared to a normal concentration of 3–5%, while muscle glycogen is not much affected. All these symptoms are rapidly reversed by the administration of adrenal cortical extracts or crystalline adrenal cortical glucocorticoids, such as corticosterone, 11-dehydro-17-hydroxycorticosterone (cortisone), or 17-hydroxycorticosterone (hydrocortisone). Excessive amounts of these compounds can induce hyperglycemia and other symptoms resembling those of diabetes; since most glucocorticoids also possess some mineralocorticoid activity, hypercorticalism is frequently accompanied by sodium and fluid retention.

III. The Gonadal Hormones

A. ANDROGENS

The male gonads (the testes), when appropriately stimulated, produce several steroid hormones—the androgens. These compounds bring about marked changes in the size and functional competence of the male genital apparatus; in the rat these changes are marked especially in the seminal vesicles and the ventral prostate. Testicular hormones are also responsible for the growth and development of the male secondary sex characteristics in a variety of animal species—the fins and spines of elasmobranch and teleost fishes, the dorsal crests of lizards and salamanders, the combs and wattles of domestic fowl, plumage in some other birds, the horns and antlers of ruminants, and the body hair and laryngeal cartilage in humans.

One of the earliest observations of a general metabolic effect of a hormone was the observation, by Kochakian and Murlin in 1935, that androgens induced nitrogen retention in dogs. These original observations have been extended to a number of other species of animals, including rats, mice, guinea pigs, and humans. In castrated rats small doses of androgens induce nitrogen retention (as measured by a decrease in urinary nitrogen excretion) and increase in body weight; although part of the latter is accounted for by an increase in the amount of accessory sex tissue, most of it is due to increased carcass (i.e., muscle) weight. Particularly sensitive to this steroid anabolic effect are organs such as the kidneys of mice and rats and one or two skeletal muscles of guinea pigs.

In rats, the anabolic effect of the steroid androgens is a temporary phenomenon; after 10 days, or so, urinary nitrogen begins to increase until nitrogen balance is restored. At this time, increasing the amount of androgen injected may again depress nitrogen excretion (Fig. 1.3).

B. ESTROGENS

Like the androgens, the estrogens, the characteristic secretory products of the vertebrate ovary, are primarily anabolic in nature. Their ranges of action are, however, considerably more restricted than those of the androgens. The primary functions of the estrogens are concerned with the maintenance of the female reproductive tract, including the oviduct, the uterus, and the vaginal epithelium. In the ovariectomized female rat the uterus atrophies and the vagina undergoes a marked involution, becoming lined with a thin layer of epithelial cells with few mitotic figures. The motilities of both the oviducts and the horns of the uterus are greatly reduced; the latter effect is due to diminished responsiveness to hormones of the posterior pituitary. Under the influence of estrogen, oviduct and uterine motility are increased

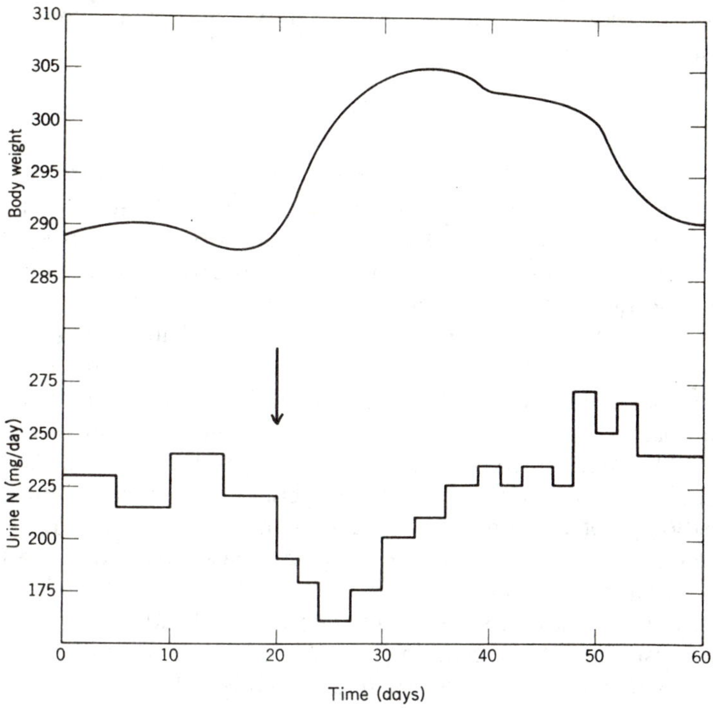

Fig. 1.3 *Effect of testosterone propionate (arrow, TP 0.5 mg/day) on the weight and urinary nitrogen of castrated male rats. Reproduced, with permission, from Frieden (1964).*

and the atrophic changes in the uterus are reversed, with accumulation of fluid and growth of glandular, stromal, and myometrial elements. The epithelial cells of the vaginal wall proliferate and are covered with a layer of cornified (nonnucleated) cells; their characteristic appearance is frequently used as an index of estrogenic activity. Although this effect is a characteristic aspect of the vaginal response to estrogen, cornification occurs to only a limited extent in some mammalian species, and not at all in others (i.e., rabbits).

Estrogens also stimulate the development of secondary sex characteristics in female animals. In combination with other hormones (progesterone and prolactin) estrogen is necessary for the development of the mammary apparatus, although, under some conditions high concentrations of estrogen may actually inhibit lactation. Estrogens can cause fluid retention in certain areas of the skin, the most sensitive area being the perineum (sex skin) of some primates. Bone resorption in birds and epiphyseal closure in mammals are also influenced by estrogens, and, like androgens, estrogens can modify feather pigmentation in some birds, e.g., pheasants. Finally, estrogen can evoke sexual receptivity (heat) in animals in which such a state is a normal periodic occurrence.

C. PROGESTOGENS

The mature ovarian follicle is generally thought to be the major source of ovarian estrogen. The corpus luteum of the ovary is the source of another gonadal steroid, progesterone. Progesterone acts upon the uterine endometrium to induce mucous secretory activity necessary for the implantation of the fertilized ovum. Progesterone is also necessary for the maintenance of pregnancy and for mammary development. For all the above actions of progesterone concomitant or prior action of estrogen is required.

An unusual action of progesterone is seen in animals in which rapid proliferation of the connective tissue elements of the uterine mucosa has been stimulated by mechanical trauma (scratching, insertion of threads, or glass beads, etc.). This phenomenon, which occurs in pseudopregnant animals, may be thought of as representing an attempt of the uterus to form the analog of a placenta in the absence of an implanted blastocyst and can result in a ten- to thirtyfold increase in uterine horn weight in a relatively short time. Progesterone is required for maintenance of the decidual response; since decidual reactions of respectable size can be supported in ovariectomized animals maintained on progesterone, estrogen is not necessary.

In addition to its action as a sex hormone, progesterone, an obvious analog of 11-deoxycorticoids, possesses some mineralocorticoid activity and can synergize with adrenal cortical hormones in maintaining life in adrenalectomized animals.

D. RELAXIN

In the guinea pig and, to a lesser extent, in some other animals an unusual adaptation to the demands of parturition results in softening and relaxation of the cartilagenous union of the pelvic bones (the symphysis pubis), permitting enlargement of the birth canal. About 50 years ago, F. L. Hisaw discovered that this process was hormonally controlled in the guinea pig and could be partially duplicated in nonpreganant estrous animals by injection of the blood serum of pregnant rabbits or guinea pigs. Subsequently, it was shown that (1) ovariectomized animals would also respond, provided that estrogen had been supplied earlier, and (2) the ovaries of some pregnant animals, especially sows, were a rich source of the active principle, which Hisaw named *relaxin*.

In addition to its effects on the symphysis pubes of guinea pigs and mice, relaxin has been implicated in a number of other physiological processes, all concerned in some way with the physiology of reproduction; it exerts a slight protein anabolic effect in the uterus of the rat and also inhibits decidual reactions induced in rats by progesterone. Cervical dilatability in both the sow and the rat increases after relaxin administration; as with the process of relaxation itself, this response is seen only if the animals are pretreated with estrogen. Finally, relaxin, as well as some closely related compounds, will inhibit spontaneous contractions of the uteri of rats and mice *in vitro* (and of guinea pigs *in vivo*). Again, this effect requires estrogen since only the uteri of estrous or estrogen-treated animals possess the necessary spontaneous motility.

Unlike the other gonadal hormones, which are all steroids, relaxin is a low molecular weight protein.

IV. Pancreatic Hormones

A. INSULIN

The vertebrate pancreas, in addition to acinar tissue which produces digestive enzymes, possesses aggregates of endocrine cells (the islets of Langerhans) which serve as the sources of two important hormones, insulin and glucagon. The discovery by von Mering and Minkowski, 1889, that removal of the pancreas gives rise to diabetes mellitus, and the subsequent demonstration by Banting and Best, in 1922, that pancreatic extracts were capable of reversing the symptoms of the disease are landmarks in the history of endocrinology.

Insulin is secreted by the β-cells of the islets of Langerhans. These cells are the most numerous of islet cell types (except in reptiles and birds) and are distinguished by the presence within them of alcohol-soluble granules. β-Cells can be selectively destroyed by the administration of alloxan; this technique has been widely used, along with pancreatectomy, as a means of assessing the effects of insulin lack, which include the following:

1. An increase in the steady state blood-glucose concentration to 300–400 mg% (normal is 80–120 mg%). Glucose may also appear in the urine, and loss of glucose via this route may approximate 3–4 gm per day.

2. Liver glycogen is abnormally low (0.045%, as compared to a normal value of 0.26%)* and no significant increase occurs after glucose feeding. Glycogen stores in other tissues (heart, kidney, etc.) are less severely affected.

3. Utilization of glucose is decreased, as indicated by reduced glucose tolerance, glycosuria, and lowered respiratory quotient. *In vitro,* tissues

* In fasted dogs.

removed from depancreatized animals also consume glucose at rates lower than normal.

4. Protein utilization and the conversion of amino acids to glucose (gluconeogenesis) is increased; glycosuria is accompanied by increased nitrogen excretion.

5. The amount of depot fat decreases and the lipid content of blood is increased. The conversion of glucose to fatty acid diminishes and the utilization of fat is increased. In advanced stages of insulin deficiency oxidation of fatty acids is incomplete, so that β-hydroxybutyric acid, acetoacetic acid, and acetone accumulate and are excreted.

6. Loss of glucose, nitrogen, and fatty acid in the urine is accompanied by increases in the amount of water and electrolytes, especially cations. Loss of base may be sufficient to cause severe acidosis and, eventually, death.

All of the above symptoms can be readily reversed by the administration of insulin.

The metabolic consequences of pancreatectomy are extremely variable from one species to another. Diabetes induced by insulin deprivation is more severe in mammalian carnivores (rats, cats, dogs, etc.) than in herbivores. Pancreatectomy in ducks results in a transient hyperglycemia; under the same conditions diabetic symptoms are observed in geese. Tortoises are also very sensitive to removal of the pancreas, but other reptiles and some birds appear to be relatively insensitive to either the presence or absence of insulin. In lizards the principal effect of pancreatectomy is hypoglycemia, perhaps as a result of the loss of glucagon (see Section IV,B). Elasmobranch and teleost fishes become hyperglycemic upon the removal of islet tissue.

Although insulin can affect the metabolism of nearly all tissues, including muscle and adipose tissue, its principal effect appears to be exerted upon the liver. The liver is necessary for the development of hyperglycemia following pancreatectomy; in fact, pancreatectomy in hepatectomized dogs results not in hyperglycemia but in hypoglycemia. Furthermore, the metabolic consequences of insulin deprivation, as well as insulin excess, are dependent upon the actions of other hormones, especially those of the pituitary and the adrenal glands. In both rats and dogs, the severity of diabetes induced by removal or destruction of islet tissue is greatly reduced by prior removal of the pituitary.

Insulin secretion is also affected by other hormones. Although the primary stimulus for increased insulin secretion is hyperglycemia, the injection of glucagon, as well as the gastointestinal hormones, secretin, gastrin, and pancreozymin–cholecystokinin will cause prompt increases in insulin secretion. In contrast, the catecholamines, even in the presence of glucose, are inhibitory.

B. GLUCAGON

Soon after insulin became available for experimental and clinical use, it was discovered that its typical hypoglycemic effect was often preceded by a transient hyperglycemia (Fig. 1.4). Kimball and Murlin (1923) separated the pancreatic hyperglycemic factor from insulin and gave it the name glucagon. Like insulin, glucagon has been isolated in crystalline form and knowledge of its chemical and physiological properties is well advanced.

Glucagon is secreted by the α-cells of the islets of Langerhans—cells characterized by the presence of large acidophilic granules which are soluble in water and alkali. Their identification as the source of glucagon secretion was accomplished by classic methods: destruction of both acinar tissue and islet β-cells leaves glucagon secretion unaffected, whereas destruction of α-cells by x-irradiation is accompanied by the disappearance of glucagon.

The immediate effect of glucagon administration is an elevation of blood glucose concentration, an effect which has been observed in a variety of vertebrates, including mammals, birds, reptiles, and amphibians. An adequate dose may double the blood sugar within 20–30 minutes. The additional glucose is derived entirely from liver glycogen; liver glycogen stores are rapidly depleted in animals injected with glucagon, while muscle glycogen is unaffected. Furthermore, the hyperglycemic action of glucagon disappears in hepatectomized animals.

Glucagon administration stimulates rapid release of insulin. In young

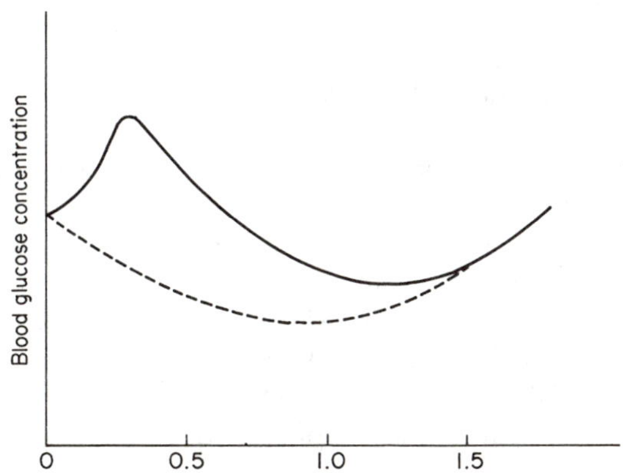

Fig. 1.4 *Effects of glucagon-contaminated (—) and glucagon-free (---) insulin upon blood glucose.*

rabbits prolonged and intensive treatment with glucagon ultimately leads to a condition which approximates true diabetes. This syndrome (metaglucagon diabetes) possibly results from the exhaustion and degeneration of β-cells as a result of overstimulation.

An inventory of the metabolic consequences of glucagon administration also suggests that it exerts a protein catabolic effect. Thus, plasma amino acid concentration is decreased, urea excretion is increased, and a negative nitrogen balance develops. It is possible that gluconeogenesis, as well as glycogenolysis, accounts for part of the observed hyperglycemia.

Although the existence of a true glucagon-deficiency syndrome has never been established unequivocally, all the available evidence suggests that this hormone is part of the complex array of mechanisms which regulate glucose metabolism. Like the catecholamines, glucagon can rapidly mobilize glucose to meet the needs of the peripheral tissues; unlike them, however, the late restoration of liver glycogen (which may be observed 24 hours after glucagon administration) does not involve depletion of muscle glycogen. Many of the other actions of glucagon, including some related only indirectly to carbohydrate or protein metabolism, are opposite to those of insulin. Thus, glucagon lowers food consumption by suppressing contractile and secretory activities of the gastrointestinal tract; it inhibits fatty acid synthesis and stimulates ketone body production. Glucagon also increases electrolyte and water excretion; alone of all the functions of glucagon these actions seem unrelated to any known function of insulin.

Glucagon secretion, like that of insulin, is regulated by blood glucose concentration, but its release is stimulated by hypo-, rather than, hyperglycemia. Pancreozymin (Section VIII,C) stimulates the secretion of glucagon as well as that of insulin, although larger quantities are required.

V. Parathyroid Hormone and Calcitonin

Hormonal regulation of calcium metabolism is provided by two substances, parathyroid hormone and calcitonin. Parathyroid hormone is produced by the parathyroid glands, a pair of glands which have a limited phylogenetic distribution. They are present in mammals, birds, reptiles, and most amphibians, but are absent in fishes. In birds, reptiles, amphibians, and fishes calcitonin is secreted by the ultimobranchial bodies, groups of cells which lie alongside the trachea and below the thyroids. In mammals these cells are anatomically part of the thyroid gland, where they are distinguished as parafollicular or "C" cells.

Removal of the parathyroid glands leads to an immediate fall in plasma calcium; conversely, the administration of parathyroid hormone (PTH) causes an increase in plasma Ca^{2+}. The principal target of PTH is the bone cell (osteoclast), where it promotes the dissolution of bone mineral and release of calcium to the plasma. Although not all the steps between the interaction of PTH with its receptor and the release of Ca^{2+} are known, one of them is undoubtedly activation of the adenyl cyclase system. PTH also exerts an anabolic effect and may alter the relative proportions of osteoblasts and osteoclasts, the bone-forming and bone-destroying cells. The hypercalcemic effect of PTH is much reduced if actinomycin D is given prior to PTH, indicating that its osteolytic activity requires prior synthesis of RNA (and probably of protein).

A second target of PTH is the kidney. The immediate renal response is increased excretion of inorganic phosphate and resorption of calcium. At one time it was supposed that phosphaturia was the primary physiological response to PTH; this view has largely been supplanted by the concept of a direct effect upon increased calcium resorption by the kidney tubule.

In contrast to PTH, the administration of calcitonin or calcitonin-containing preparations to experimental animals results in hypocalcemia, an effect which is insensitive to actinomycin D. While the action of PTH is relatively slow, persisting for many hours, that of calcitonin is rapid and transient. The only known target of calcitonin is bone, which responds to calcitonin by a diminished flow of Ca^{2+} into plasma. In contrast to parathyroid removal, however, destruction or elimination of the "C" cells does not significantly affect either the calcium content of plasma, the rate of bone turnover, or bone composition. The only demonstrable effect in calcitonin-deprived animals is a slower return of plasma Ca^{2+} to normal following an acute calcium load; some patients with "C" cell adenomas, having high circulating calcitonin concentrations, display normal plasma Ca^{2+} levels.

VI. The Pituitary Hormones

In most vertebrates the pituitary gland may be recognized as consisting of at least three cytologically distinct elements: the neurohypophysis (posterior lobe), the pars distalis (anterior lobe), and the pars intermedia (intermediate lobe). The relative amounts of each kind of tissue and their anatomical arrangement vary widely. In birds no intermediate lobe is identifiable, and in some fishes (teleosts and elasmobranchs) the delineation between the neurohypophysis and other parts of the pituitary is very diffuse. Each glandular component possesses its characteristic complement of hormones; in the mammalian pituitary two hormones are elaborated by the posterior lobe, two by the intermediate lobe, and six by the anterior lobe. Nearly all of the acute metabolic sequela of hypophysectomy are attributable to the loss of anterior pituitary function.

A. ANTERIOR LOBE HORMONES

Probably the most important physiological consequence of hypophysectomy (or the congenital absence of the pituitary) is cessation of growth in young animals and loss of weight in adults. This phenomenon may be seen in almost all vertebrates. In very young animals, hypophysectomy may be followed by a period of near-normal growth (especially under favorable dietary conditions), but thereafter dwarfism becomes increasingly prominent. In addition, hypophysectomized mammals are much more sensitive than intact ones to the hypoglycemic action of insulin, and the effects of fasting (hypoglycemia, ketonemia, and depletion of liver glycogen) are much more severe. Nitrogen excretion usually increases immediately after hypophysectomy; subsequently, nitrogen loss is reduced.

All these symptoms are reversed upon the administration (to hypophysectomized animals) of growth hormone (somatotropin, GH); a general increase in body size occurs, accompanied by nitrogen retention and increase in total body protein. Although nearly all tissues are affected in some degree (the brain is a notable exception) those most readily affected include skeletal muscle and the long bones of immature animals.

Hypophysectomy in mammals also results in rapid atrophy of the adrenal cortex, the thyroid glands, and the gonads. Atrophy of the adrenals under these conditions involves primarily the innermost layers of the cortex (including the zona fasciculata and the zona reticularis) and is accompanied by nearly complete loss of secretion of glucocorticoids. Neither the zona glomerulosa of the cortex nor the adrenal medulla is affected; further, the tonic secretion of the most potent mineralocorticoid, aldosterone, also appears to be independent of pituitary function. *Adrenocorticotropic hormone* (ACTH), like somatotropin, a secretion of the anterior pituitary, restores the cytology of the shrunken zones as well as glucocorticoid secretion. Most of the physiologic and metabolic actions of ACTH are secondary to its stimulatory effect upon the adrenal cortex. There are, however, some effects of this hormone which appear to result from its action directly upon extra adrenal tissue. Thus, ACTH-stimulated lipolysis in adipose tissue occurs in the absence of the adrenal, and the direct action of ACTH preparations upon melanocytes has been recognized for a generation.

Failure of thyroid function in animals deficient in pituitary function is due to the absence of another anterior pituitary hormone, *thyroid stimulating hormone* (TSH). In the absence of TSH, synthesis of triiodothyronine and thyroxine in thyroid tissue is incomplete, proceeding only as far as the iodination of tyrosine. The secretory epithelium becomes flattened and colloid accumulates in the follicles. Complete restoration of all phases of thyroid function accompanies the administration of TSH, including iodination, thyroid hormone formation, and release of stored hormone. The cells of the secretory epithelium become characteristically columnar and colloid is lost from the follicles. When TSH secretion is augmented, as during periods of decreased availability of iodine or following the use of antithyroid agents, there occurs a compensatory increase in the size of the thyroid gland, leading to the condition known as goiter. This enlargement involves both hypertrophy and hyperplasia of the secretory cells; part of the increase in size is due also to the increased vascularity of the gland.

In immature animals one of the results of loss of anterior pituitary function is failure of the gonads to develop beyond their original infantile states. In mature animals the comparable result is a gradual loss of function; germ cells soon cease to form and the secretion of gonadal hormones (androgens and estrogens) in both males and females stops. As an indirect result, therefore, the accessory sex tissues may also lose their functional integrity.

Maintenance of gonadal function is the primary role of a triad of anterior pituitary hormones, the gonadotropins. These include the *follicle stimulating hormone* (FSH), the *luteinizing hormone* (LH or *interstitial cell stimulating hormone,* ICSH), and the *leutotropic hormone* (LtH or prolactin). While each of these substances exhibits characteristic biological activities, normal reproductive function requires the concerted action of all three. Thus, while FSH stimulates the development of immature follicles, complete follicular development (and estrogen secretion) requires the presence of LH as well. The conversion of mature ovarian follicles to corpora lutea requires LH (hence the name luteinizing hormone), while secretion of progesterone by functional corpora lutea requires the concerted action of both LH and prolactin.

In males, FSH stimulates the seminiferous tubules (and hence spermatogenesis), but the Leydig cells of the testis remain atrophic in a hypophysectomized animal treated with FSH. Since the Leydig cells serve as the site of androgen production, the accessory sex organs (prostate, seminal vesicles, etc.) do not respond to FSH alone, even though testicular enlargement occurs. When LH is given along with FSH, the Leydig cells are stimulated to produce testosterone and as a consequence, the accessory sex organs enlarge.

LH also possesses the unusual property of controlling the plumage of some birds, especially finches. This effect does not require the presence of the gonads, and thus appears to be a direct action of the hormone.

The biological action of prolactin, except for some possible antigonadal effects in birds, is directed exclusively toward the female. As noted above, prolactin synergizes with LH to develop and maintain a functional corpus luteum. It is responsible for the initiation of milk secretion in the mammary gland, a process which depends upon the prior action, on this tissue, of estrogen and progesterone. In birds, especially pigeons, prolactin stimulates hyperplasia of epithelial cells of the crop gland, resulting in increase in "crop milk." Finally, two unusual behavioral responses in quite different species are attributed to the actions of prolactin. In domestic birds prolactin initiates brooding behavior, while in the spotted newt (*Triturus*) it induces, within a period of a few days, migration of this normally terrestrial species to water, preparatory to mating and egg laying.

B. INTERMEDIATE LOBE HORMONES

A number of lower vertebrates, including amphibians, fishes, and lampreys, possess the ability to change color in response to changes in their surroundings. Thus, for example, a frog placed upon an illuminated white (or light) background will become distinctly paler within a period of hours; conversely, placed upon a dark background, its skin darkens rapidly. These responses are due to concentration and dispersion, respectively, of pigment granules (melanin) within groups of epithelial cells, the melanophores. It has been clearly established that this process is at least partly under hormonal control; the hormone* in question derives from the intermediate lobe of the pituitary gland and was originally called *intermedin* by Zondek and Krohn, its discoverers. The most commonly used term at present is melanocyte-stimulating hormone (MSH). Similar dispersion of pigment by pituitary factors occurs in vertebrates as primitive as the cyclostomes, although the chemical identity of the substance(s) involved is uncertain.

Intermediate lobe extracts will also affect other types of pigment cells. The erythrophores of *Fundulus* are dispersed by MSH, although the melanophores in this species are not affected. In amphibians, MSH condenses the pigment in guanophores, even as melanophores are dispersed.

Prolonged administration of extracts rich in MSH leads to an absolute increase in the melanin content of frog skin (*R. catesbiana*). Similarly, persistent pigmentary changes in humans have been reported as a result of treatment with massive doses of MSH-active preparations.

C. POSTERIOR LOBE (NEUROHYPOPHYSEAL) HORMONES

Posterior pituitary extracts exert four principal actions in vertebrates.

1. *Pressor Effect*

This results from a combination of peripheral vasoconstriction and increased cardiac output. Although the pressor effect represents the first physi-

* Or hormones; two peptides with MSH activity have been isolated from mammalian pituitaries.

ological role demonstrated for the pituitary gland, and still finds utility as an assay method, the amount required to produce a significant response is considerably larger than that normally released by the gland. It seems likely, therefore, that the pressor effect is rather unimportant as a significant contributor to the mechanisms normally regulating blood pressure.

2. *Antidiuretic Effect*

This phenomenon is observable in almost all vertebrates; marine fishes are an exception. The antidiuretic effect is the result of an increase in permeability to water. In mammals, the result is an increase in tubular reabsorption; in amphibians, in addition to the kidney, two other organs, the skin and bladder, are also affected. Both tissues respond to neurohypophyseal hormones by increasing the flow of water in response to an osmotic gradient.

3. *Muscle-Contracting (Oxytocic) Effect*

This action is exerted mainly upon the mammalian uterus and upon the oviducts of birds and reptiles. The neurohypophysis thus plays a role in parturition; it has also been implicated in the transport of spermatozoa to the site of fertilization.

4. *"Galactobolic" or Milk-Ejection Effect*

Following completion of the secretory phase of lactation, ejection of milk by engorged alveoli is induced by neurohypophyseal activity. This effect appears to be exerted principally upon the myoepithelial cells lining the alveoli.

The pressor and antidiuretic properties of the mammalian posterior pituitary are referable to a single peptide hormone, vasopressin. As noted above, the pressor effect is of limited physiological significance. Vasopressin is, therefore, frequently referred to as the *antidiuretic hormone* (ADH). Another related peptide, oxytocin, is responsible for both the oxytocic and galactobolic effects of pituitary preparations. In most nonmammalian vertebrates a single octapeptide, vasotocin, exerts both oxytocic and antidiuretic functions. Vasotocin is the only neurohypophyseal hormone found in cyclostomes and elasmobranch fishes; It is also present, along with oxytocin, in the pituitaries of birds and amphibians.

In mammals, birds, and reptiles the neurohypophyseal peptides are secreted by the superoptic and paraventricular nuclei of the hypothalamus; in fish and amphibians they originate in the preoptic nuclei. The hormones are transported through the nerve fibers of the pituitary stalk to the posterior lobe of the pituitary, where they are stored in granules in association with a group of proteins known as neurophysins.

VII. Hypothalamic-Releasing Hormones

The idea that secretions of the anterior pituitary, as well as those of posterior pituitary, are under hypothalamic control, arose out of experiments which indicated that electrical stimulation of, or lesions produced in, the hypothalamus would affect gonadal, adrenocortical, or thyroid secretion. Unlike the posterior pituitary, however, there are few direct neural connections between the hypothalamus and the anterior pituitary. On the other hand, the blood supply from the ventral hypothalamus to the anterior pituitary is direct and plentiful. Perhaps the clearest early evidence for hypothalamic control of adenohypophyseal function was the demonstration by Harris and Jacobsohn (1952) that pituitary grafts placed under the median eminence in hypophysectomized rats rapidly acquired vascular connections with the primary plexus of the hypophyseal portal vessels. In these animals normal gonadal and thyroidal function was retained. In contrast, transplants placed under the temporal lobe, or into the hypophyseal capsule itself, failed to develop vascular connections and were unable to maintain function.

Final proof that the link between the hypothalamus and the anterior pituitary was hormonal came with the isolation, from hypothalamic tissue, of specific substances which modify pituitary secretion. As of now, nine such factors have been identified: (1) thyrotropin-releasing hormone (TRH); (2) a gonadotropin (FSH and LH)-releasing hormone (gon-RH); (3, 4) growth hormone-releasing and releasing-inhibiting hormones (GH-RH, GH-RIH); (5) corticotropin-releasing hormone (CRH); (6, 7) prolactin-releasing and release-inhibiting hormones (PRH, PRIH); (8, 9) MSH-releasing and release-inhibiting hormones (MRH, MRIH). Progress toward the isolation and chemical characterization of TRH, gon-RH, GH-RH, and GH-RIH has been rapid, but detailed information concerning the other hormones has been accumulated more slowly.

In addition to the releasing hormones, the hypothalamus also contains relatively high concentrations of catecholamines (epinephrine and norepinephrine). Evidence is accumulating that substances which are able to modify the synthesis, release, or metabolism of catecholamines can influence secretion of anterior pituitary hormones; direct evidence implicates especially the gonadotropins. This kind of regulation is a two-way street; the presence or absence of gonadal hormones can modify the dynamics of catecholamine metabolism in the hypothalamus. Although insufficient data are as yet available to define clearly the role of catecholamines in hypothalamic function, a number of possible mechanisms have been recognized (Wurtman, 1970). Catecholamines may serve as the neurotransmitters which stimulate hypothalamic cells either to secrete or release "releasing hormones"; they may modify the response of the anterior pituitary to releasing hormones; they may act directly upon the anterior pituitary.

The release of hypothalamic hormones is also subject to "negative feedback" control by gonadal steroid hormones, especially estradiol. Castration of male rats or ovariectomy in females increases the concentration of FSH-RH in the hypothalamus, while the direct application of estradiol to the median eminence or the anterior hypothalamus, or the systemic administration of either estradiol or testosterone reduces the FSH-RH content of hypothalamic tissue (Motta *et al.*, 1970). Since hypothalamic estrogen implants also reduce the amounts of FSH and LH in the peripheral plasma, the release of gon-RH from the hypothalamus appears also to be inhibited. Progesterone administration also decreases the hypothalamic concentration of FSH-RH.

Evidence for specific steroid (i.e., estrogen) receptor cells in the hypothalamus is based upon (1) changes in the electrical activity of hypothalamic neurons in response to the intravenous administration of estradiol and (2) the accumulation of radioactive estradiol (and testosterone) in the hypothalamus to a greater extent than in other areas of the brain. A macromolecule (probably a protein) with high affinity for estradiol-17β has been isolated from the hypothalamus of ovariectomized rats.

Inhibition of gon-RH secretion by the hypothalamus, with resulting inhibition of LH secretion and ovulation, has been suggested as a probable mechanism of action of antiovulatory steroids.

VIII. Gastrointestinal Hormones

These hormones comprise a group of four or five substances which have several unique characteristics. They are all produced in that section of the digestive tract which includes stomach, duodenum, and jejunum. Their actions are also confined to elements of the digestive tract (stomach, duodenum, pancreas, and liver). Finally, the action of each is independent of that of the others, despite their restricted loci of action.

A. GASTRIN

Although occasional doubts may still be raised about the identity of gastrin as a distinct hormone, careful studies appear to have firmly established its existence. Gastrin is produced in the pyloric mucosa when a food bolus is present. The hormone is carried by the blood to other areas of the stomach, in particular to the fundus, where it stimulates the secretion of gastric juice. This phenomenon may be reproduced by the systemic injection of stomach extracts.

In addition to the gastric antrum, gastrin has been found in the mucosa of the small intestine and in the pancreas. Normally, the amount of gastrin secreted by the pancreas is small compared to that in the stomach or duodenum, but large amounts may be released from islet-cell gastrinomas (Zollinger–Ellison syndrome).

B. SECRETIN

This substance bears the distinction of being the first for which the term hormone was used. About 70 years ago Bayliss and Starling showed the perfusion of the denervated dog jejunum with weak acid resulted in an increase in the flow of pancreatic juice; they also showed that an extract of acid-treated intestinal mucosa, injected intravenously, would engender a similar response. The action of secretin upon the flow of pancreatic juice is confined to water and bicarbonate; the secretion of pancreatic enzymes is unaffected. Secretin also stimulates the flow of bile from the liver.

C. PANCREOZYMIN

The pattern of hormonal control of pancreatic secretion was completed by the discovery of pancreozymin by Harper and Raper in 1943. Although it had clearly been established that secretin had no effect upon the secretion of pancreatic enzymes, Harper showed that introduction of food material into the duodenum nevertheless increased the flow of pancreatic digestive enzymes. Subsequently, he was able to show that in addition to secretin, another substance, also originating in the duodenum, was involved. This substance, which he called pancreozymin, increased the concentrations of pancreatic enzymes (amylase, trypsin, and chymotrypsin) in pancreatic secretion as much as sixfold, with no change in the volume of fluid or its electrolyte content.

D. CHOLECYSTOKININ

The entry of the acid contents of the stomach into the duodenum results, not only in acceleration of pancreatic secretion, but also in the evocation of rhythmic contractions of the gallbladder and the discharge of bile into the small intestine. In 1928, A. C. Ivy and his collaborators were able to show that the gallbladder response was under hormonal control, since the denervated gallbladder was fully responsive, and feeding one of a pair of dogs in parabiosis evoked a gallbladder response in both. Ivy also extracted a substance from intestinal mucosa which contracted the gallbladders of dogs (*in vivo*) and also caused shortening (contraction) of gallbladder strips (*in vitro*). The new hormone was given the name cholecystokinin; as might be expected, considering its source, it shares many of the properties of secretin and pancreozymin. In fact, cholecystokinin and pancreozymin have not been separated and are now considered to represent different responses to the same chemical entity. It is of interest that the horse, which lacks a gallbladder, also has no cholecystokinin in its duodenal mucosa. The hormone has, however, been extracted from the intestines of cattle, dogs, pigs, and humans.

E. ENTEROGASTRONE

This still hypothetical substance also has its presumed origin in the duodenum. Its principal action appears to be inhibition of hydrochloric acid secretion in the stomach, and, possibly, diminution of gastric motility. Enterogastrone secretion occurs in response to a fatty meal; the introduction of fats, oils, or hypertonic sugar solutions directly into the duodenum stimulates its formation.

Dogs subjected to an anastomosis of the jejunum and the stomach, so that the acidic stomach contents drain directly into the jejunum and remain unneutralized, frequently develop chronic peptic ulcers of the jejunum. Enterogastrone preparations have been reported to prevent or cure ulcers in such animals.

IX. Erythropoietin

The stimulation of red blood cell formation by plasma obtained from anemic rabbits is a phenomenon that was described very early in the history of endocrinology (Carnot and Deflandre, 1906). The real significance of their original observations remained obscure for several decades. Evidence accumulated during the past 15 years, however, indicates quite clearly that a humoral factor capable of stimulating erythropoiesis does, in fact, exist. After a period of rather confusing terminology, the name erythropoietin seems generally to have been accepted.

Formation of erythropoietin occurs readily in response to hypoxia; hypoxia, in turn, may result from a reduction in the oxygen-carrying capacity of the blood (due to anemia caused by repeated bleeding or the injection of hemolytic agents) or from reduced interstitial oxygen tension resulting from exposure to lowered barometric pressure. Other factors will also affect the response, and experiments which demonstrated that starvation or hypophysectomy reduced erythropoietin production while metabolic stimulants, such as thyroxine or dinitrophenol, increased it have given rise to the hypothesis that the rate of formation of this hormone is determined by the relation between the partial pressure of oxygen in the blood and the oxygen of the tissue (Fried *et al.*, 1957).

Another agent which effectively stimulates erythropoietin formation is divalent cobalt. As little as 5 μM of $CoCl_2$, injected on each of 2 successive days, occasions a significant erythropoietic response in rats (Fig. 1.5). The mechanism whereby cobalt exerts its effect is unknown; it may be related to the ability of cobalt to inhibit some oxidative enzymes (e.g., succinoxidase) in liver and kidney. Removal of oxygen from hypoxic blood used to perfuse dog kidneys is slower if cobalt is present, than if it is absent.

The ability of cobalt to raise the erythropoietin titer of the plasma of a recipient animal within 12 hours of its administration has enabled Goldwasser *et al.* (1968) to establish that the major site of formation of erythropoietin in rats is the kidney. Bilateral nephrectomy suppressed or eliminated the response to cobalt, or to acute hemorrhage, while removal of 85–90% of the liver was without effect. Although extrarenal sites for erythropoietin synthesis have been suggested for rabbits and humans, no certain information concerning their locations exists.

Repeated injections of erythropoietin-rich extracts into normal adult rats causes a sustained (during 3 weeks) increase in the number of red blood

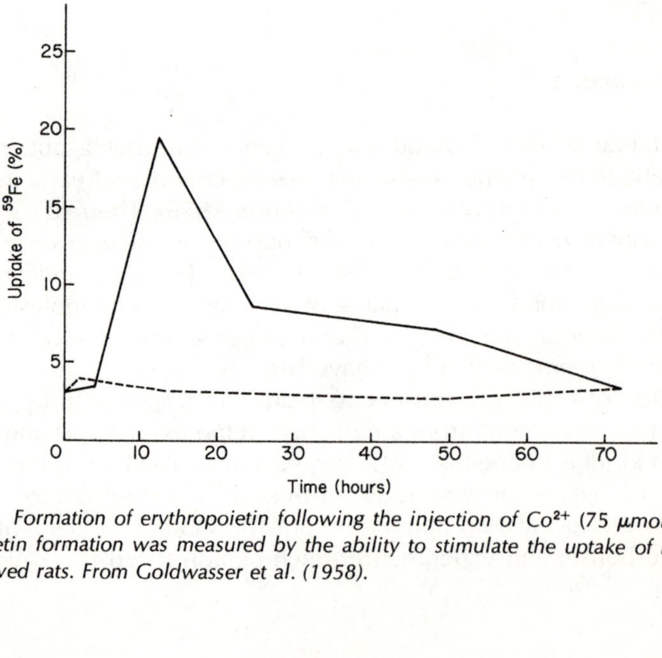

Fig. 1.5 *Formation of erythropoietin following the injection of Co^{2+} (75 μmoles) in rats. Erythropoietin formation was measured by the ability to stimulate the uptake of radioactive iron in starved rats. From Goldwasser et al. (1958).*

cells, in the hemoglobin content of the blood, in the hematocrit, and in the reticulocyte content of peripheral blood. Experimental animals were found to have somewhat larger blood volumes so that the total red cell mass and hemoglobin were substantially increased (50–60%). Both rats and rabbits (Linman and Bethell, 1956; Erslev, 1953) receiving erythropoietin responded with increased numbers of erythrocytic elements in bone marrow. The effect on the marrow appears to be at the level of the stem cell, accelerating the differentiation of primitive stem cells first into pronormoblasts and subsequently into reticulocytes. It has been shown that the addition of erythropoietin to bone marrow cells in tissue culture results in a marked increase in heme synthesis.

In addition to increasing the rate of red blood cell formation and of hemoglobin production, erythropoietin can, in some animals at least, modify the nature of the hemoglobin produced. The blood of sheep and goats contains two kinds of hemoglobins (A and B) which differ in electrophoretic mobility, oxygen affinity, and amino acid composition. Individual animals may be heterozygous (AB) or homozygous for either variant (AA, BB). Heterozygous sheep, or those which are homozygous for hemoglobin A, respond to phenylhydrazine or phlebotomy-induced anemia by producing a new hemoglobin variant—hemoglobin C, which may completely replace hemoglobin A (van Vliet and Huisman, 1964; Gabuzda *et al.*, 1968). A similar phenomenon has been observed in anemic goats (Huisman *et al.*, 1967), except that in goats hemoglobin B is also partly replaced by hemoglobin C.

In nonanemic sheep the same "switching" phenomenon can be induced by the injection of anemic sheep plasma or human urinary erythropoietin (Thurmon *et al.*, 1970). A similar effect of erythropoietin has been demonstrated in bone marrow cells, from sheep or goats, maintained in tissue culture (Adamson and Stamatoyannapoulos, 1973; Barker *et al.*, 1973). Since the switch from Hgb A to Hgb C involves an alteration in the amino acid sequence of the β-globin chain, the effect of erythropoietin appears to be exerted at the mRNA level.

2

The Measurement of Hormone Concentration

A prime prerequisite for the isolation of a hormone (indeed, any biologically active substance) from tissues, and for its subsequent purification and characterization is the availability of a method for its quantitative, or at least qualitative, determination. Indeed, the strategy and tactics of an isolation procedure are sometimes dictated by the methods of assay available. The assay must obviously be based upon some unique property of the compound being studied. Once a compound has been chemically characterized it is often possible to devise a chemical procedure for its quantitative determination. Within the past 2 decades extremely sensitive methods for the estimation of most nonprotein hormones have been worked out; many of these methods take advantage of the unique possibilities associated with spectrophotometric, fluorometric, chromatographic (especially gas–liquid chromatography), or radioisotopic procedures. The art of the protein chemist, however, is not yet equal to the task of quantitatively measuring the concentration of one protein or polypeptide, present at very low concentration, in a mixture of others of more abundant occurrence, unless the former possesses some property unshared by the others present (e.g., a heme-, flavo-, or metalloprotein). The determination of protein or polypeptide hormones, therefore, depends most often upon their special biological properties.

Even for those hormones for which chemical procedures of sufficient discrimination and sensitivity are available, bioassays continue to be indispensable tools, especially for the evaluation of the biological properties of synthetic analogs of the naturally occurring hormones. Thus, while the functional state of the thyroid gland may readily be assessed by chemical determinations of thyroxine or protein-bound iodine in plasma or serum, a variety of bioassay procedures are necessary to evaluate the therapeutic possibilities which may be lodged in synthetic compounds resembling thyroxine or triiodothyronine.

The first hormone assays were essentially qualitative in nature, the presence of the hormone being indicated by its ability to restore functional or morphological normality in situations of endocrine deficiency, or to exaggerate a hormone-dependent response (e.g., precocious metamorphosis in amphibians). The first quantitative assays were quantal in nature, measuring essentially the occurrence or nonoccurrence of a response, usually within a group of animals. Later, responses were selected which were more amenable to quantitative assessment—size or weight of an animal or of an anatomical unit, concentration of a metabolite, etc.

I. Units and Standards

If a chemical assay is available, the comparison of two different preparations of a hormone rarely presents a problem. It is only necessary that some well-defined stoichiometric or nonstoichiometric relationship exists between the amount of hormone present and the end point selected. Comparison by means of bioassays, on the other hand, requires that the effects of different preparations be referred to some standard. The standard may be defined in terms of a particular biological response, or it may be defined in terms of the effect of an arbitrarily selected quantity of an available preparation of the hormone. For example, in the early work which led to the isolation of insulin a "unit" of insulin activity was defined as the amount which would lower the blood sugar of a 2-kg rabbit to 45 mg% within 4 to 5 hours. It was possible to compare two different insulin samples by titrating each to this end point. On the other hand, the International Unit (IU) of oxytocin or vasopressin was originally defined as the activity contained in 0.5 mg of the dried defatted powder obtained from bovine posterior pituitary lobes. An oxytocin or vasopressin sample of unknown activity could then be compared with the standard by determining the amount of each needed to produce the same oxytocic or pressor responses.

Isolation (or synthesis) of the pure hormone permits the replacement of the arbitrary standard by a preparation of known chemical composition. It also permits the "unit" of activity to be defined in terms of a definite quantity of material. For example, the unit of insulin activity is now defined as the activity present in 0.0417 mg of a mixture of crystalline porcine and bovine insulins. Pure oxytocin turned out to be 225 times as active as the International standard preparation, and thus contains 450 IU/mg.

II. Types of Bioassays for Adrenocorticotropin

Adrenocorticotropin (ACTH) will serve to illustrate some of the end points that have been employed for bioassays. Shortly after Smith (1930) showed that hypophysectomy in the rat was followed by atrophy of the adrenal cortex, Collip *et al.* (1933) suggested using hypophysectomized, unilaterally adrenalectomized rats for ACTH assay; the amount of hormone required to restore the normal histological appearance of the remaining adrenal gland when given during 1 week was defined as a "unit" of ACTH activity. Quantitation of this kind of assay rests upon the fraction of positive responses in a population of assay animals; even with a large number, however, the precision is relatively low.

Subsequently, as more was learned about the effects of ACTH in hypophysectomized animals, other indices of ACTH action were adapted to assay use. Figures 2.1–2.4 represent dose–response curves obtained in ACTH assays in which four different responses were measured in hypophysectomized animals. Figure 2.1 indicates the change in adrenal weight which occurred when young (40-day-old) rats were treated with ACTH for 4 days, beginning shortly after hypophysectomy. Figure 2.2 displays a different response—the change in adrenal ascorbic acid 1 hour after the injection of the sample. In Fig. 2.3 the independent variable is the amount of corticosteroid discharged into adrenal vein blood after the parenteral injection of ACTH. Figure 2.4 shows how the amount of corticosteroid secreted into the medium by adrenal tumor slices is influenced by the amount of ACTH present.

The four assays shown represent, in principle, the major phenomena upon which essentially all hormone assays are based: change in weight of a target tissue, decreased (or increased) concentration of a cellular component, increased output of a metabolite, and measurement of one of these responses in an isolated tissue *in vitro*. It is evident that, although the various assays differ in respect of the amount of ACTH which calls forth a response, all share a common property, i.e., a region in which the response is linearly proportional to the logarithm of the concentration (or amount) of the hormone. For each assay, there exists a minimum dose, or concentration, below which the response is indistinguishable from that of an untreated animal; likewise, for most assays a sufficiently large dose results in a maximal

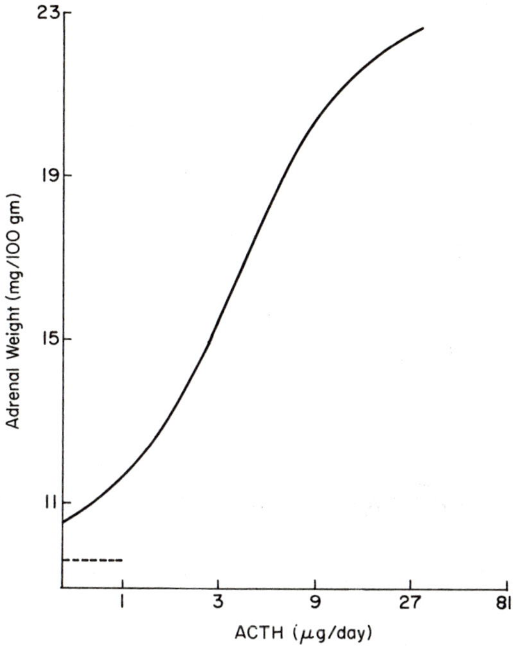

Fig. 2.1 *Changes in the adrenal weights of hypophysectomized rats in response to the injection of ACTH. Data of Li et al. (1957).*

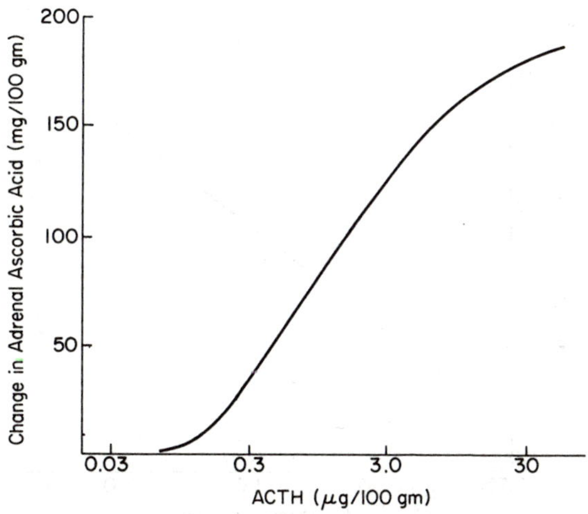

Fig. 2.2 *Effect of ACTH upon adrenal ascorbic acid in hypophysectomized rats. Ascorbic acid was determined 1 hour after ACTH injection. Data of Sayers et al.*

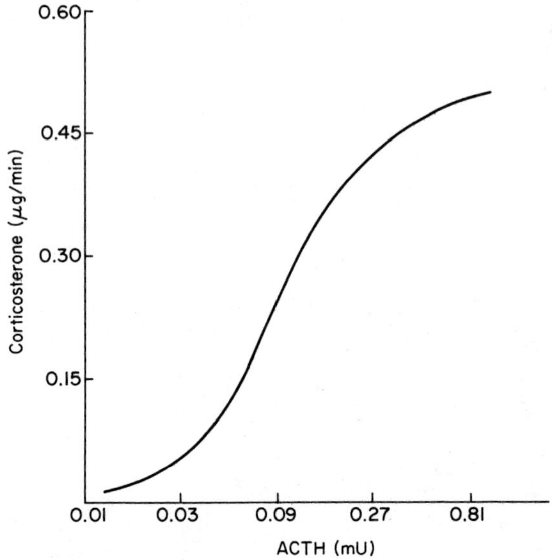

Fig. 2.3 *Effect of ACTH upon the secretion of corticosterone into the adrenal vein of hypophysectomized rats. Data of Liddle et al. (1962).*

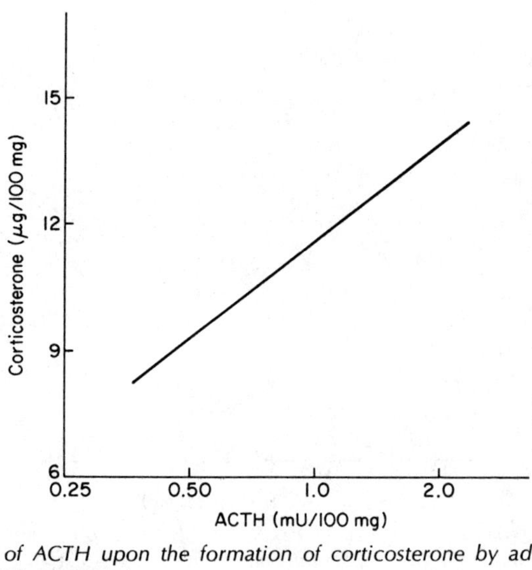

Fig. 2.4 *Effect of ACTH upon the formation of corticosterone by adrenal tumor slices. Data of Cohen and Furth (1959).*

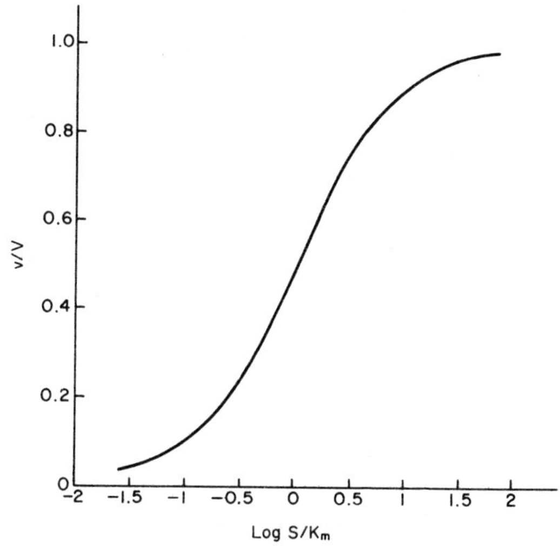

Fig. 2.5 *Logarithmic form of the Michaelis–Menten equation. V, maximum velocity; v, velocity.*

response which is not further increased by increasing the dose. Conventionally, comparisons of standards and unknowns require at least two different doses or concentrations of the latter, so that the slopes as well as the ordinates of bioassay curves may be compared.

Complete dose–response curves for many hormones, therefore, are sigmoid in shape when the appropriate response parameter is plotted as a semilogarithmic function of the dose or concentration of the hormone. Such curves bear at least a formal resemblance to the logarithmic form of the Michaelis–Menten equation (Fig. 2.5). This resemblance is consistent with the supposition that expression of hormone action is dependent upon interaction with specific protein receptors, analogous to the formation of a substrate–enzyme complex in enzyme action. Recent progress toward the isolation and characterization of some receptor proteins, especially those specific for steroid hormones, offers direct support for this view (see, however, Stetten, 1956).*

III. Hormone Assay by Specific Ligand Binding

The need for assay methods sensitive enough to detect the minute concentrations of hormones in blood and other body fluids has resulted in the

* Note however that the Michaelis expression predicts a linear relationship between *v* (analogous to response) and log *S* (dose) which is limited to a range of *S* which is less than 2 log units wide. Dose–response curves for some assays are significantly wider than this.

development, during the past 15 years, of two extremely versatile and sensitive analytical techniques. Both methods depend upon the unique affinities of certain proteins for specific ligands; the latter may be a peptide or protein hormone, a nonprotein hormone, or a nonprotein hormone conjugated to a nonhormonal protein. For one group of assays (immunoassays) the binding proteins are antibodies; for the other, the binding proteins are plasma or cellular proteins which have been found to possess special affinities for small molecules (e.g., steroids). In the most elegant applications of both, hormones labeled with radioisotopes are used to achieve extreme sensitivity and reliability.

A. IMMUNOASSAY

In recent years, the biological assay of many hormones has been replaced by various kinds of immunoassays; because of their exquisite sensitivity such assays have been particularly useful for clinical studies and for the elucidation of taxonomic relationships. All immunoassays depend fundamentally upon the detection of a reaction between an antigen (the hormone) and an antibody induced in an appropriate animal by injections of the antigen. Most macromolecules, such as protein hormones, can act as antigens under appropriate circumstances. Nonprotein hormones can be made antigenic by coupling them with a suitable protein.

Three principal techniques are used to quantitate immunochemical responses: hemagglutination, complement fixation, and radioimmunological methods.

1. *Hemagglutination*

These assays depend upon the fact that antigen-coated erythrocytes will be agglutinated by antibody specific for the bound antigen. The addition of an excess of "free" antigen (i.e., not bound to cells) will compete with coated cells for antibody, thus inhibiting agglutination. In many methods, sheep red blood cells are treated successively with formaldehyde, tannic acid, and the antigen. Antiserum is produced in rabbits. Mixtures of antigen, antiserum, and coated cells are incubated 1–2 hours and the pattern of agglutination observed.

2. *Complement Fixation*

Complement is a heat-labile mixture of substances which is required for the hemolysis of red blood cells by hemolysin [anti-red blood cell (anti-RBC) antiserum]. In the absence of complement, anti-RBC antiserum will agglutinate erythrocytes but will not hemolyze them. Complement is also bound by many antigen–antibody complexes, including soluble ones. The existence of such complexes can be determined indirectly by mixing antiserum, antigen, and complement at 40° for 18 hours. A mixture of "sensitized" erythrocytes (erythrocytes mixed with hemolysin) is added, and the extent of hemolysis is noted. If carefully measured amounts of complement are used, the assay may be quantified by spectrophotometric determination of the amount of hemoglobin released into the solution.

Arquila and Stavisky (1956) found that hemolysis of insulin-sensitized erythrocytes by rabbit anti-insulin serum was inhibited by prior incubation of the antiserum with insulin solutions; the degree of inhibition was linear when plotted against the logarithm of the insulin concentration. Yalow and Berson (1961) greatly improved the sensitivity of immunoassays by employing the competition between radioactive (*indicates labeled with ^{131}I) and unlabeled insulin for specific binding sites on the antibody:

$$\text{Ab-Ins} \longleftarrow \text{Ins} + \text{Ab} + {}^{*}\text{Ins} \longrightarrow \text{Ab-}{}^{*}\text{Ins}$$

If a mixture of anti-insulin antibody, ^{131}I-labeled insulin and unlabeled insulin, is incubated, part of the radioactive hormone will be bound to the antibody and part will remain free in the solution. If the amount of labeled antigen and antibody are kept constant, and the amount of unlabeled antigen is increased, the ratio of bound to free radioactivity (B/F) will decrease. Using known concentrations of insulin, a standard curve relating insulin con-

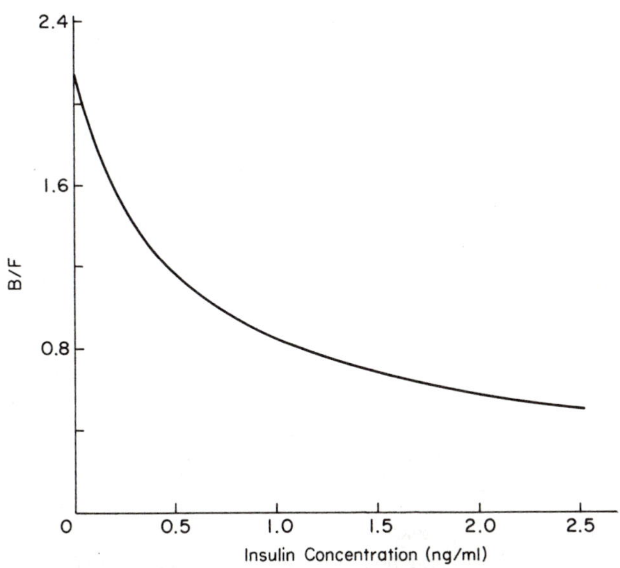

Fig. 2.6 *Radioimmunoassay of insulin in plasma. Ordinate, ratio of bound to free insulin in solution. Data of Yalow and Berson (1960).*

centration and B/F ratio may be prepared (Fig. 2.6), from which the concentration of insulin in an unknown solution may be estimated.

The determination of the B/F ratio in an experiment such as that described above requires that some means of separating free and antibody-bound radioactivity be devised. In some circumstances, when the antigen–antibody complex is insoluble, simple centrifugation may suffice. More often, however, the antibody is nonprecipitating, and some other procedure must be used. Yalow and Berson originally used chromatoelectrophoresis (electrophoresis on paper strips) at pH 8.6 in Veronal buffer for the separation of free and bound insulin. In their studies, insulin remained bound to the paper at the point of application, while the insulin–antibody complex moved toward the anode. Quantitative data were provided by scanning the strip in an automatic scanner equipped with an integrating recorder (Fig. 2.7). With the amounts of antibody and labeled insulin properly adjusted, the addition of 5×10^{-7}mg of unlabeled insulin diminished the fraction of bound labeled insulin from 100 to 50%.

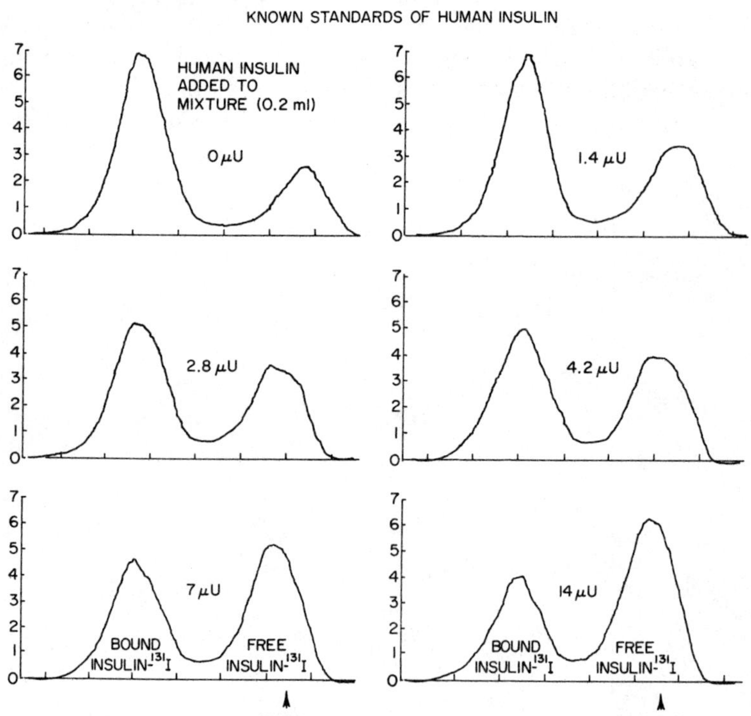

Fig. 2.7 *Separation of free and bound ^{131}I-insulin by chromatoelectrophoresis. Reproduced, with permission, from Yalow and Berson (1960).*

Several other methods for separating antigen and antigen–antibody complex have been described. The "double antibody" method uses a second antibody (prepared using homologous γ-globulin) to precipitate the first. Thus, if guinea pig antiserum is used, the addition of rabbit anti-guinea pig γ-globulin precipitates the antigen–antibody complex along with unreacted antibody. The precipitate can then be collected by centrifugation or filtration and counted (Hales and Randle, 1963). Salt precipitation and gel filtration (on Sephadex G-75) have also been used. Other separation methods include the use of dextran-coated charcoal (which absorbs free, but excludes antibody-bound antigen) and ion-exchange resins.

In principle, the technique of radioimmunoassay can be used for any peptide or protein hormone which (1) is available in pure form, (2) is antigenic, and (3) can be labeled with a suitable radioisotope. The most critical feature is the availability of a sufficiently pure protein preparation to serve as antigen. As rapidly as success has attended efforts to isolate each peptide and protein hormone in a pure state, radioimmunological methods for its determination have been developed and are now available for nearly all the protein or peptide hormones. In some instances, cross reaction between antibodies to the hormone prepared from one animal and the same hormone isolated from another is sufficiently extensive to obviate the need for isolating pure hormones from both.

3. *Radioimmunoassay of Nonprotein Hormones*

Although nonprotein (e.g., steroid) hormones are not antigenic, it has been possible to use radioimmunoassay methods for steroid hormone analysis by taking advantage of the fact that steroid-specific antibodies are produced when chlorocarbonates or hemisuccinates of various steroids are linked to plasma albumin; the products are then used to induce antibody formation in rabbits or guinea pigs. To increase the specificity of the reaction, the antibody is treated with native plasma albumin to absorb nonspecific antibody.

4. *Radiobioassay*

It has been known for many years that plasma proteins play important roles in the transport of many substances; interactions between proteins and steroid hormones or between proteins and iodothyronines not only increase the apparent solubility of the original compounds in plasma but also may prevent their loss via the usual excretory routes. More recently, it has been found that some plasma proteins possess high affinities for several steroid hormones and thyroxine. At about the same time, receptor proteins specific for estrogens, androgens, and mineralocorticoids were identified in a number of "target" tissues. The exploitation of the specific steroid-binding properties of these proteins for the assay of androgens, estrogens, corticoids, and progesterone in plasma and other body fluids has been accomplished successfully by a number of investigators; it seems safe to predict that such methods will replace much of the older analytical technology in the near future.

The basic principles of radiobioassay using ligand-specific proteins are entirely analogous to those of the radioimmunoassay of protein hormones. A mixture of tracer (usually ^{3}H)-labeled and unlabeled ligand is added to a sample of the protein; provided that the total amount of ligand in both forms exceeds the binding capacity of the protein present, the fraction of labeled material bound to the protein at equilibrium will depend upon the amount of unlabeled hormone present. As with immunoassays, comparison of B/F ratios after addition of a sample of unknown concentration, with ratios obtained for a series of standards, offers an estimate of the concentration of the unknown.

Corticosteroids are assayed with the aid of plasma corticosteroid-binding proteins (abbreviated CBG, since the proteins are globulins) which are present in the plasmas of various animals. The steroid selectivity of CBG is relatively low; in addition to cortisol and corticosterone, for which it has maximum affinity, human CBG will bind 21-deoxycortisol, prednisolone, progesterone, and deoxycorticosterone. To achieve specificity in the assay of any one of these compounds in plasma, an alcoholic extract of plasma is fractionated chromatographically into steroids of various polarities. CBG's from other vertebrates (dogs, monkeys, chickens) which differ in intrinsic steroid-binding capacity from human CBG, may be preferable for certain kinds of assays. Thus, canine CBG, which has an especially high affinity for cortisol, is useful for measurement of the extremely low concentrations of cortisol in cerebrospinal fluid.

Along with CBG, human plasma contains another β-globulin which binds 17-hydroxy estrane or androstane derivatives. Since testosterone and estradiol are among the steroids which are tightly bound, Murphy (1969) has called this protein the sex hormone-binding globulin (SHBG); it has been used as the ligand-binding agent in determinations of both these hormones. The concentration of SHBG is highest during late pregnancy, and pregnancy plasma is often used as its source.

In addition to various steroid-binding proteins, plasma contains at least three proteins which bind thyroxine. Binding of thyroxine to two of these (prealbumin and albumin) is relatively weak. The affinity of the thyroxine-binding globulin is much higher. Plasma thyroxine can be measured by competitive protein binding even in the presence of triiodothyronine, and triiodothyronine itself can be measured if a preliminary separation of T_3 and T_4 is carried out.

Tissues other than plasma have also been found to contain proteins with characteristic affinities for steroid hormones. The uterotrophic action of estradiol, for example, is initiated by binding of low concentrations of the steroid to a specific extranuclear "receptor." In rat uteri the receptor has been identified as a protein with a sedimentation constant of 4 S (molecular weight approximately 70,000). The estrogen-receptor complex is translocated from the cytoplasm into the nucleus of the cell, simultaneously undergoing a transformation to a more rapidly sedimenting (5 S) molecule. The latter binds to uterine chromatin and initiates the process (RNA synthesis) which leads to eventual tissue growth (Jensen and De Sombre, 1973). A similar hormone-mediated transformation of a protein receptor for dihydrotestosterone has been demonstrated in rat ventral prostate, and a receptor protein specific for progesterone has been identified in the cytoplasm of rat and rabbit uteri.

Assays for steroid hormones using hormone-specific proteins from uteri of pregnant animals and from rat ventral prostates (see Chapter 5, Section I, A) are subject to less interference from other steroids and are more sensitive than those using SHBG.

3

The Thyroid Hormones

I. Assay

Chemical methods are commonly employed for the determination of thyroid hormone concentrations in blood and other tissues. These methods, which depend upon sensitive techniques for the determination of organically bound iodine, following a preliminary chromatographic separation to increase specificity, are sensitive to 0.01–0.05 μg of iodine. Recently, the technique of competitive protein binding has been applied to the determination of thyroxine in nanogram amounts (Murphy, 1965). The protein used was thyroxine-binding globulin (TBG), a plasma α-globulin which possesses a very high affinity for thyroxine. Serum for assay was deproteinized with alcohol; an aliquot of the thyroxine-containing supernatant was evaporated and the residue dissolved in a mixture of diluted pooled plasma and ^{131}I- or ^{125}I-labeled thyroxine. After incubation with TBG, the bound thyroxine was separated on an anion-exchange resin and the filtrate, containing displaced radioactive thyroxine, was counted. Figure 3.1 shows the useful range of the assay to be 5–30 ng of T_4.

Churchill and Tapley (1964) successfully prepared an antibody, specific for tetra- and triiodothyronines and their propionic and acetic acid analogs, by coupling tetraiodothyropropionic acid to bovine serum and using the

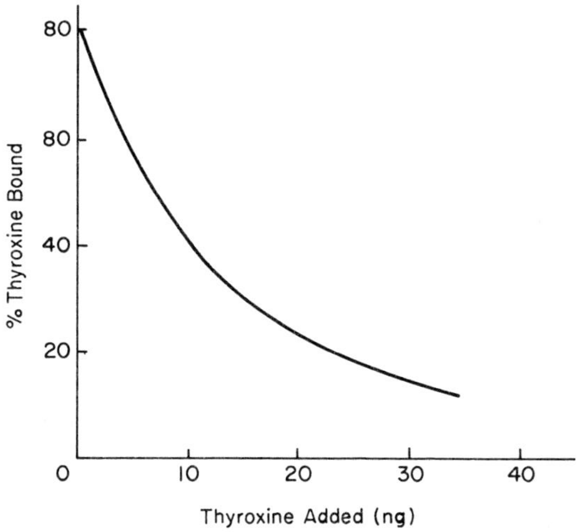

Fig. 3.1 *Determination of thyroxine in serum by radio-ligand binding. Data of Murphy (1965).*

product as antigen. The reported specificity seems adequate to permit its use in an immunoassay for thyroid hormone in plasma, although it does not seem to have been used for this purpose, thus far.

The use of thyroid hormone bioassays is confined almost exclusively to the determination of thyroactive compounds in bulk (thyroid powders or iodinated proteins) or to the determination of the thyroxine-like activity of analogs of the native hormones.

Methods for the bioassay of thyroid hormones may be grouped into three categories: (a) methods which are based upon the ability of the hormone to cause premature metamorphosis in amphibian larvae, usually tadpoles; (b) methods which depend upon the ability of these compounds to increase oxygen consumption in intact animals or isolated tissues; and (c) anti-goitrogenic methods, which measure the ability of the compound to reduce thyroid enlargement or thyroidal accumulation of iodine in animals rendered hypothyroid by administration of a goitrogen.

The use of amphibian metamorphosis as an index of thyroid hormone activity has been common practice ever since the original observations of Gudernatch in 1912. The earliest quantitative application of this effect was made by Gaddum in 1927. As modified by Frieden and Winzler (1948), groups of *Bufo* tadpoles were kept in solutions of thyroxine or thyroxine-like compounds for 7 days at 25°. The larvae decreased in length at a rate which was proportional to the concentration of thyroid hormone present. With DL-thyroxine, body length decreased 65% when the concentration was 0.5 μg/ml (Fig. 3.2). Quantitatively similar results were obtained by

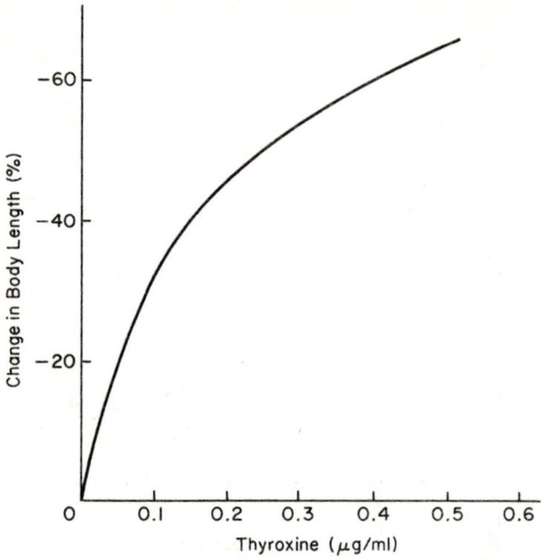

Fig. 3.2 *Effect of thyroxine upon body length of Bufo tadpoles. Data of Frieden and Winzler (1948).*

Bruice *et al.* (1954) and by Shellabarger and Godwin (1954) using *Rana* tadpoles.

Calorigenic (oxygen consumption) methods for the assay of thyroid hormone activity are significantly less sensitive than tadpole assays. Measurable increases in oxygen consumption of thyroidectomized rats can be observed within 6 days after beginning daily injections of 24 μg/kg of thyroxine (Holtkamp *et al.*, 1955). Using intact mice, Maclagen and Sheahan (1950) found that oxygen consumption increased 80–90% after 2 days with relatively large (1 mg/kg) doses of DL-thyroxine; the response was essentially linear up to 4 mg/kg (120% increase).

A simplified form of the oxygen consumption assay was proposed by Smith *et al.* (1947), based upon the survival time of mice in closed containers. For normal mice, death occurred when the oxygen concentration reached 5 volumes % and carbon dioxide, 13 volumes % (2 hours in a vessel of 870 ml capacity at 23°); thyroxine-treated animals showed less resistance to anoxia and expired at oxygen and carbon dioxide concentrations of 8% and 10%, respectively. The survival time for thyroxine-treated mice was about half that of untreated mice; the range of effective action corresponded to 0.075–0.50 mg T_4/kg of body weight every other day for 3 days (Tomich and Woolett, 1954).

Tissues isolated from animals which have been treated with thyroid hormone also show increased oxygen consumption *in vitro*. For rats, after 4 days on 2.0 mg T_4/kg/day, increases in Q_{O_2} varied from 30 (skeletal muscle) to 160% (heart) (Barker, 1956). A more rapid response was obtained with ventricular slices from cockerels which had been made hypothyroid with thiouracil (Newcomer and Barrett, 1960). With a single injection of 10 μg T_4/kg of body weight, Q_{O_2} increased from 4.0 to 9.6 μl/hour/mg within 9 hours.

If thyroxine secretion by the thyroid is inhibited, either by making iodine unavailable to the gland, or by administering a substance which blocks thyroxine synthesis (a goitrogen), the secretion of thyroid-stimulating hormone (TSH) is increased. This, in turn, induces thyroid hyperplasia, as indicated by an increase in thyroid weight. At the same time, the uptake of circulating iodide by the thyroid is increased. The administration of exogenous thyroxine inhibits TSH secretion and thus blocks both responses.

For assays of thyroid hormone by goiter prevention, mice, rats, or chicks have been used. In the modification described by Tomich and Woolett (1954), 150–250 gm rats were fed a diet containing 0.1% thiouracil for 10 days. Thyroid weights at the end of this period averaged 29.0 mg, compared to those of control animals which usually weigh 10.3 mg. Three and one-half micrograms of T_4 per day, given subcutaneously during this experimental period, reduced the average thyroid weight to 14.1 mg, while twice this dose restored it, essentially, to control values (9.9 mg).

A convenient way of measuring the antigoitrogenic properties of a preparation is to determine its ability to reduce or eliminate the accumulation of radioiodine by goitrous thyroids. Money *et al.* (1958) showed that 10–15 μg of thyroxine daily was sufficient to reduce the uptake of ^{131}I, by thyroids of thiouracil-treated rats, to values characteristic of euthyroid animals.

II. Comparative Biochemistry of the Thyroid Hormones

Thyroxine (3,5,3′,5′-tetraiodothyronine) was identified as a thyroid hormone in 1915; another, even more active compound, 3,5,3′-triiodothyronine, was isolated from thyroid tissue in 1952. Although five other organic iodine compounds have been isolated from thyroid tissue, only one, 3,3′-diiodothyronine, has any significant activity in mammals. The term "thyroid hormone" is generally reserved for thyroxine (T_4) and triiodothyronine (T_3).

Thyroid glands, or their homologs, are found only in vertebrates. In all of these animals, from cyclostomes to mammals, the only thyroid-active compounds present are T_4 and T_3. However, many vertebrate tissues other than the thyroid (or the ammocete endostyle) can concentrate iodine; these include the notochord, gills, stomach, ovary, adrenal cortex, salivary glands, and skin (Roche *et al.*, 1963). In some instances, e.g., in milk, formation of iodoproteins occurs, but in no instance has a compound more complex than diiodotyrosine been found either in the tissue or in its hydrolytic products.

The evidence for the existence of thyroxine and triiodothyronine in protochordates (amphioxus and tunicates) is more impressive. Amphioxus possesses an endostyle which serves as a thyroid anlage; in addition to concentrating iodine, this organ secretes a substance with the histochemical characteristics of thyroglobulin, the characteristic iodoprotein of the thyroid. Furthermore, implantation of amphioxus endostyles into axolotls will induce metamorphosis, and the isolation of thyroxine from an extract of the endostyle region has been reported. Good chromatographic evidence exists for the formation of thyroxine and triiodothyronine in tunicates, although there is no indication that they play a physiological role in the metabolism of any tunicate species. Again, thyroglobulin, or an allied protein, is elaborated.

Occasional reports of the existence of thyroid hormones in other invertebrates (insects, mollusks, worms) have not been confirmed. On the other hand, iodinated proteins are of widespread occurrence in invertebrates; indeed, the dry protein of some corals, anemones, and sponges may contain as much as 8% iodine. However, again there is no evidence for the existence of any iodinated component more complex than the simple iodotyrosines.

As noted above, thyroxine (Fig 3.3, III), triiodothyronine (Fig. 3.3, II), and diiodothyronine (Fig. 3.3, I) are the only naturally occurring thyroid-active compounds. However, a large number of compounds related to the iodothyronines and possessing activity in one or another kind of bioassay has been synthesized. Tables compiled from the data available in the literature have been assembled by Selenkow and Asper (1955), by Bruice *et al.* (1956) and by Frieden (1968).

Until 1952, no compound more active than thyroxine was known. In that year, Gross and Pitt-Rivers isolated triiodothyronine, and discovered it to be 5–10 times as active as thyroxine by assays in both amphibians (induction of metamorphosis) and mammals (O_2 consumption, goiter prevention). Later, Money *et al.* (1958, 1959) reported that some deamino analogs of the principal hormones, tri- and tetraiodothyroacetic (Fig. 3.3, IV, $n = 1$), thyropropionic (Fig. 3.3, IV, $n = 2$), and thyrobutyric (Fig. 3.3, IV, $n = 3$) acids were 8–30 times as active in inducing metamorphosis in tadpoles as T_4. These same compounds were found by Stasilli *et al.* (1963) to possess only a fraction of the activity of T_4 in antigoitrogenic and calorigenic assays. The anomalously high activity in tadpoles was later (Frieden and Westmark, 1961) shown to be an artifact of the immersion method for testing compounds for metamorphic activity; when the same compounds were tested by injection in tadpoles, their relative effectiveness

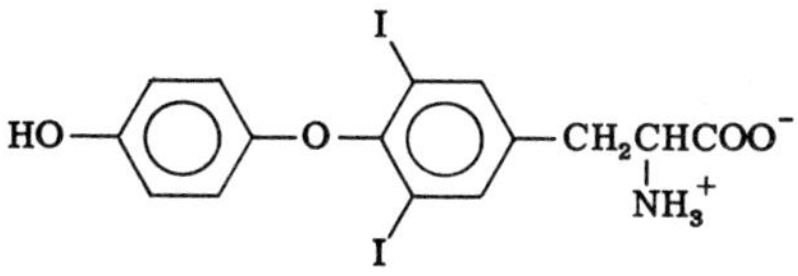

(I)

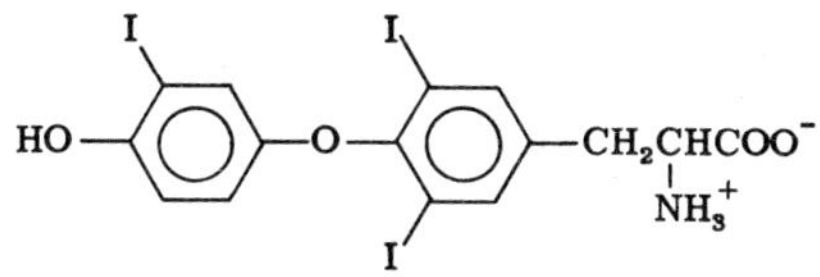

(II)

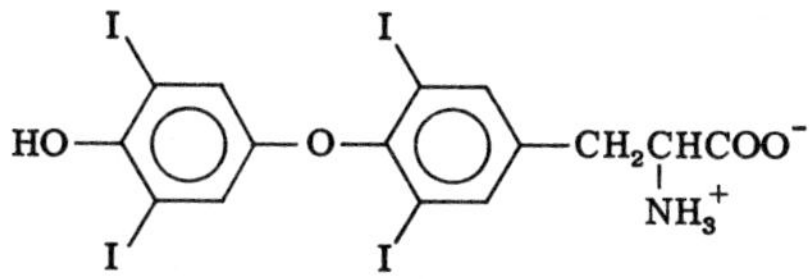

(III)

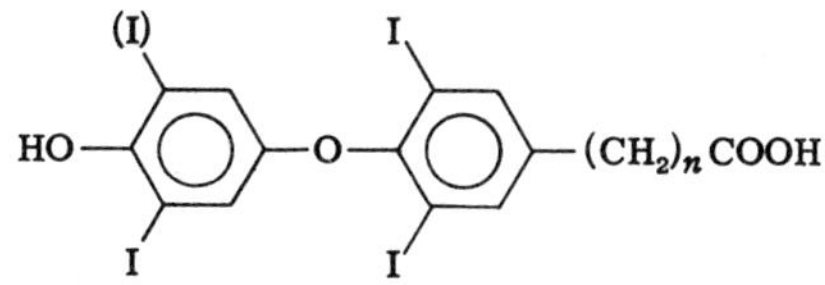

(IV)

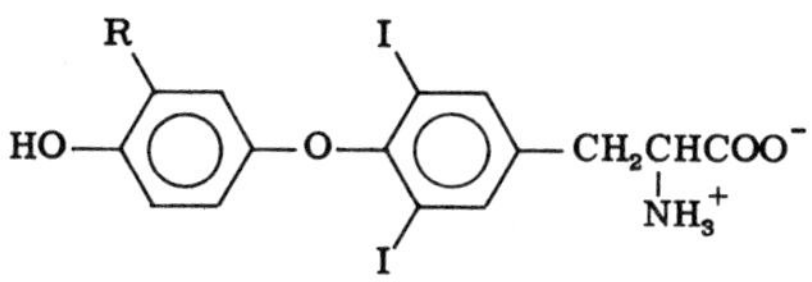

(V)

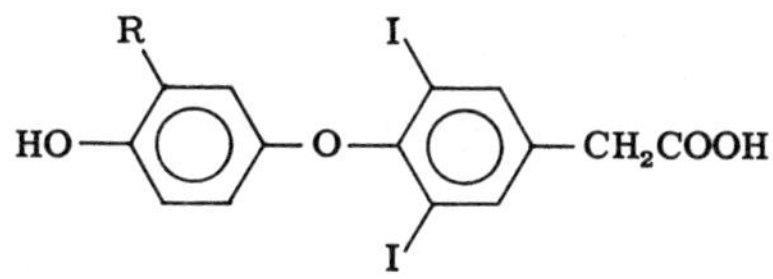

(VI)

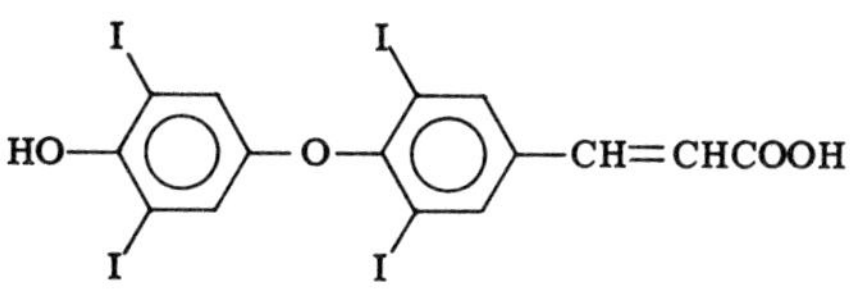

(VII)

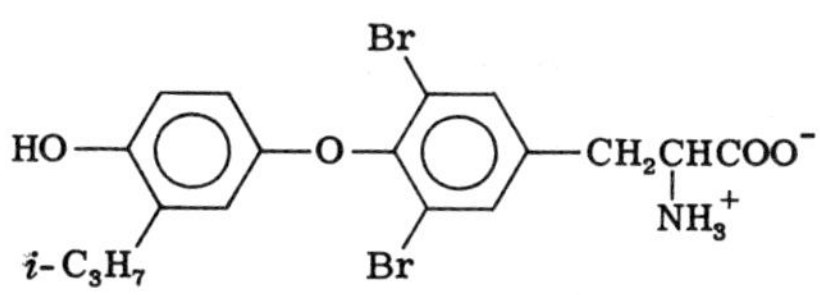

(VIII)

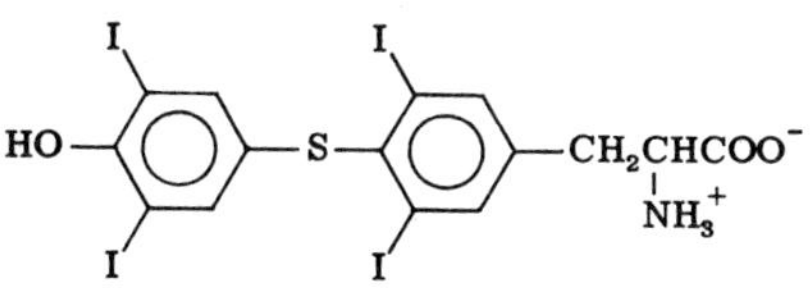

(IX)

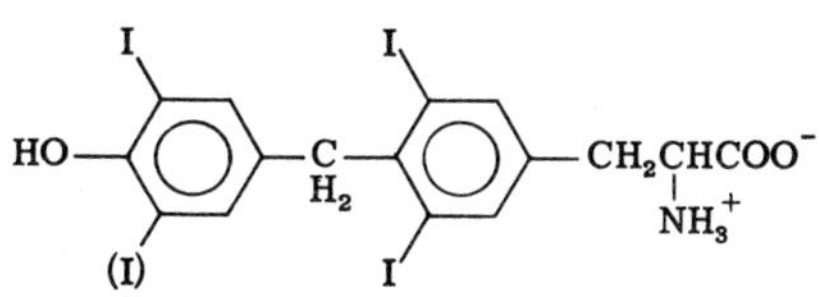

(X)

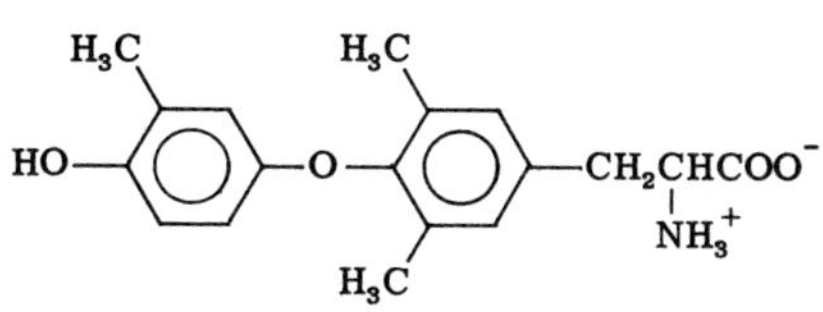

(XI)

Fig. 3.3 *Structures of thyroxine analogs.*

was substantially reduced (from three- to tenfold). Other compounds which have substantial activity in the tadpole include the 3′-ethyl (Fig. 3.3, V, $R = C_2H_5$) and 3′-methyl (Fig. 3.3, V, $R = CH_3$) analogs of T_3, the 3′-isopropyl derivatives of diiodothyronine and diiodothyroacetic acids (Fig. 3.3, V, VI, $R = CH(CH_3)_2$), and tetraiodothyroacrylic acid (Fig. 3.3, VII). Of these, only the methyl, ethyl, and isopropyl diiodothyronines are as active as T_4 in mammals.

The D-isomers of both thyroxine and triiodothyronine have substantially reduced activities in all assays.

3,5-Dibromo-3′-isopropylthyronine (Fig. 3.3, VIII), which is more active than T_4 in both amphibian and mammalian assays, is one of the few examples of an active compound which contains no iodine. Thyroid activity is also displayed by the thioether (Fig. 3.3, IX) and methylene (Fig. 3.3, X,XI) analogs of T_3 or T_4. 4-Thiothyroxine possesses about one-fifth the activity of the parent compound and displays typical T_4-like activity. Methylene bridged thyroxine [3,5-diiodo-4(3,5 diiodo-4-hydroxybenzyl)phenylalanine] has about one-tenth the activity of T_4 in the assay used (Psychoyos *et al.*, 1973).

Recently, an active nonhalogenated thyronine, L-3,5,3′-trimethylthyronine (Fig. 3.3, XII) was synthesized by Jorgensen and Block (1973). This compound was 2% as active as L-T_4 in the rat antigoiter assay, while L-3,5,3′,5′-tetramethyl thyronine was inactive at a dose equivalent to 100 times the effective dose of T_4.

4

Hormones of the Adrenal Medulla

I. Assay

The chemical determination of epinephrine and norepinephrine has reached a state of sophistication rivaled by few hormone assays. The separation of epinephrine (E) from norepinephrine (NE), and their fluorometric estimation, is applicable to fractions of a nanogram (10^{-9}gm); despite this, however, the amounts found in blood are so small that several milliliters of plasma may be required for reliable determinations (Haggendal, 1966; Callingham, 1967; Weil-Malherbe, 1968).

Bioassays of epinephrine and norepinephrine employ both whole animals and isolated tissues. In one of the earliest bioassays, blood pressure changes in the anesthetized cat resulting from the intravenous injection of E or NE were recorded. Approximately 100 ng of NE sufficed to produce a distinct increase in blood pressure. About twice as much E as NE was usually required for a comparable response.

Blood pressure changes in rats also may be used to assay E and NE. Both hormones are equally effective, about 2 ng of either representing the lower limit of detection. If the rat's spinal cord is destroyed, a single preparation may be used for repeated assays during a period of 10 hours.

When a small amount of adrenaline is injected into the central artery of the ear of a denervated rabbit, the ensuing constriction is clearly visible. The test is extremely sensitive, and a rough estimate of quantity is possible, since the duration of the effect is proportional to the dose. Thus, the injection of 0.1 ml of plasma containing 1 ng of epinephrine produces a vasoconstriction lasting about 90 seconds, whereas one-tenth this amount also produces a clearly observable response, lasting, however, for but 30 seconds.

For *in vitro* assays of the catecholamine hormones, the rat stomach, the rat or rabbit ileum, and the fowl cecum have been used. Specificity was achieved by prior separation of E from NE (or from other substances) by chromatography. The rat uterus is also fairly specific for epinephrine if, after spontaneous contractions have been abolished, the unknown is titrated against a predetermined quantity of acetylcholine or carbachol. These agents restore rhythmic contractions of the uterus, while epinephrine inhibits the response. As little as 0.1 ng E in 5 ml of fluid is needed. Norepinephrine is much less effective, the index of discrimination being 100–200.

Like the rat uterus, the fowl cecum is relatively insensitive to NE *in vitro;* on the other hand, rat and rabbit intestine respond similarly to both.

In the bioassay of adrenaline, only rarely is a complete dose (or log dose) response curve plotted. Instead, two solutions of the unknown, differing by a factor of 1.5 or 2 in concentration, are sought, which will bracket the effects of a standard preparation. By this means, estimates of unknown concentrations reliable to ±20% are sometimes possible.

Very recently, the differences in sensitivity, between the rat stomach strip and fowl cecum, to E and NE have been exploited by Vane (1964; 1966) for continuous measurement of both hormones in circulating blood. Carotid blood from an experimental animal was pumped successively through a chamber containing a strip of rat stomach, then through one containing a fowl cecum, before being returned to the circulation. From the responses of the two muscles, rapid changes in the concentrations of both E and NE could be followed. Injection of as little as 0.6 μg/kg of epinephrine into an experimental animal caused a recognizable change in the tone of each muscle.

II. Chemical Nature; Occurrence

Epinephrine and norepinephrine are both catecholamines, derived from the amino acid tyrosine.

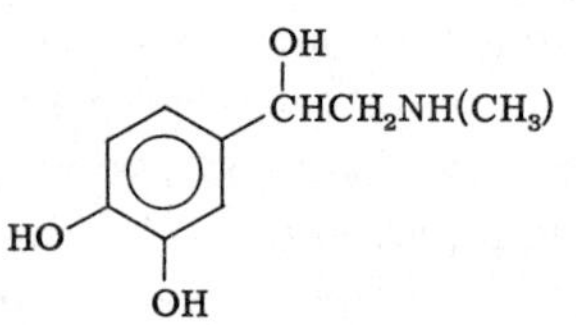

Epinephrine

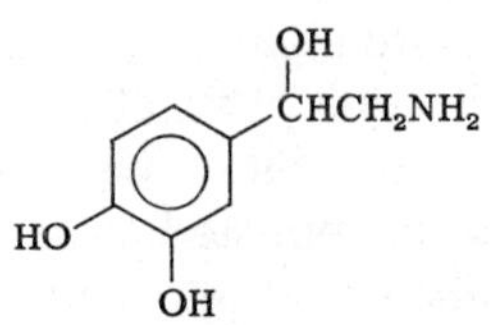

Norepinephrine

The naturally occurring form (of epinephrine) is the D(−) isomer; the L(+) form has only 5% of the activity of its stereoisomer.

Both epinephrine and norepinephrine have been identified in the tissues of a large number of homiothermic and poikilothermic vertebrates. Aside from the adrenal glands and their homologs, the largest concentrations (10–20 μg/gm for norepinephrine) are found in splenic nerves of mammals; in general, the catecholamine content of most tissues is correlated with the degree of adrenergic innervation. The proportions of epinephrine to norepinephrine vary widely, but in most vertebrate tissues, only a small fraction of the total is epinephrine. Exceptions include the ventricles of both *Myxine* (hagfish) and *Rana* (frogs).

Östlund *et al.* (1960), and later von Euler (1961), looked for catecholamines in representatives of eight invertebrate phyla. Measurable amounts were found in four groups. From 0.3–2.0 μg/gm of norepinephrine was reported to be present in the larva and imagos of earwigs, beetles, houseflies, bees, and butterflies; some of these contained smaller quantities of epinephrine. In earthworms both amines were concentrated in the ganglionic chain, and the salivary glands of *Octopus* contained a considerable quantity of NE. Little is known of the functions of catecholamines in invertebrates, and pharmacodynamic data for the actions of epinephrine on the heart and other muscles of invertebrates are quite contradictory (see Gabe *et al.*, 1964).

III. Structure and Biological Activity

The complexity of the physiological responses to epinephrine and norepinephrine makes it difficult to carry out any extended studies of the relationship of structure to physiological activity, unless such a survey is confined to one or, at most, two aspects of sympathomimetic action. From the earliest of such studies, beginning in the early 1900's, the pressor response has generally been selected as a principal index of comparison. More recently, Pruss *et al.* (1965) have used induction of contraction in a strip of rabbit aorta *in vitro* to compare the properties of aromatic congeners of epinephrine and norepinephrine.

Epinephrine and norepinephrine are approximately equally effective in increasing blood pressure in the cat, rabbit, or rat. Norepinephrine is somewhat more (approximately 20%) active than epinephrine on the rabbit aorta *in vitro.* Although a very large number of compounds have been tested for epinephrine-like pressor activity, few can claim to be even remotely as effective. A good many phenylethylamines are active, but the doses required are from four to several hundred times the effective dose of epinephrine. Some of the compounds which possess activity, however, also have proper-

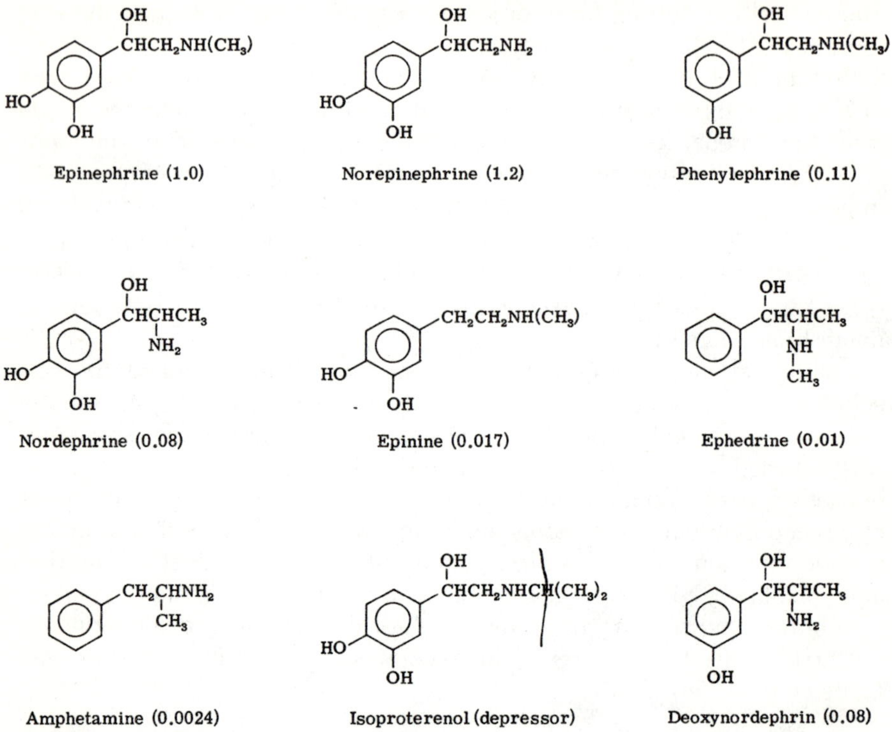

Fig. 4.1 *Compounds with epinephrine-like (pressor) activity. The numbers in brackets represent the relative pressor activity (epinephrine = 1.0). Data of Hartung (1945).*

ties such as prolonged activity, or enhanced stability, which make them useful therapeutically. Some representative compounds with epinephrine-like action are shown in Fig. 4.1.

The key to significant pressor activity apparently lies in the basic phenylethylamine structure. Hydroxylation of the benzene ring is an important amplifier of pressor activity; phenylephrine (3-OH) is one-fifth to one-tenth as active as epinephrine, while ephedrine and amphetamine, which are nonphenolic, are less than one-hundredth as active as the standard. More extensive data on the relationship between structure and activity in this series of compounds are to be found in Hartung's paper (1945).

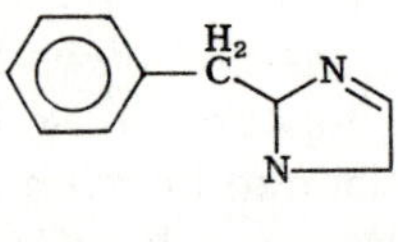

2-Benzylimidazoline

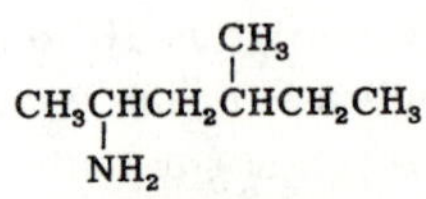

2-Amino-4-methylhexane

In addition to the phenylethylamines, two other classes of compounds possess adrenergic activity. One group includes some substituted imidazolines, especially benzylimidazoline. In a sense, these are phenylethylamines in which the ethylamine moiety has become part of a heterocyclic ring. The other class of compounds, which possess activities between 0.001–0.005 times that of epinephrine, are primary alkylamines with six or more carbon atoms.

5

The Steroid Hormones

I. Estrogens

A. ASSAY

In recent years, sensitive nonbiological techniques for the quantitative determination of a number of steroids, including the steroidal hormones, have been developed. The most sensitive of these depend heavily upon isotope derivative, fluorometric, or gas chromatographic techniques, and have enjoyed increasing popularity, especially for the determination of steroid hormones and their metabolites in body fluids. Nevertheless, in this area, as in so many others, bioassays continue to be widely employed, both for situations which require the utmost sensitivity and when studies of comparative biological effectiveness are required.

The most sensitive bioassays for estrogens are based upon the appearance of cornified cells in the vaginal epithelium of ovariectomized rats or mice. This is also one of the oldest assays, the basic technique having been introduced by Allen and Doisy in 1923. In mice the systemic injection of 0.1 μg of estradiol benzoate, or 0.35 μg of estrone (both dissolved in an oily vehicle) induces positive responses in about half the animals injected, as shown in vaginal smears prepared 48–56 hours later. A similar response in

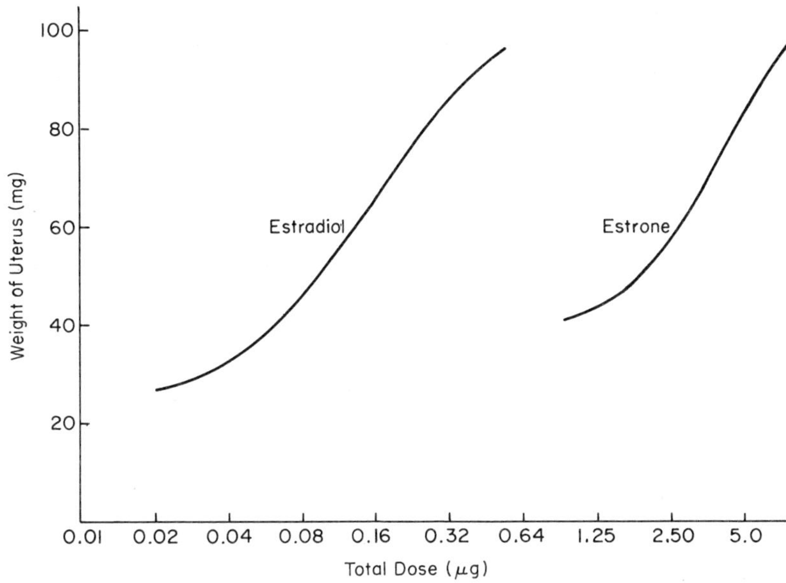

Fig. 5.1 *Estrogen assay. Immature rats were treated twice daily for 3 days and killed on the fourth day. Data of Lauson et al. (1939; quoted by Emmens, 1962b).*

rats requires 0.3 μg of estradiol benzoate or 2–3 μg of estrone (Pincus, 1948).

Efforts to improve the sensitivity, reliability, or precision of the Allen–Doisy assay have resulted in the introduction of modifications in the basic technique by literally scores of investigators. These include variations in the vehicle used, the route of administration, and frequency of injection. Marked improvement in the sensitivity of the assay is achieved by introducing the sample directly into the vagina; the effective dose of estrone under these conditions is only 0.003 μg. A further tenfold increase in sensitivity occurs if the number of mitoses in vaginal sections is used as an index of response (Emmens, 1962a).

Quantitative determinations of estrogen content may also be made by measuring the increase in weight of the uterus of the immature rat after multiple injections. In the modification described by Lauson (Emmens, 1962b) a total dose of 0.05 μg estradiol for 4 days will double the uterine weight (Fig. 5.1). An assay which requires only 6 hours, and which depends upon the rapid increase in hydration of the immature rat uterus was described by Astwood in 1938. The response is linear with the logarithm of the dose over a wide range (0.07–1.2 μg estrone; 0.006–0.10 μg estradiol).

The application of radiobioassay techniques to the determination of estrogen concentrations in body fluids has been alluded to earlier. Methods for the determination of plasma estradiol using pregnancy plasma as a source of sex hormone-binding globulin (SHBG) (see Chapter 2, Section III, A, 4) have been described by Mayes and Nugent (1970) and by Dufau *et al.* (1970). These methods differ principally in the way plasma estradiol is first separated from other sterols and in the final separation of free and bound estradiol; the applicable concentration range was 1–5 ng (Fig. 5.2).

Improved specificity and sensitivity in estrogen assays may be achieved if estrogen-binding proteins (isolated from uteri of various pregnant animals—rabbits, cows, horses, sheep, rats, and humans) are used as the source of the ligand-binding protein in place of plasma proteins. These proteins display considerably more specificity than does plasma SHBG; they will bind the natural estrogens (estradiol, estrone, estriol), as well as other compounds with estrogenic activity (stilbestrol, ethinylestradiol, and estrone acetate). Other steroids, such as testosterone, progesterone, and cortical steroids are bound feebly, if at all.

Korenman *et al.* (1970) used a crude estrogen-binding protein fraction obtained from the cytoplasm of pregnant rabbit uteri. The basis of the assay was, as before, displacement of either tritiated estradiol or tritiated estrone from the estrogen-binding protein by unlabeled estradiol, estrone, or estriol. Samples to be assayed were first extracted with ether, then the ethereal extract was fractionated on celite; this procedure not only separated estrogens from other steroids, but separated the three phenolic estrogens from each

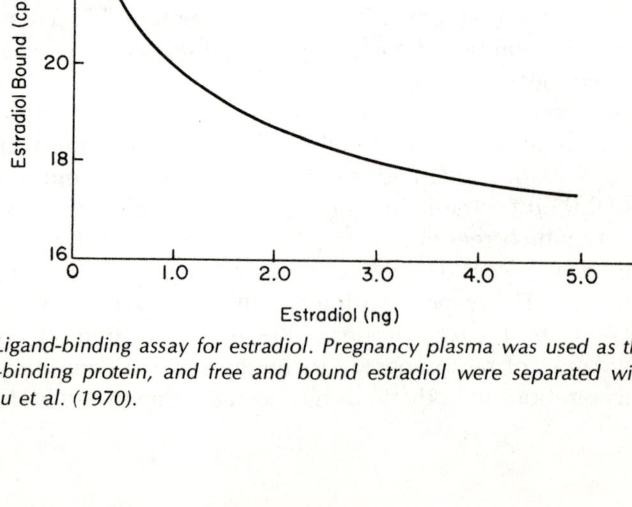

Fig. 5.2 *Ligand-binding assay for estradiol. Pregnancy plasma was used as the source of the estrogen-binding protein, and free and bound estradiol were separated with charcoal. Data of Dufau et al. (1970).*

other. After incubation of protein, labeled steroid, and sample, free and bound steroids were separated by treatment with dextran-treated charcoal. The minimum detectable amount of estradiol was 10–20 pg (1 pg = 10^{-12}gm); for estrone and estriol, the minima were somewhat higher (25–50 pg). Corker and his associates have described a procedure similar in many details except that plasma estrogens were separated by thin-layer chromatography on alumina before assay (1970).

Lieberman, Goodfriend, and others, several years ago, showed that various steroids would serve as haptens when conjugated with plasma albumin (Lieberman *et al.*, 1959; Goodfriend and Sehon, 1960), and that antibodies to such steroid-protein complexes would cross react specifically with the steroid used as the hapten, as well as its derivatives and near homologs. To prepare the antigens, the 3-, 17-, or 21-hydroxy groups of steroids were coupled through the hemisuccinate or chlorocarbonate with the ε-amino groups of plasma albumin. Ketonic steroids could also be used; they were first allowed to react with *O*-carboxymethyl hydroxylamine; the resulting acid oxime was then conjugated to protein.

Immunochemical assays of various estrogens have been reported to be capable of detecting 50–400 pg (Abraham *et al.*, 1970; Mikhail *et al.*, 1970).

B. OCCURRENCE, CHEMISTRY, AND BIOLOGICAL ACTIVITY

In addition to their universal occurrence in vertebrates, extracts with estrogenic activity have been prepared from protozoans, coelenterates, worms, mollusks, crustaceans, arachnids, insects, and echinoderms. Indeed, the ubiquity of estrogens is not confined to the animal kingdom, since thirty families of higher plants have been discovered to have estrogen-like activity. The chemical nature of most of these substances is unknown; however, estradiol has been identified in plant extracts as well as in starfish ovaries. A nonsteroidal compound, genistein (Fig. 5.3, I), which possesses potent activity as an estrogen, has been isolated from Australian subterranean clover. Estradiol (Fig. 5.3, II) and estrone (Fig. 5.3, III) have been identified in the ovaries or placentas of humans, cattle, pigs, and horses. Among mammals, estriol (Fig. 5.3, IV) has so far been found only in humans. Estradiol-17α (Fig. 5.3, V) has been isolated from cattle placentas and appears to be the only identifiable estrogen in sheep and goat placentas. Pregnant mares excrete estrogens with additional unsaturation in ring B—equilen (Fig. 5.3, VI) and equilenin (Fig. 5.3, VII); whether these compounds are metabolites of other steroids is not known.* Hydroxyestradiol-6α (Fig. 5.3, VIII) has been found in the follicular fluid of pregnant mares.

* However, Heard *et al.* (1956) showed that ^{14}C-labeled estrone does not give rise to labeled equilin or equilenin in horses.

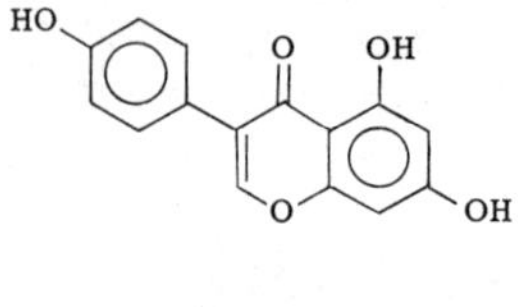

Genistein
(I)

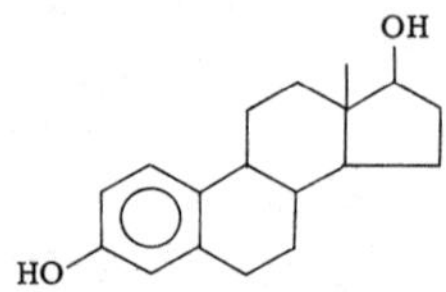

Estradiol
(II)

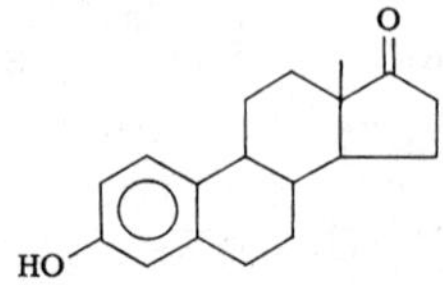

Estrone
(III)

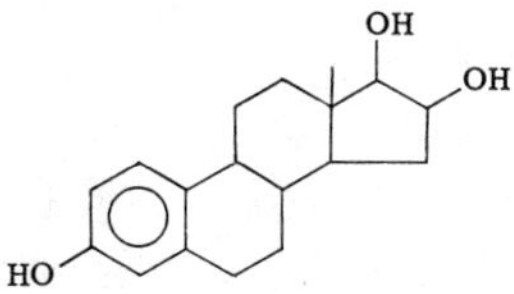

Estriol
(IV)

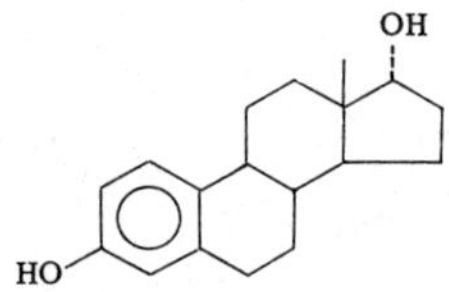

Estradiol-17α
(V)

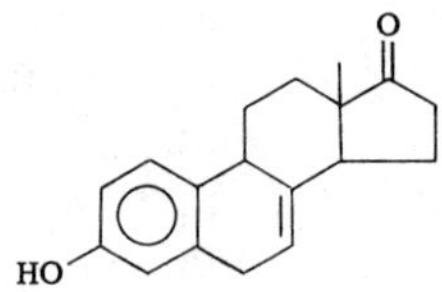

Equilenin
(VI)

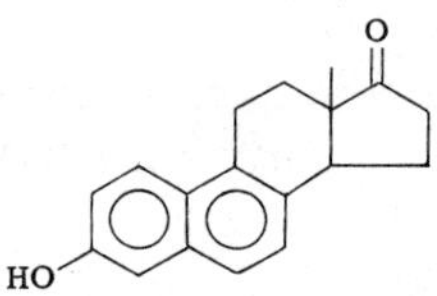

Equilenin
(VII)

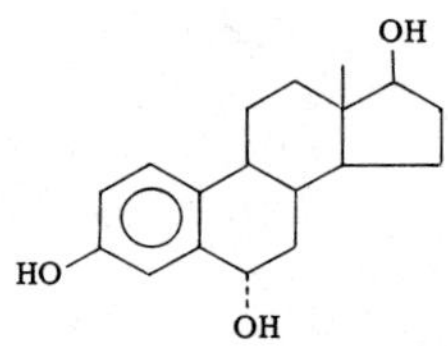

Hydroxyestradiol-6α
(VIII)

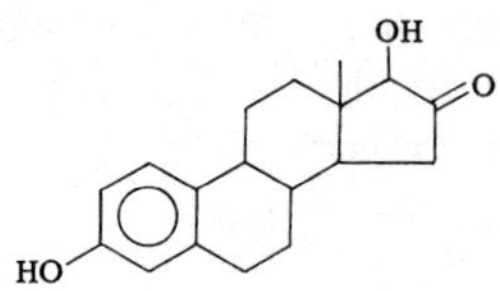

16-Ketoestradiol
(IX)

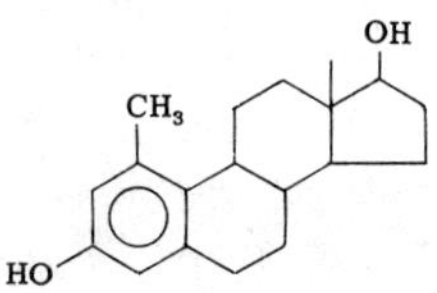

1-Methylestradiol
(X)

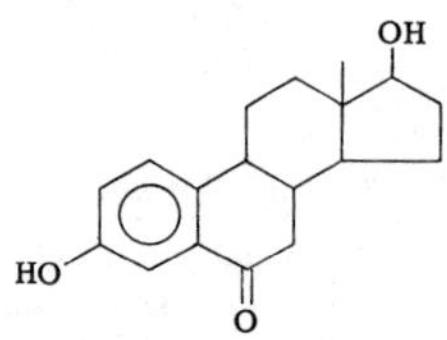

6-Ketoestradiol
(XI)

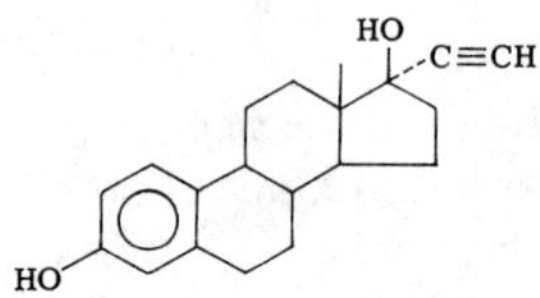

17α-Ethinylestradiol
(XII)

Fig. 5.3 *Structures of some naturally occurring estrogens and related compounds.*

Among nonmammalian vertebrates, estrone and estradiol have been found in ovaries and plasma of the domestic hen, in amphibians, in reptiles, in the ovaries and/or plasma of a number of species of fish (dogfish, cod, salmon), and in the ovaries of the sea urchin and a mollusk (Botticelli *et al.*, 1961). Fish plasma has also been shown to contain estriol, *epi*-estriol, estradiol-17α, and 16-ketoestradiol (Fig. 5.3, IX).

The relative activities of a number of naturally occurring estrogens are shown in Table 5.1. These data are based on responses in the Allen–Doisy (vaginal cornification) test (Shoppee, 1964).

TABLE 5.1 Biological Activities of Naturally Occurring Estrogens

Compound	Relative activity[a]
Estradiol-17β	1.00
Estrone	0.125
Dihydroequilen-17β	0.10
Equilin	0.08
Estradiol-17α	0.025
Estriol	0.010
Dihydroequilenin	0.008
Equilenin (*dextro*)	0.006
Dihydroequilen-17α	0.0025
17α-Ethinylestradiol	0.100

[a] *Relative activity* $= \dfrac{\textit{minimum dose of estradiol}}{\textit{minimum dose of compound}}$.

Estrogen activity is critically dependent upon the presence of at least one benzene ring; estrane derivatives with only one or two double bonds are essentially inactive. Insertion of alkyl groups or oxygen atoms onto the steroid nucleus [1-methylestradiol (Fig. 5.3, X), 6-ketoestradiol (Fig. 5.3, XI), 16-ketoestradiol (Fig. 5.3, IX)] result in products that are significantly less active than the parent compound. However, 17α-ethinylestradiol (Fig. 5.3, XII) is as active as estradiol parenterally, and considerably more active orally.

Ever since the discovery (by Dodds *et al.*, in 1938) that diethylstilbestrol (*trans*,-4,4′-dihydroxy-α, β-diethylstilbene) was a potent estrogen, a search for other compounds with estrogenic activity has been pursued. Hogg and Korman (1956) have summarized the comparative estrogenic potencies of approximately 2000 compounds as determined by vaginal cornification assay. Representatives of the major classes of compounds which are estrogenic, parenterally or orally, in doses of fractions of a microgram to a few micrograms in rats are shown in Fig. 5.4.

The naturally occurring estrogens, taken orally, are relatively inactive. For example, the orally effective dose of estradiol in rats is 100 times the subcutaneous dose. A potent stimulus for research into new estrogens has therefore been to discover compounds which are orally active. One example of success in this search is ethinylestradiol; in contrast to estradiol, the ratio of orally effective vs. subcutaneously effective doses is only 10:1.

Among the groups of compounds which display relatively high oral activity are the stilbestrols, hexestrols, and doisynolic acids. Recently a new group of compounds, the 11β-nitro-9α-hydroxy analogs of estrone and estradiol, have been discovered to possess high oral:subcutaneous effectiveness ratios. Thus, 9α-hydroxy-12β-nitroestrone is as active as estrone by

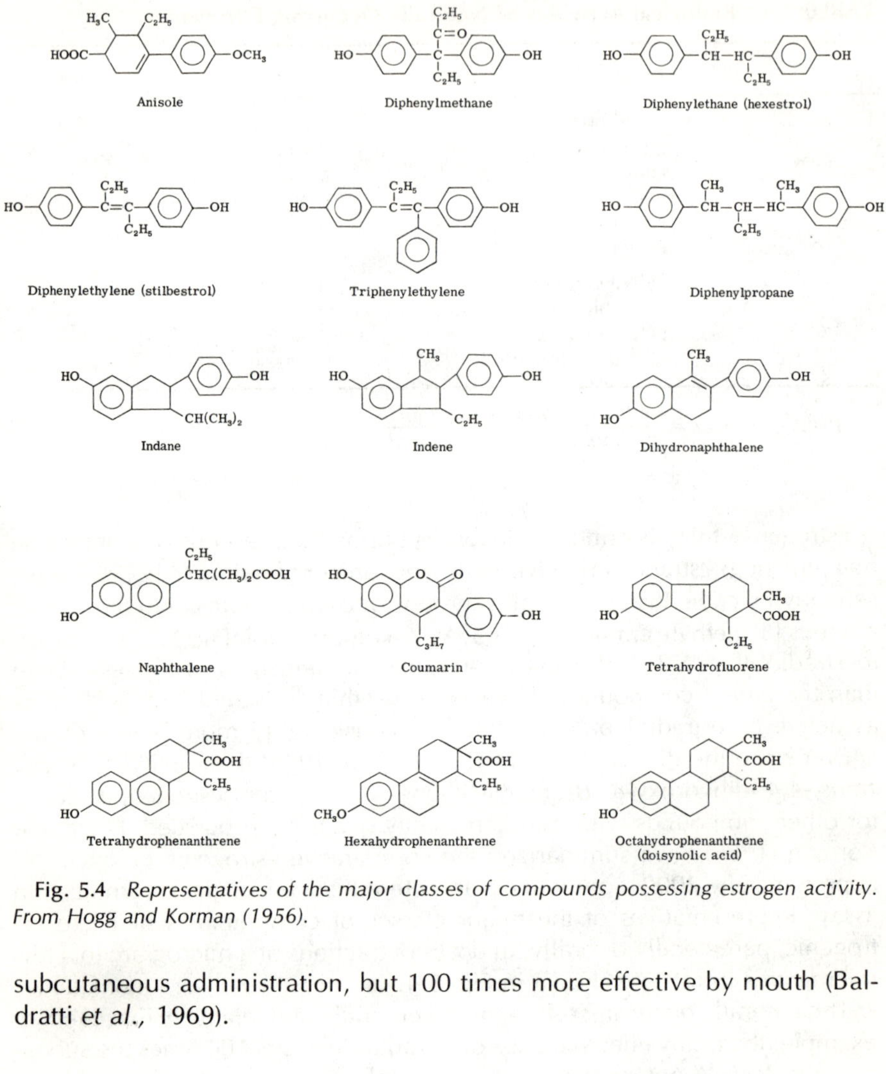

Fig. 5.4 *Representatives of the major classes of compounds possessing estrogen activity. From Hogg and Korman (1956).*

subcutaneous administration, but 100 times more effective by mouth (Baldratti *et al.*, 1969).

II. Progestins

A. ASSAY

Most of the bioassays of progesterone are based upon the original observation of Corner and Allen, in 1929, that progesterone would cause progestational proliferation in the uterus of a rabbit that had been spayed after mating. Clauberg (1930) used immature rabbits that had received estrogen priming for 6 days. A total of 0.75 mg of progesterone in divided doses during the ensuing 5 days produced a definite transformation of the endometrium.

In 1939, McGinty described a modification of the Clauberg test in which the progestational substance was injected directly into the lumen of one uterine horn of an immature, estrogen-primed rabbit. The other horn served as a control. The uteri were sectioned for histological examination 3 days

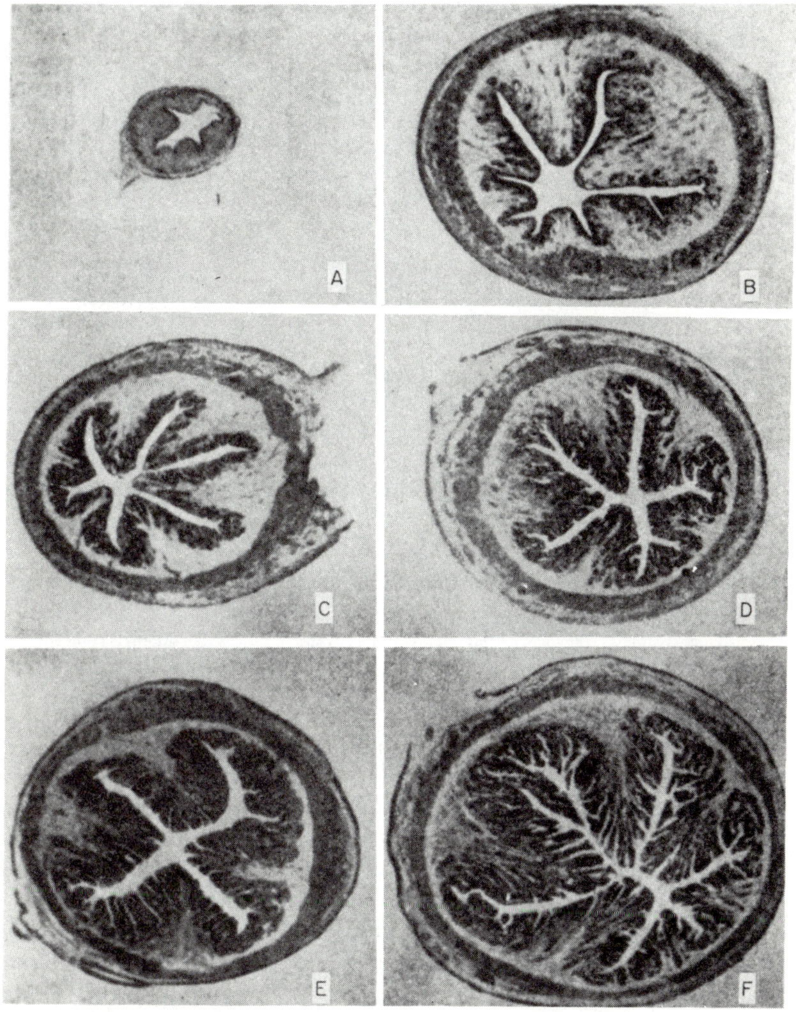

Fig. 5.5 *Clauberg assay for progesterone. The photographs are of uterine sections from rabbits treated with increasing amounts of progesterone. Reproduced, with permission, from Miyake (1962).*

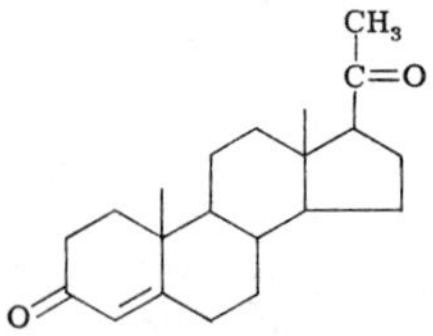

Progesterone
(1.0)
(I)

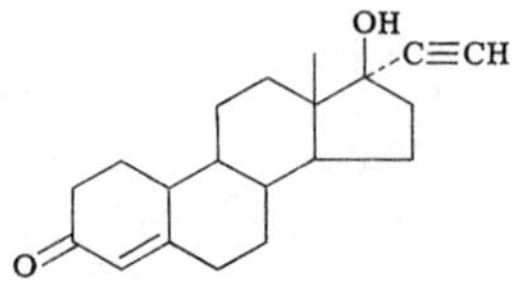

17α-Ethinyl-19-nor-
testosterone (0.5-1.5)
(II)

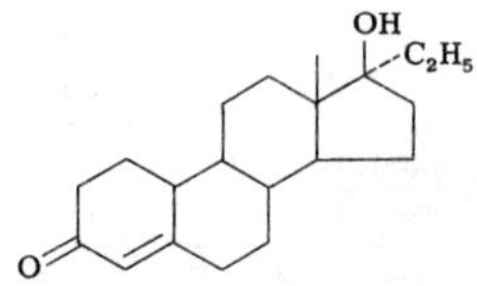

17α-Ethyl-19-nor-
testosterone (5-10)
(III)

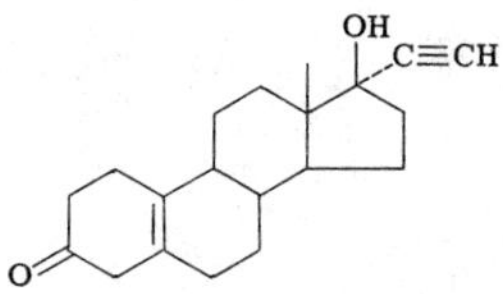

17α-Ethinyl-$\Delta^{5(10)}$-
androsten-17-ol-3-one
(IV)

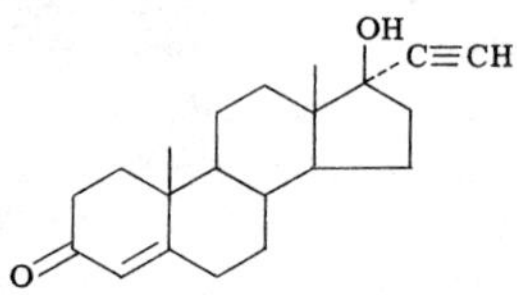

17α-Ethinyl-
testosterone (0.3)
(V)

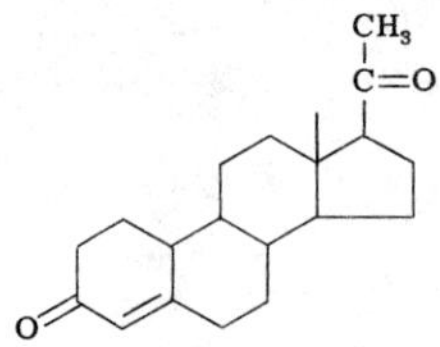

19-Norprogesterone
(4-8)
(VI)

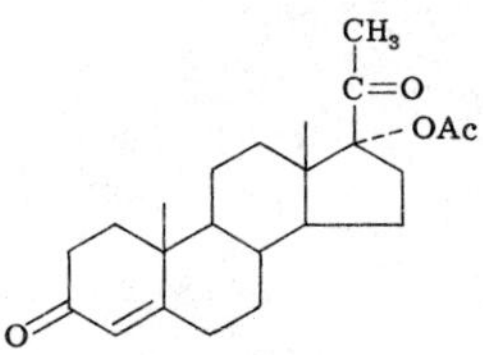

17α-Hydroxyproges-
terone acetate (10)
(VII)

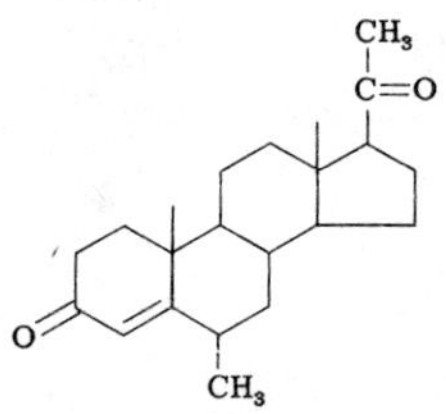

6α-Methylprogesterone
(5)
(VIII)

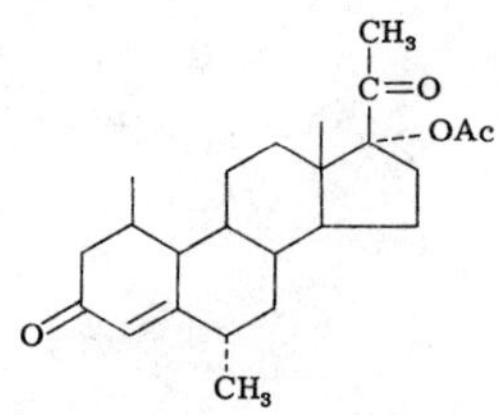

6α-Methyl-17-hydroxy-
progesterone acetate (10-20)
(IX)

Fig. 5.6 *Some synthetic progestins. The arabic numbers in parentheses represent progestational activity, compared to progesterone (=1).*

after the injection (Fig. 5.5). The McGinty test is sensitive to 0.5–10 μg of progesterone and a dose–response curve can be constructed by grading each response according to an arbitrary scale. The sensitivity of progesterone assays was vastly improved by Hooker and Forbes (1947), who showed that minute amounts (0.2–1.0 ng) of progesterone injected into the lumen of a ligated segment of the uterus of an ovariectomized mouse resulted in hypertrophy of the stromal nuclei of the endometrium within 48 hours after the injection. This test possesses high specificity as well as sensitivity; its principal disadvantage is its all-or-none character, which makes it difficult to quantitate.

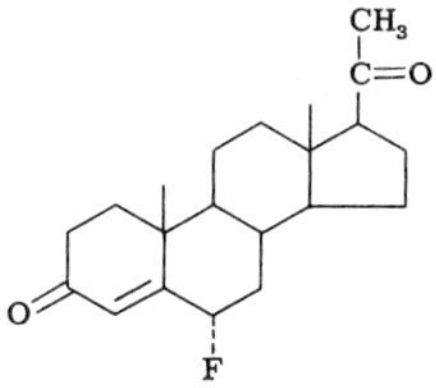

6α-Fluoroprogesterone (5-10)

(X)

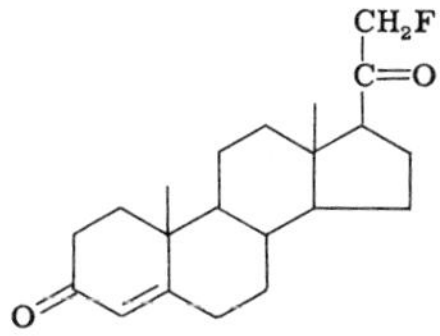

21-Fluoroprogesterone (6)

(XI)

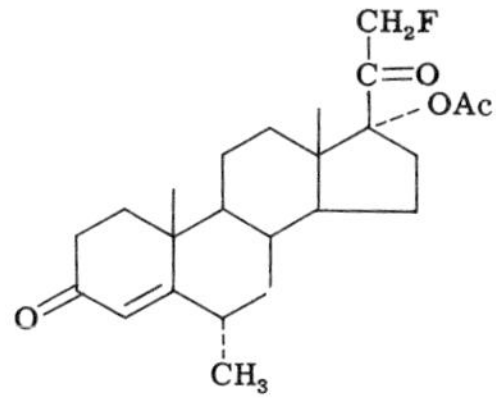

6α-Methyl-17α-acetoxy-21-fluoroprogesterone (50)

(XII)

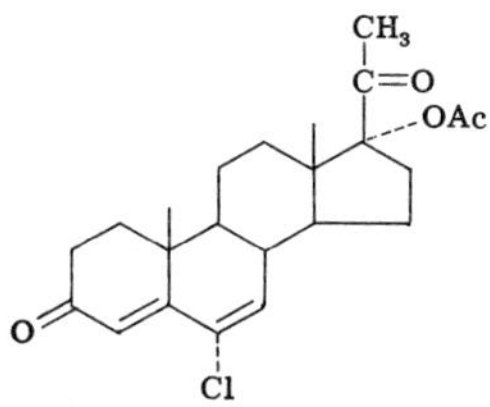

6-Chloro-Δ^6-17α-acetoxy-progesterone (50)

(XIII)

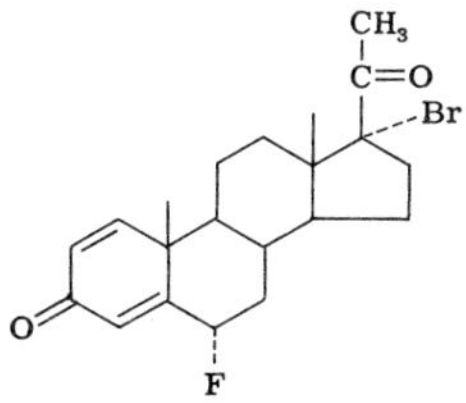

Δ^1-6α-Fluoro-17α-bromo-progesterone (12)

(XIV)

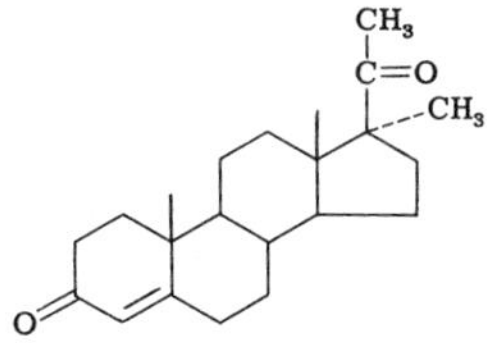

17α-Methylprogesterone (3)

(XV)

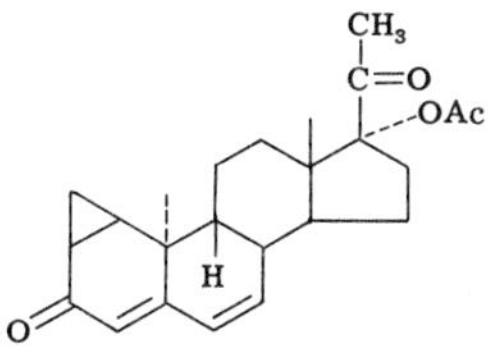

1, 2β-Methylene-Δ^6-9β, 10α-17α-acetoxyprogesterone (30)

(XVI)

Fig. 5.6 *(Continued)*

Other bioassays for progesterone are based upon the ability of this substance to increase carbonic anhydrase activity in rabbit endometrium and its ability to induce decidual responses in traumatized uteri of ovariectomized cervically stimulated rats. Both assays give responses that can be quantitated; however, their sensitivities are several orders of magnitude less than the Hooker–Forbes assay, requiring, as they do, amounts of progesterone ranging from 0.5–5.0 mg per animal.

The application of radiobioassay methods to the determination of progesterone has been described by Yoshimi and Lipsett (1968). They used plasma from estrogen- and dexamethasone-treated women (see Section IV, A) as a source of steroid-binding globulin. A small column of Sephadex G-25 was used to separate free and bound ^3H-progesterone. For the assay of progesterone in plasma, the plasma was extracted with ether and the extract was subjected to thin-layer chromatography and column chromatography on alumina. Losses during the extraction and fractionation were estimated by adding a small amount of tritiated progesterone to the original plasma sample. (This amount of tracer was too small to interfere in subsequent steps in which tritiated progesterone was again used.)

B. OCCURRENCE, CHEMICAL NATURE

Progesterone has been isolated from corpora lutea of nearly a dozen mammalian species, including humans, cattle, elephants, guinea pigs, rats, and whales. Nonmammalian sources include the ovaries of birds, dogfish, lungfish, starfish, sea urchins, and scallops. No other progestationally active compounds have been identified with certainty, except for the 20α- and 20β-hydroxy analogs isolated from human reproductive tract tissue by Zander *et al.* (1958).

The first synthetic compound which was found to have progestational activity was a testosterone derivative, 17α-ethinyl testosterone (Fig. 5.6, V), which was only about half as active as progesterone subcutaneously, but was active orally (progesterone is not). A considerable number of parenterally and orally active progestins have since been discovered. These fall into three principal categories: derivatives of 19-nortestosterone (Fig. 5.6, II, III); derivatives of testosterone (Fig. 5.6., V); and modifications of progesterone itself (Fig. 5.6, VI–XV). The latter group includes 19-norprogesterone (Fig. 5.6, VI), compounds into which additional unsaturation has been introduced at positions 1 (Fig. 5.6, XIV), and 6 (Fig. 5.6, XIII), and those which bear substituents at C-6, C-17, and C-21.

Although ethisterone (17α-ethinyltestosterone, Fig. 5.6, V) is relatively inactive parenterally, its 19-norderivative is about five times as active as the parent compound. It is also active orally. None of the 17α-hydroxyprogesterone derivatives are active; however, the esters (acetates) of 17α-hydroxyprogesterones are 10–50 times as active as the alcohols. The relative inactivity of the free 17-alcohols, as compared to the esters, is also true for testosterone derivatives; 17α-ethinyl 19-nortestosterone acetate is 30 times as active as norethisterone.

Introduction of halogen atoms, and additional unsaturation in rings A or B increases biological activity; the size of the halogen atom does not appear to be critical, as is the case for the corticoids. Although 21-fluoroprogesterone (Fig. 5.6, XI) is more active than 21-chloroprogesterone, the reverse is true when the 17α-hydroxy-21-haloprogesterone acetates are compared.

The halogenated, methylated, and 1,2- or 6,7-dehydroprogesterone derivatives, as well as the 19-nortestosterones, are effective oral progestogens, a fact which is important for their selection as oral contraceptive agents. Other orally effective progestogens are the 17-methyl, 17-ethyl, or 17-ethinyl derivatives of $\Delta^{5(10)}$-androstenolones. Among the most active are fluoroprogesterone (Fig. 5.6, XI) and 6α-methyl-17α-acetoxy-21-fluoroprogesterone (Fig. 5.6, XII), which are approximately 150 and 25 times as active, respectively, as the same amount of subcutaneously administered progesterone (Drill and Riegel, 1958; Drill, 1959; Ringold, 1961; Briggs and Botherington, 1970).

Another group of compounds with high progestational activity are those in which a 1,2 β-methylene bridge has been introduced into 6-dehydro-9β, 10α-(retro) progesterone. The parent compound 1,2β-methylene Δ^{6}-9β,10α-17α-acetoxy progesterone (Fig. 5.6, XVI), is some 30 times more effective when given orally than is progesterone (Halkes *et al.*, 1972). Its 6-chloro and 6-fluoro derivatives were even more active (110 and 430 times as active as progesterone, respectively).

Miyake and Rooks (1966) have catalogued some 450 steroids which have been tested for progestational activity by various routes in different kinds of animals.

III. Androgens

A. ASSAY

The original methods used for the determination of the biological activities of testicular steroids were based upon the increase of comb size in castrated birds (capons) and upon changes in the weights of seminal vesicles and ventral prostates in castrated rats. The discovery that androgens also had nitrogen-retaining activity in mammals aroused wide interest in the general anabolic properties of these compounds. Since the two kinds of activities do not always parallel each other, separate assays for each have been developed.

For the assay of androgens in birds, either caponized cockerels or 6-day old chicks are used. The sensitivities to androgens of various breeds of chicks varies tremendously; white leghorn chicks are fifty times as sensitive as the barred rock variety. The steroid may be administered either intramuscularly or by inunction. The latter technique increases the sensitivity to androgen some two hundredfold. Quantification of the assay may be achieved by measuring the size (sum of the length and height of individual combs, averaged over 10–20 animals) or, less frequently, on the basis of weight. In the modification described by Munson and Sheps (1958), 0.20 μg of androsterone in ethanol, applied daily for 7 days to the combs of day-old chicks, resulted in a significant increase in the ratio of comb weight to body weight (from 3 mg/100 gm to 5 mg/100 gm) (see also Dorfman, 1948b).

In castrated adult rats the seminal vesicles and ventral prostate regress in size; in prepuberally castrated rats the accessory sex tissues fail to grow. Both organs are stimulated by the injection of androgens. Figure 5.7 shows data collected by Hershberger *et al.* (1953) using rats castrated at 21 days of age and given seven daily injections of testosterone. These animals responded to as little as 0.50 mg of testosterone per day. Androsterone is more effective in stimulating the seminal vesicles than is testosterone; the reverse is true for stimulation of the ventral prostate.

The original study of the nitrogen-retaining activity of androgens was done in dogs (Kochakian and Murlin, 1935). No convenient and quantitative assay for nitrogen-retaining activity in smaller animals has found general application. Instead, the suggestion (by Eisenberg and Gordan in 1950) that the effects of steroids on the growth of the rat levator ani muscle represented an index of anabolic (as opposed to androgenic) activity has been the basis for most of the quantitative determinations of this property. Confidence in levator ani assays is based principally upon a reasonably good correlation with nitrogen-retaining effects in humans. In immature, castrated rats, 0.05 mg/day of testosterone will increase levator ani weight by 75% in 7 days (Fig. 5.7). Only a marginal effect is obtained with even ten times this dose of androsterone.

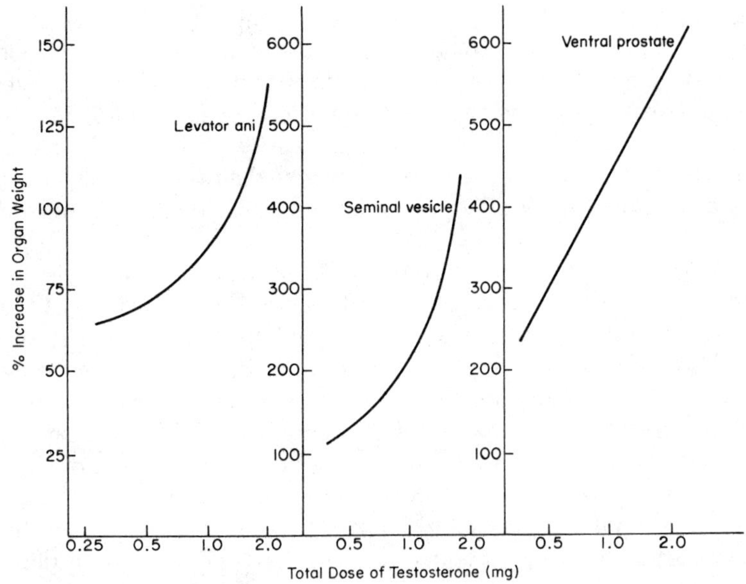

Fig. 5.7 *Effects of testosterone upon organ weights in castrated rats. (For details see text.)*

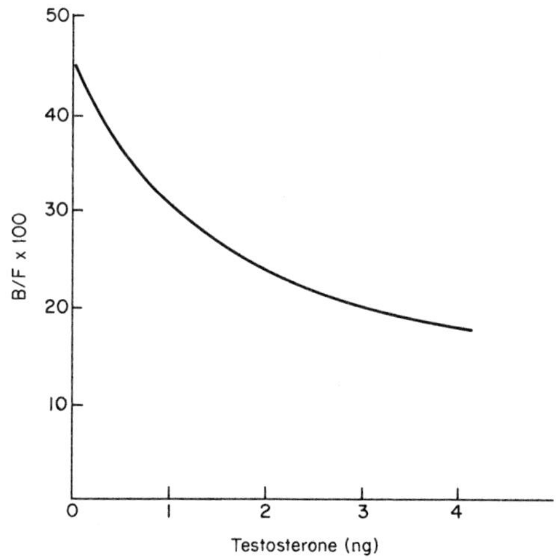

Fig. 5.8 *Testosterone assay by ligand binding. The ordinate represents the ratio of bound to free testosterone. Data of Murphy (1969).*

Testosterone assays using SHBG (see Chapter 2, Section III, A, 4) have been described by Murphy (1969) and by Vermuelen and Verdonck (1970). Murphy used late pregnancy plasma as the source of the binding protein and florisil to separate free and bound steroid; testosterone in plasma was extracted into ether and the ethereal extract was used without further purification. Vermuelen used plasma from estrogen-treated males or females and separated protein-bound testosterone by half-saturation with ammonium sulfate. Testosterone in plasma was extracted with methylene chloride and then isolated by chromatography on paper. Both methods were sensitive to 0.5–4.0 ng testosterone (Fig. 5.8).

Steroid-specific antibodies have also been exploited for the estimation of androgen concentrations in biological fluids. Midgley and Niswender (1970) displaced steroid derivatives of proteins, tyrosine copolymers, or tyrosine methyl ester (all labeled by iodination with radioactive iodine) from steroid-specific antibody by the addition of free steroid. In turn, the antibody-bound steroid complex was precipitated by addition of anti-γ-globulin serum. When applied to the determination of plasma and serum testosterone, the results by this method compared favorably with those obtained by gas–liquid chromatography.

B. OCCURRENCE, CHEMICAL NATURE, AND BIOLOGICAL ACTIVITY

The predominant testicular androgen in mammals is testosterone; this compound has been isolated from the testes of humans, dogs, rabbits, cattle, stallions, rams, and hogs. In rats, no testosterone can be found; instead,

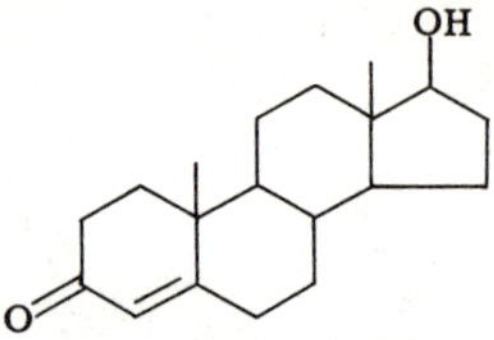

Testosterone (100)
(I)

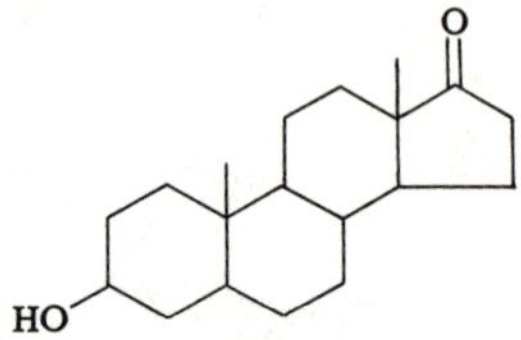

Androsterone (15)
(II)

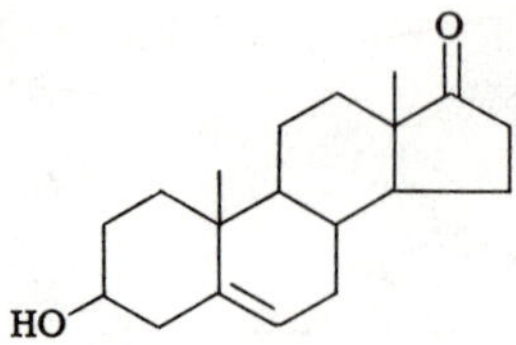

Androstenolone (5-7.5)
(III)

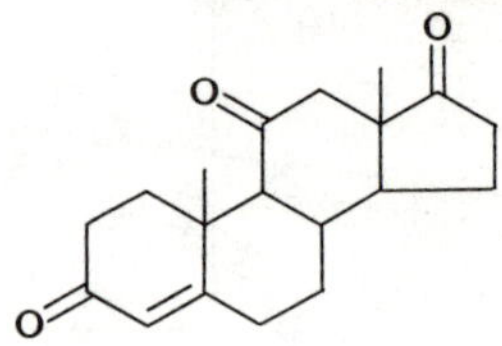

Andrenosterone (3)
(IV)

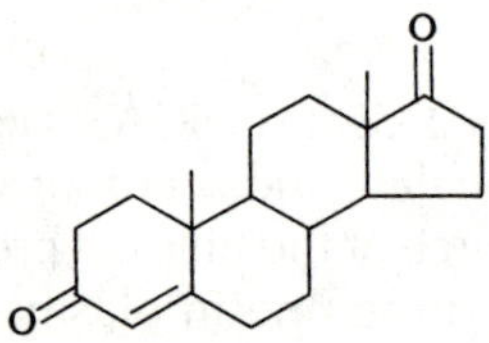

Androstenedione (12-15)
(V)

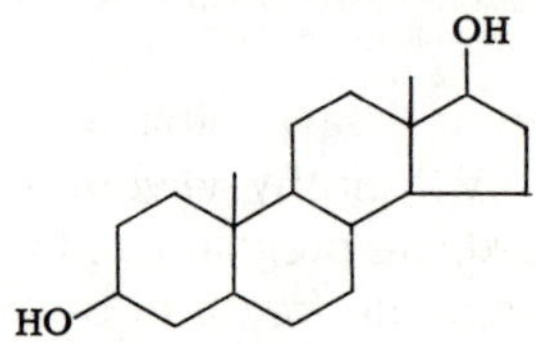

Androstanediol (60-75)
(VI)

Fig. 5.9 *Some representative naturally occurring androgens. The arabic numbers in parentheses indicate relative activities (testosterone = 100).*

androstenedione is the predominant androgen. Although testosterone has not been isolated (or otherwise identified) from bird testes, it has been shown that avian testicular homogenates can convert progesterone into testosterone and androstenedione. The same two sterols have also been identified in plasma or tissues of amphibians, reptiles, and fishes; in addition, androsterone has been found in some nonmammalian vertebrates.

Other compounds which possess some measure of androgenic activity (2 IU or more/mg)* have also been isolated from mammalian testes, urine, or adrenal cortex. With a few exceptions, these substances are 19 carbon atom steroids, with oxo or hydroxyl groups at carbons 3, 17, and (rarely) 11 and double bonds at 3,4, 4,5, or 5,6 positions. The structures of the most important naturally occurring androgens, together with their relative activities (testosterone = 100), are shown in Fig. 5.9. The activity figures are based upon comb assays in capons (Dorfman, 1948a; Fieser and Fieser, 1959).

* The International Unit (IU) of androgen activity is the activity of 100 μg androsterone.

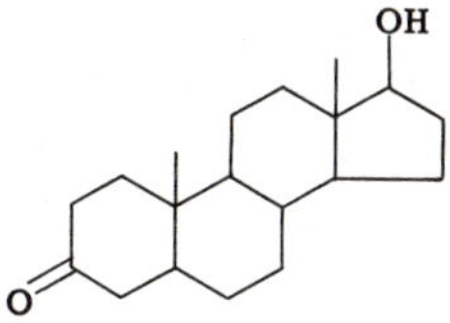

Dihydro-
testosterone (268)
(I)

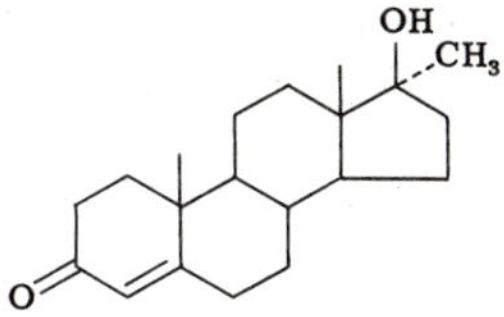

17α-Methyl-
testosterone (103)
(II)

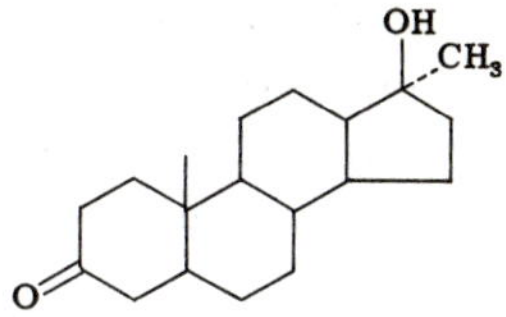

17α-Methyldihydro-
testosterone (254)
(III)

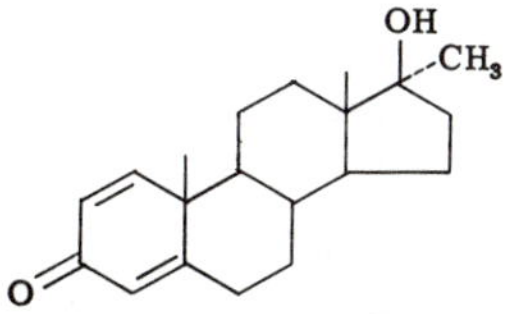

Δ^1-Dehydro-17α-methyl-
testosterone (55)
(IV)

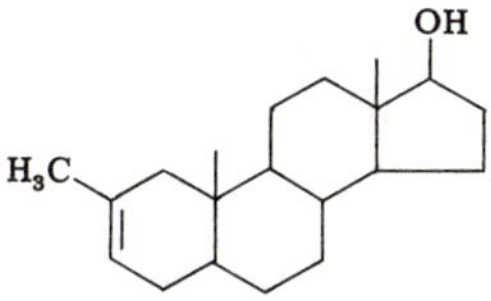

2-Methyl-Δ^2-5α-
androsten-17β-ol (127)
(V)

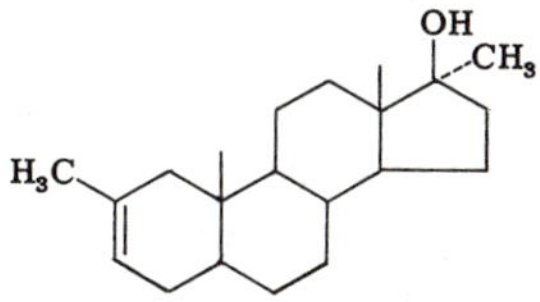

2, 17α-Dimethyl-Δ^2-
androsten-17β-ol (64)
(VI)

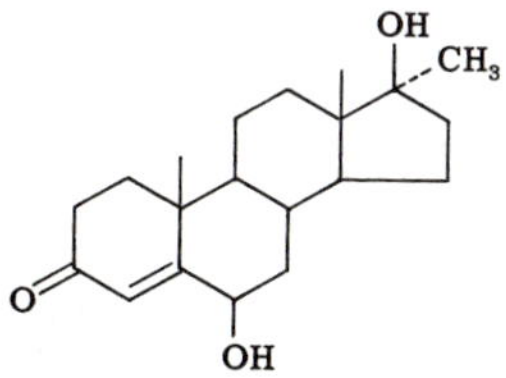

6-Hydroxy-17α-methyl-
testosterone (60)
(VII)

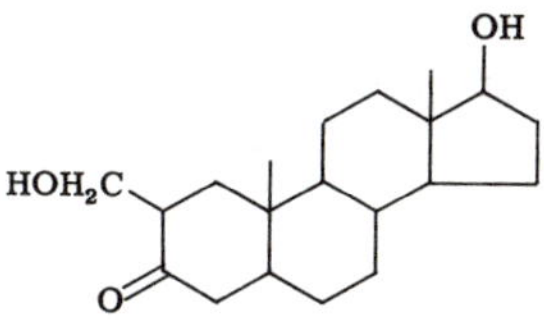

2α-Hydroxymethyl-
dihydrotestosterone (35)
(VIII)

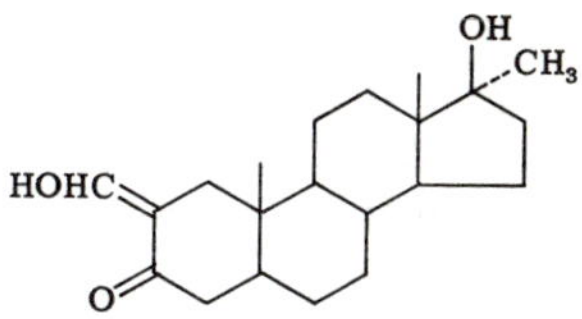

2-Hydroxymethylene-17α-
methyldihydrotestosterone (100)
(IX)

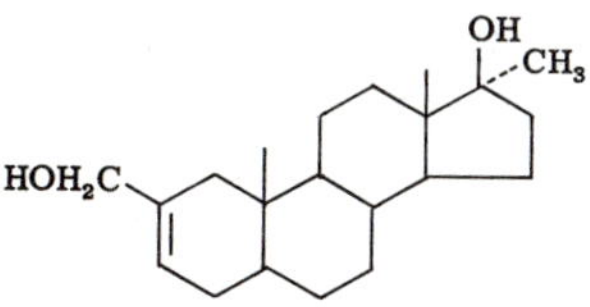

2-Hydroxymethyl-17α-methyl-
Δ^2-5α-androsten-17β-ol (45)
(X)

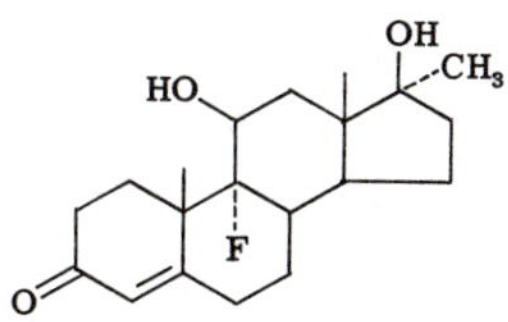

9α-Fluoro-11β-hydroxy-17α-
methyltestosterone (75)
(XI)

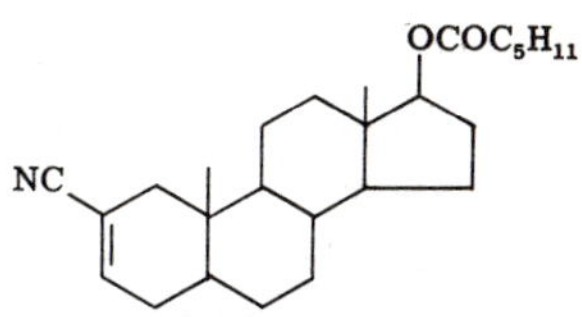

2-Cyano-Δ^2-5α-androsten-
17β-ol caproate (125)
(XII)

Fig. 5.10 *Synthetic analogs of testosterone. The arabic numbers in parentheses represent activities relative to testosterone (=100).*

Although testosterone is the most active naturally occurring androgen, a number of synthetic modifications have been synthesized which are more active than testosterone when assayed in castrated rats. Figure 5.10 shows the structures of 12 of these compounds, and compares their activities to that of testosterone (= 100).

Dorfman and Kincl (1963, 1964) have determined the biological activities of a number of androstane derivatives given either orally or subcutaneously (sometimes both) to castrated rats.* The criteria for activity included increases in the weight of ventral prostates, seminal vesicles, and levators ani; the data, expressed as percent of the response induced by testosterone (for subcutaneous administration) or 17α-methyltestosterone (for oral administration), are tabulated in Table 5.2. Although compounds that are more (or less) effective than testosterone in stimulating the growth of ventral prostates are, also, usually more (or less) effective than the standard androgen in stimulating growth of seminal vesicles, this is not always so. Thus, dihydrotestosterone (Fig. 5.10, I) and its 17-methyl derivative (Fig. 5.10, III) are both relatively more effective on the prostate than on seminal vesicles, while the reverse is true for 2-methyl-Δ^2-androsten-17β-ol (Fig. 5.10, V), 2-cyano-Δ^2-androsten-17β-ol, and 9α-fluoro-11β-hydroxy-17α-methyltestosterone (Fig. 5.10, XI). A similar increase in sensitivity of the seminal vesicle response may be seen when 17-methyl- or 2,17-dimethyl-Δ^2-androsten-17β-ol is given orally.

Esterification of testosterone with acetic acid does not significantly alter its biological activity. In contrast, esterification with either propionic, dichloracetic or chlorofluoracetic acids increases androgenic activity by 65%, 88%, and 200%, respectively (average of prostatic and vesicular effects). Few other changes in the testosterone or androstanol molecule consistently increase androgenic activity, although changes in one or another index occur upon reduction of the 4,5 double bond, introduction of a double bond at 2,3 or a methyl (or cyano) group at C-2, or introduction of a fluorine atom at C-6 or C-9.

Testosterone is relatively ineffective orally. Table 5.2 lists several compounds with considerably greater oral activity, including 17α-methyltestosterone, 9α-fluoro-11-hydroxy-17α-methyltestosterone, and two or three androstan-17-ol derivatives.

Aside from their use in the treatment of testicular deficiency and as an estrogen antagonist in mammary cancer, the major interest in the clinical use of androgens is their function as an anabolic agent in some debilitating syndromes and in osteoporosis. A desirable feature for compounds that are so used is high activity as an anabolic agent combined with relatively low

* A more extensive list, covering the literature through 1967, and including data on about 650 compounds, has been compiled by Vida (1969).

TABLE 5.2 Activities of Androgenic and Anabolic Steroids[a]

Compound	Relative activity							
	Subcutaneous[b]			Oral[c]			A/M Index[d]	
	V.P.	S.V.	L.A.	V.P.	S.V.	L.A.	S.C.	Oral
Testosterone (Fig. 5.9, I)	100	100	100	28	50	36	1.0	1.1
Dihydrotestosterone (Fig. 5.10, I)	268	158	152	—	—	—	1.4	—
17α-Methyltestosterone (Fig. 5.10, II)	103	94	115	100	100	100	0.85	1.0
17α-Methyldihydrotestosterone (Fig. 5.10, III)	254	78	107	—	—	—	1.5	—
Δ^1-Dehydro-17α-methyltestosterone (Fig. 5.10, IV)	55	50	125	6	12	30	0.42	0.30
2-Methyl Δ^2,5α-androsten-17β-ol (Fig. 5.10, V)	127	240	117	—	—	—	1.6	—
2,17α-Dimethyl Δ^2-androsten-17β-ol (Fig. 5.10, VI)	64	87	310	97	320	1040	0.25	0.20
4-Hydroxy-17α-methyltestosterone (Fig. 5.10, VII)	61	42	134	—	—	—	0.39	—
2α-Hydroxymethyldihydrotestosterone (Fig. 5.10, VIII)	35	50	152	—	—	—	0.28	—
2-Hydroxymethylene-17α-methyldihydrotestosterone (Fig. 5.10, IX)	100	64	230	19	44	320	0.36	0.14
2-Hydroxymethyl-17α-methyl Δ^2,5α-androsten-17β-ol (Fig. 5.10, X)	45	62	203	19	44	218	0.26	0.15
9α-Fluoro-11β-hydroxy-17α-methyltestosterone (Fig. 5.10, XI)	75	188	89	118	757	1740	1.5	0.25
2-Cyano-Δ^2,5α-androsten-17β-ol caproate (Fig. 5.10, XII)	125	170	870	—	—	—	0.17	—
17α-Ethyl 19-nortestosterone	94	118	710	—	—	—	0.15	—
6α-Fluorotestosterone	123	128	206	—	—	—	0.61	—
2-Hydroxymethyl Δ^2-androsten-17β-ol	66	50	457	—	—	—	0.13	—
2-Cyano,17α-methyl Δ^2,5α-androsten-17β-ol	—	—	—	20	73	800	—	0.06
2-Methylene-17α-methylandrostan-17β-ol	37	40	73	75	146	205	0.53	0.54
17α-Methyl Δ^2-androsten-17β-ol	70	88	362	119	218	437	0.22	0.39

[a] *Data from Dorfman and Kincl, 1963, 1964.*

[b] *Testosterone = 100.*

[c] *Methyltestosterone = 100.*

[d] *A/M Index* $= \dfrac{V.P. + S.V.}{2 \times L.A.}$.

androgenicity. The last two columns of Table 5.2 include calculations of the "androgenic:myotropic" ratio, a figure arrived at by dividing the average androgenic effect (V.P. + S.V.)/2 by the effect upon the levator ani. A low ratio usually indicates a compound with the desired property. Although the several esters of testosterone are effective myotropic agents, their A/M ratios are not far from that of testosterone. With some exceptions, other testosterone derivatives also display relatively high ratios (Figs. 5.10, I, III), whereas 3-deoxytestosterones are generally much lower (Fig. 5.10, VI, X) as well as 2-hydroxymethylandrost-2-en-17β-ol and 2-cyano-17α-methylandrost-2-en-17β-ol). Several of these compounds have the additional advantage of being effective orally.

All of the compounds considered heretofore have been androstane derivatives, containing the typical tetracyclic steroid nucleus. A series of tricyclic analogs of androstanol, lacking ring A, have been prepared by Zanati and Wolff (1973); the parent compound (1,4-*seco*-2,3-bisnor-5α-androstan-17β-ol), its acetate, its 17α-methyl, and its 7α-methyl derivatives were about 10% as active as testosterone in the ventral prostate and seminal vesicle assays, but were half as active in myotropic assays. Their *A/M* index was, thus, about 0.2. These compounds represent the most active nonsteroid androgens yet described.

IV. Adrenal Cortical Hormones

A. ASSAY

The many effects that accompany ablation of the adrenal cortex in laboratory animals has led to a corresponding array of potential bioassays for adrenal cortical hormones, their analogs, and antagonists. Assays that have received serious attention include assessment of life maintenance, electrolyte excretion, alterations in carbohydrate or protein metabolism, protection against thermal, mechanical, or chemical stress, changes in the formed elements of the blood, and tests for antiinflammatory activity. In this section we can do no more than to examine the characteristics of the most frequently used bioassays.

Immature male rats, adrenalectomized and maintained on a standard laboratory diet (including tap water) have a mean survival time of about 8 days. This period may be extended by the injection of mineralocorticoids, survival periods reaching 21 days with 0.18 mg/day of deoxycorticosterone (Fig. 5.11). The total time required for the assay may be shortened by comparing weight changes in the 6 days after adrenalectomy with those in animals receiving daily hormone injections. Weight increases (0.5–4.0 gm/day) are a

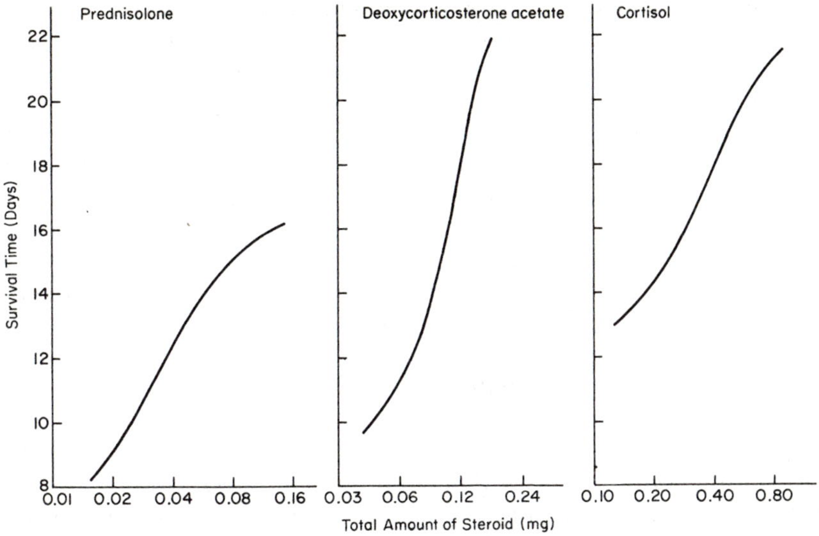

Fig. 5.11 *Life prolongation assay of adrenal corticoid activity. Data of Tolksdorf et al. (1956).*

linear function of the logarithm of the dose of mineralocorticoid; with 0.15 mg DOC/day, the weight increase approximates 3.6 gm/day.

Adrenalectomized rats, given a relatively large dose of sodium chloride (35 μg/gm of body weight) will excrete most of the sodium during a 6-hour period following injection of the salt load. If one microgram of DOC is given along with the salt solution, excretion of sodium is significantly reduced. Determination of sodium excretion is facilitated by using radioactive sodium (^{24}Na) as a tracer; when this is done, sodium excretion may be expressed as the fraction of the total radioactivity which appears in the urine during the test period (Dorfman *et al.*, 1947). Chemical or photometric estimation of sodium in the urine allows this principle to be used when access to the short-lived ^{24}Na is limited. In normal rats, less than 1% of the ^{24}Na dose appears in the urine during the ensuing 6-hour period. After adrenalectomy, this figure increases variably (2–7%).

Simpson and Tait (1952) measured the sodium/potassium ratio in urine and found this number could be used as an index of mineralocorticoid activity. The animals were first given a salt mixture high in potassium and relatively low in sodium. The urinary Na/K ratio was high (2.25) in adrenalectomized animals but could be reduced (to 1.10) by giving mineralocorticoid. The useful range was 0.8–4.0 μg of DOC. Simpson and Tait used ^{42}K as well as ^{24}Na, thus simplifying estimation of the Na:K ratio.

The ability of cortical steroids to influence glycogen deposition in the liver has been used extensively for bioassay, especially to compare the relative glucocorticoid potencies of various compounds. Both rats and mice have been used. In adrenalectomized rats, fasted 24 hours, liver glycogen is reduced to less than 0.1%. One milligram of cortisol, given in divided doses on the fifth postoperative day (and following a 24-hour fast) will restore the glycogen concentration to nearly 2%, and the effect of less than one-half a milligram is readily observed. Other naturally occurring glucocorticoids have similar, if quantitatively less striking, effects. Examples of typical responses are shown in Fig. 5.12. Immature (21-day-old) rats are several times as sensitive to cortisone as are older animals; a significant increase in liver glycogen may be obtained in younger animals with as little as 10 μg of cortisone. Adrenalectomized mice also respond to small amounts of cortisone given in divided doses during a period of several hours, the total liver glycogen increasing from 0.7 to 6.0 mg/10 gm of body weight.

Experimentally, the simplest measure of the anti-inflammatory property of a steroid hormone rests upon diminution of the size of the granuloma induced by the insertion of a foreign object (a small pellet of cotton is most often used) under the skin of an adrenalectomized rat. Approximately 1 mg of cortisol, given in divided doses, during the 7 days after implantation will reduce the weight of the granuloma formed by somewhat more than 50%. When used as a means of ranking naturally occurring and synthetic cortical steroids in order of effectiveness, the "granuloma pouch" method correlates

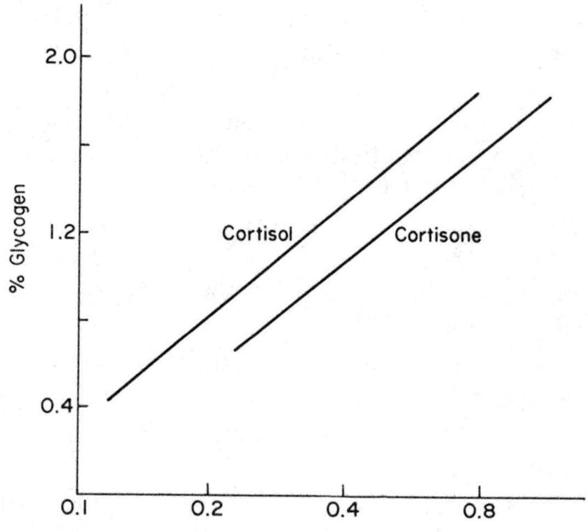

Fig. 5.12 *Glycogen deposition assay of glucocorticoid activity. Fasted, adrenalectomized rats received the indicated amount of steroid during 6 hours. Liver glycogen was determined 8 hours after the first injection. Data of Pabst et al. (1947; quoted by Dorfman, 1962).*

well with the procedure in which diminution of thymus weight is determined in adrenalectomized rats receiving glucocorticoid.

Another useful index rests upon the ability of cortisone to prolong the survival time of adrenalectomized rats exposed to low temperatures. A single dose of 320 μg of 11-dehydrocorticosterone will prolong the survival time, at 8.3°, from 9.7 to nearly 15 hours. In this test, cortisone is three times as effective as 11-dehydrocorticosterone.

The first application of the ligand-binding technique to the problem of steroid hormone assay took advantage of the affinity of plasma corticosteroid-binding globulin (CBG, see Chapter 2, Section III, A, 4) for cortisol to measure the concentration of this metabolite (Murphy *et al.*, 1963). Diluted human plasma was mixed with ^{14}C-labeled cortisol and an extract of the unknown plasma sample; after incubation, the ratio of bound to free cortisol was determined by equilibrium dialysis. Subsequently, the sensitivity of the procedure was improved by using tritiated corticosterone, and separation of free and bound steroid was made easier by adding florisil, which adsorbs free, but not protein-bound corticoid (Murphy, 1967; Hsu and Bledsoe, 1970). Plasma from estrogen-treated women, treated also with dexamethasone to reduce their endogenous corticoid levels, proved to be the best source of the binding protein. Under these conditions it was possible to detect 1–100 ng of cortisol, the principal corticoid of human plasma. The method was sensitive to ±5 ng.

The corticosteroid binding globulin of human plasma has maximum affinity for cortisol and corticosterone. Other steroids, including 21-deoxycortisol, prednisolone, progesterone, 17α-hydroxyprogesterone, and deoxycorticosterone will also bind. These and similar substances can be measured separately by chromatographic fractionation of a steroid mixture. Corticosteroid-binding globulins from animals (dogs, monkeys, and chickens) whose steroid-binding affinities differ from those of human plasma may also be used; as noted earlier (in Chapter 2, Section III, A, 4), dog plasma has been used to measure the extremely low concentrations of cortisol in cerebrospinal fluid.

Robinson and Fanestil (1970) separated a mineralocorticoid-binding protein from the kidneys of adrenalectomized rats and applied it to the assay of aldosterone in blood. Although good reproducibility was obtained with each protein preparation, the variability encountered with different samples as well as the instability of the aldosterone-binding fraction has thus far limited its application. Sensitivity to 1 ng was claimed.

B. OCCURRENCE, CHEMICAL NATURE, BIOLOGICAL ACTIVITY

Figure 5.13 shows the structures of seven compounds that possess either glucocorticoid or mineralocorticoid activity and that have been isolated

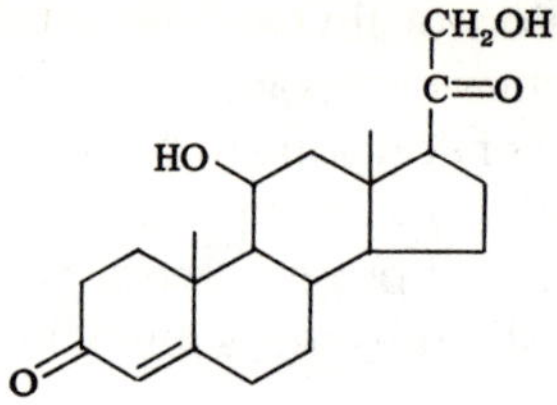

Corticosterone

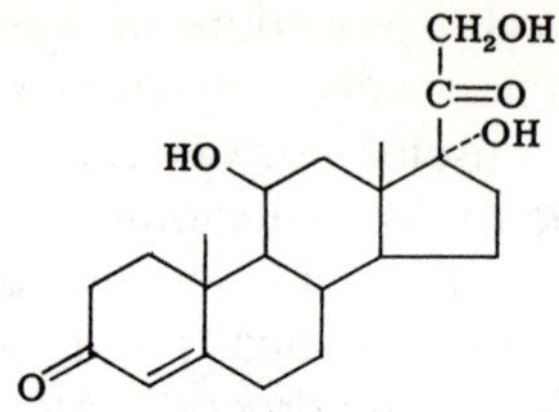

Hydrocortisone
(17-hydroxycorticosterone)

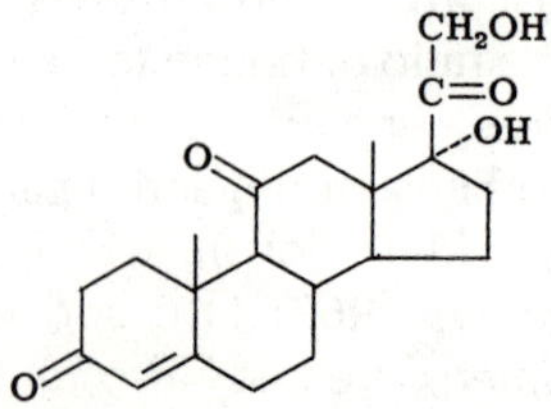

Cortisone (11-dehydro-
17-hydroxycorticosterone)

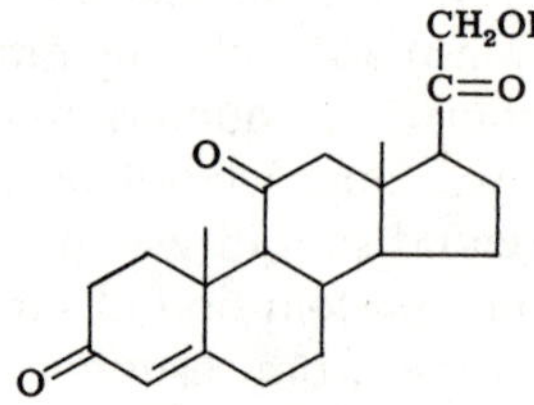

11-Dehydro-
corticosterone

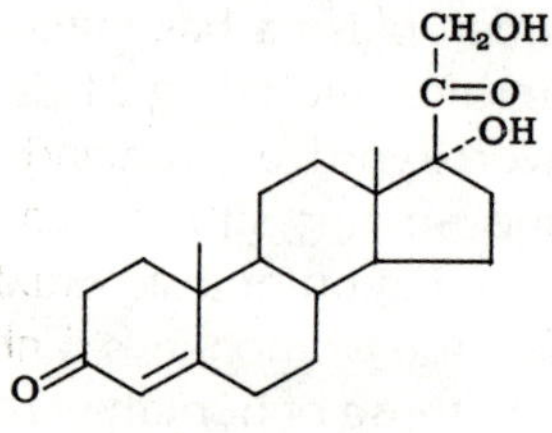

11-Deoxy-17-hydroxy-
corticosterone

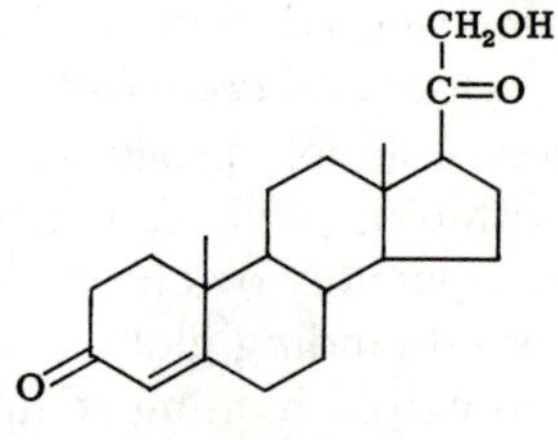

11-Deoxy-
corticosterone

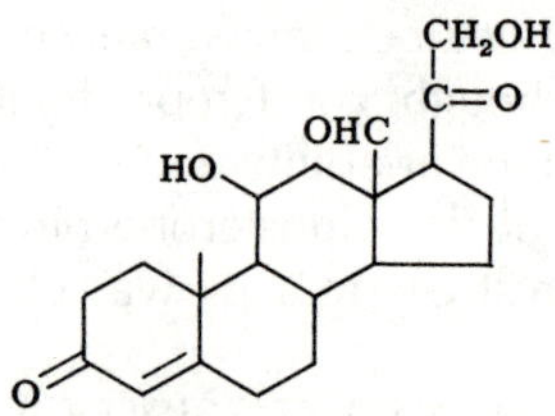

Aldosterone
(18-oxocorticosterone)

Fig. 5.13 *Naturally occurring adrenal corticoids.*

TABLE 5.3 Corticosteroids in Vertebrate Classes

Class	Corticosterone	Cortisol	Cortisone	Aldosterone
Cyclostomes	+	+		
Elasmobranchs	+	+		+
Actinopterygii	+	+		+
Amphibians	+	+		+
Reptiles	+	+	+	+
Birds	+	+	+	+

from bovine adrenals. Many of these compounds, as well as 18-hydroxycorticosterone, and 18-hydroxy, 11-deoxycorticosterone, have been isolated from the adrenals of other mammals as well.

Steroid-producing cells are found in all sub-mammalian vertebrate species, from cyclostomes to birds. In chicken adrenals the principal steroids are corticosterone, 11-dehydrocorticosterone, 18-hydroxycorticosterone, and aldosterone. Corticosterone and aldosterone are found in the adrenals of reptiles and in the steroid-producing tissue of amphibians. The "head kidneys" of teleost fishes (eels, salmon, etc.) produce a rich array of steroids, including nearly all those characteristic of mammalian adrenals except aldosterone. On the other hand, the interrenal tissue of elasmobranch fishes produces aldosterone, as well as cortisol, corticosterone, and 1α-hydroxycorticosterone. It appears that aldosterone and corticosterone are the principal steroids secreted by those species which inhabit nonsaline aquatic or terrestrial environments, while in saline aquatic environments cortisol and corticosterone are the major products (Nandi, 1967). Table 5.3, after Barrington, summarizes the distribution of steroids in the principal vertebrate classes. 11-Deoxycorticoids (11-deoxycorticosterone, 11-deoxycortisol) are also present in most classes of nonmammalian vertebrates.

The relative biological activities, using several bioassays, of six of the corticosteroids shown in Fig. 5.13 are summarized in Table 5.4.

The discovery, by Hench and Kendall of the antirheumatic properties of cortisone led to many attempts to prepare biologically active analogs of adrenal steroids (Fig. 5.14). The simplest compounds with adrenocortical activity are derivatives of indane: 1-glycoyl indane and its hexahydro derivative;

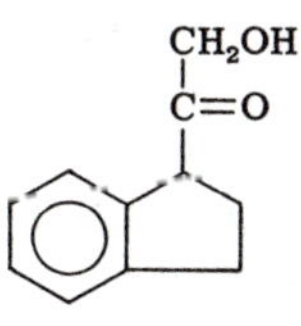

1-Glycoloyl indane

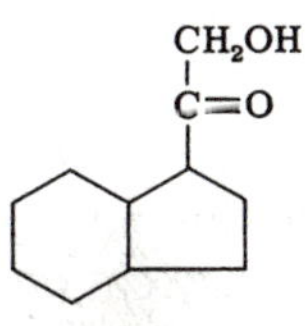

1-Glycoloyl hexahydroindane

TABLE 5.4 Biological Activities of Adrenal Cortical Steroids[a]

	Relative activity			
Compound	Life maintenance	Glycogen deposition	Sodium retention	Antiinflammatory response
Cortisone	1.00	1.00	1.00	1.00
Corticosterone	0.75	0.54	2.55	0.03
11-Dehydrocorticosterone	0.58	0.48	—	0.00
Cortisol (Hydrocortisone)	1.00	1.55	1.50	1.25
11-Deoxycorticosterone	4.0	0.0	30	0.0
Aldosterone	(80)	0.30	600	0.0

[a] *In rats. Data taken from White et al. (1973).*

On a molar basis, these compounds possess 6% and 10%, respectively, of the life-maintaining activity of deoxycorticosterone (Linnel *et al.*, 1951). Both substances may be considered to be analogs of 11-deoxycorticosterone with rings A and B missing. Another compound which extended the survival time of adrenalectomized rats subjected to cold stress is the α,β unsaturated ketone.

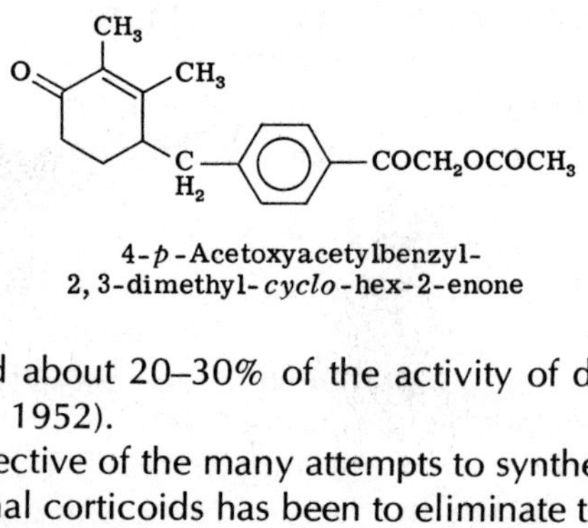

4-*p*-Acetoxyacetylbenzyl-
2, 3-dimethyl-*cyclo*-hex-2-enone

This compound had about 20–30% of the activity of deoxycorticosterone acetate (Dyer *et al.*, 1952).

The principal objective of the many attempts to synthesize new chemical analogs of the adrenal corticoids has been to eliminate the undesirable side effects which accompany the use of the natural corticoids (cortisone, hydrocortisone) at dose levels sufficient to provoke an antiinflammatory response. In practical terms, this means reducing the mineralocorticoid response while maintaining or intensifying the glucocorticoid response. In general, success in this endeavor has been achieved by modifying the basic 17-hydroxycorticosterone structure by introducing: (a) additional unsaturation in ring A; (b) methyl groups at C-2, C-6, and C-16; (c) halogen at C-6 and C-9; and (d) additional hydroxyl groups at C-16. Figure 5.14 shows a number of active corticosterone analogs, the biological activities of which are summarized in Table 5.5. Introduction of a double bond at C-1 (Δ^1) increases glucocorticoid and antiinflammatory activities three- to fivefold

TABLE 5.5 Biological Activities of Corticosterone Analogs[a]

	Substituents on 11-deoxycorticosterone nucleus							Relative activity[c] as measured by			
No.[b]	1	2	6	9	11 (β)	16	17 (α)	Life maintenance	Glycogen deposition	Sodium retention	Anti-inflammatory
I	Δ'				—OH		—OH		3–5		3–4
II		—$CH_3(\alpha)$			—OH		—OH		6	5–10	5
III				—F(α)	=O			18–36[d,e]	2.3	26.2	2.7
IV				—F(α)	—OH		—OH	9[d,e]; 1	12[d]	5[d]	7[d]
V				—Cl(α)	—OH		—OH	2.3–4.5[d,e]	2.4[d]	10.8[d]	3.4[d]
VI					—OH	—$CH_3(\alpha)$	—OH				3
VII	Δ'		Δ^6		—OH		—OH		1.1		
VIII	Δ'		—$CH_3(\alpha)$		—OH		—OH		10	Excreted	6
IX	Δ'			—F(α)	—OH		—OH	20–40	14	2.5	20
X	Δ'				—OH	—$CH_3(\alpha)$	—OH				12
XI		—$CH_3(\alpha)$		—F(α)	—OH		—OH		32	90	9
XII			—$CH_3(\alpha)$		—OH	—OH/α)	—OH		1	0	
XIII			Δ^6	—F(α)	—OH		—OH		2.5	25	
XIV				—F(α)	—OH	—OH(α)	—OH		3–5	Excreted	1
XV				—F(α)	—OH	—$CH_3(\alpha)$	—OH				36
XVI	Δ'		—$CH_3(\alpha)$	—F(α)	—OH		—OH		120[d]	0.1[d]	24[d]
XVII	Δ'		—F(α)	—F(α)	—OH		—OH		44		20
XVIII	Δ'			—F(α)	—OH	—$CH_3(\alpha)$	—OH				190
XIX	Δ'			—F(α)	—OH	—OH(α)	—OH		13	Excreted	4

[a] *Taken from Fried and Borman (1958); some data from Steelman and Hirschman (1967); and from Briggs and Brotherton (1970).*

[b] *Roman numerals correspond to those in Fig. 5.14.*

[c] *Activity standards: life maintenance, sodium retention, deoxycorticosterone acetate = 1.0; glycogen deposition, antiinflammatory, hydrocortisone = 1.0.*

[d] *Acetates.*

[e] *In adrenalectomized dogs; all other data are for adrenalectomized rats.*

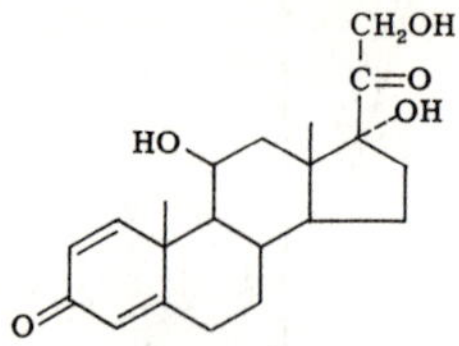

Δ^1-Dehydrocortisol (prednisolone)

(I)

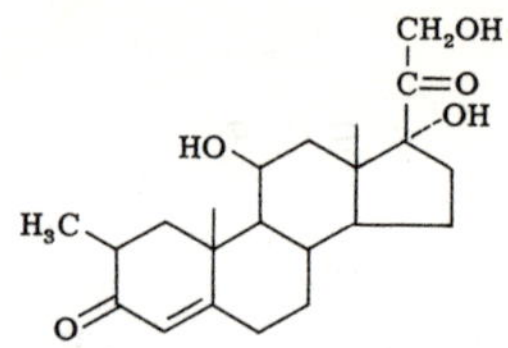

2α-Methylcortisol

(II)

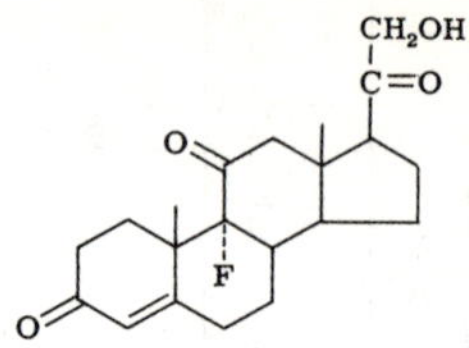

9α-Fluorodehydro-corticosterone

(III)

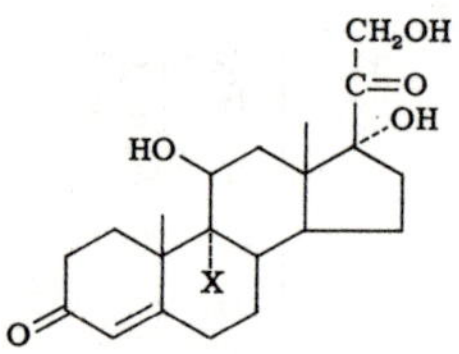

9α-Halocortisol

(IV) X = F
(V) X = Cl

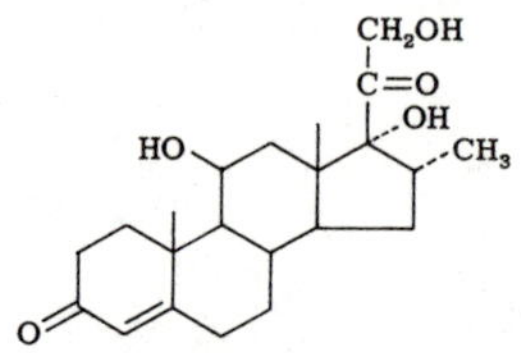

16α-Methylcortisol

(VI)

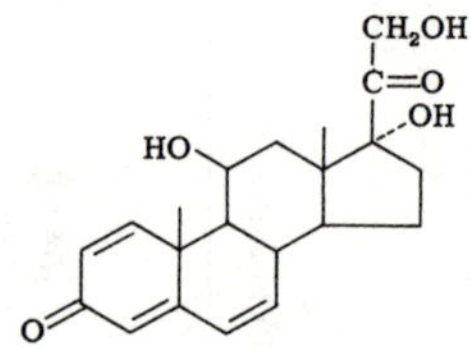

$\Delta^{1,6}$-Didehydro-cortisol

(VII)

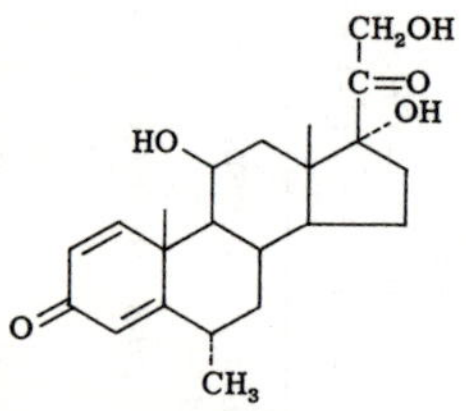

Δ^1-Dehydro-6α-methylcortisol

(VIII)

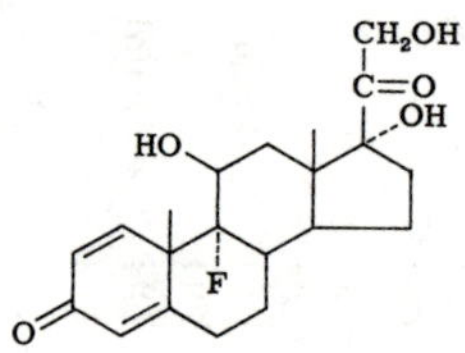

Δ^1-Dehydro-9α-fluorocortisol

(IX)

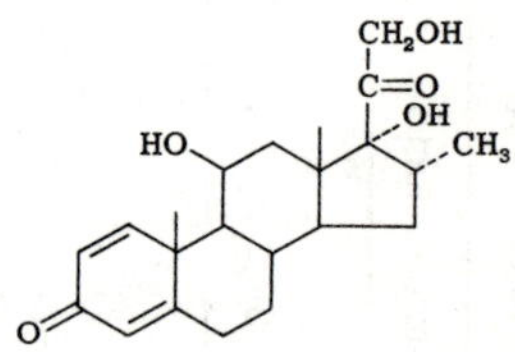

Δ^1-Dehydro-16α-methylcortisol

(X)

Fig. 5.14 *Synthetic analogs of corticosterone.*

(Fig. 5.14, I, IX), while suppressing mineralocorticoid activity; 6,7 dehydrogenation (Δ^6) has opposite effects (Fig. 5.14, VII, XIII). 2α-Methyl groups also increase both glycogen deposition and sodium retention (Fig. 5.14, II, XI). Antiinflammatory properties are also enhanced. 6α-Methyl derivatives are generally more potent glucocorticoids, while salt retention is suppressed, (Fig. 5.14, VIII, XVI). Substitution of hydrogen by a halogen (F, Cl) at C-9 (Fig. 5.14, III, IV, V, XI) enhances glucocorticoid, mineralocorticoid, and antiinflammatory responses; while the 9α-fluoro derivatives are better glucocorticoids than the 9α-chloro compounds, the reverse is true for mineralocorticoid activity (Fig. 5.14, IV, V).

Salt retention is also suppressed by introduction of an OH group at C-16

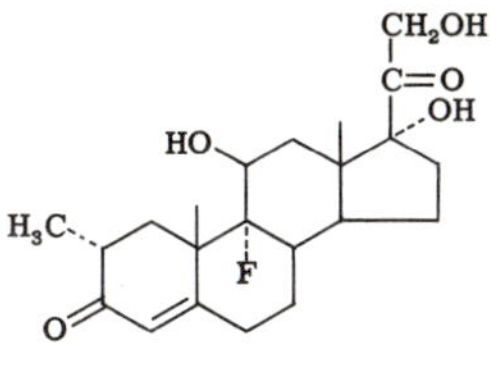

2α-Methyl-9α-fluorocortisol

(XI)

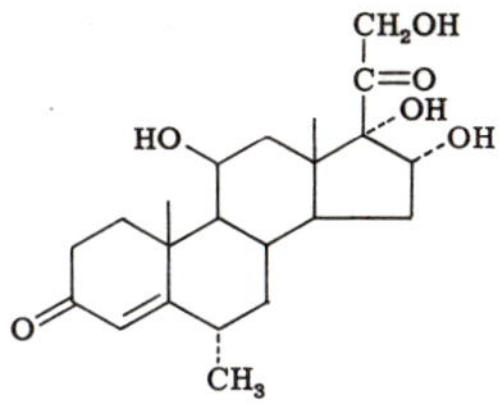

6α-Methyl-16α-hydroxycortisol

(XII)

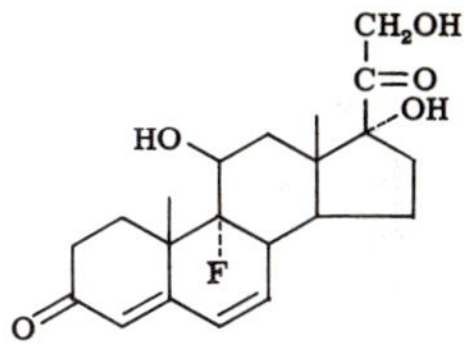

Δ^6-Dehydro-9α-fluorocortisol

(XIII)

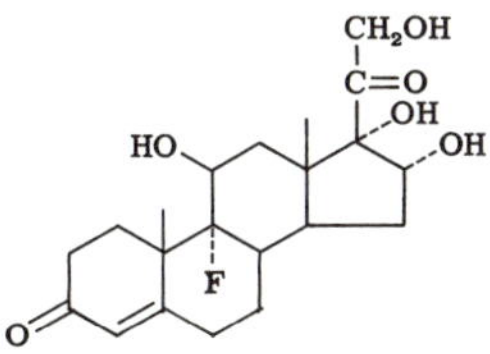

9α-Fluoro-16α-hydroxycortisol

(XIV)

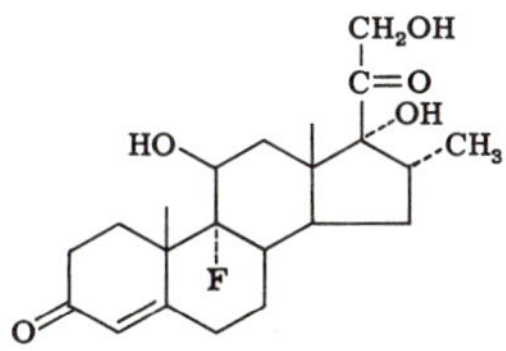

9α-Fluoro-16α-methylcortisol

(XV)

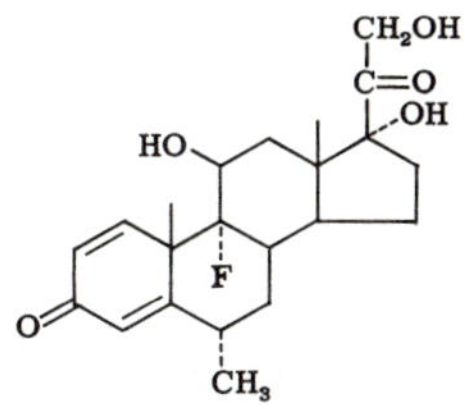

Δ^1-Dehydro-6α-methyl-9α-fluorocortisol

(XVI)

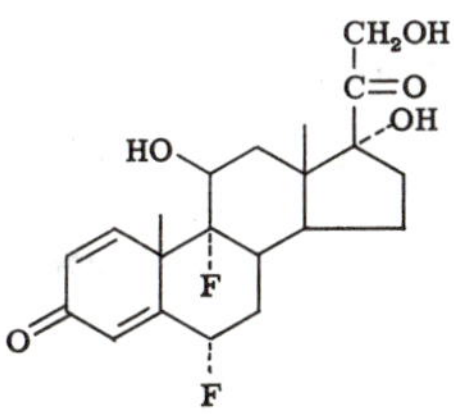

Δ^1-Dehydro-$6\alpha,9\alpha$-difluorocortisol

(XVII)

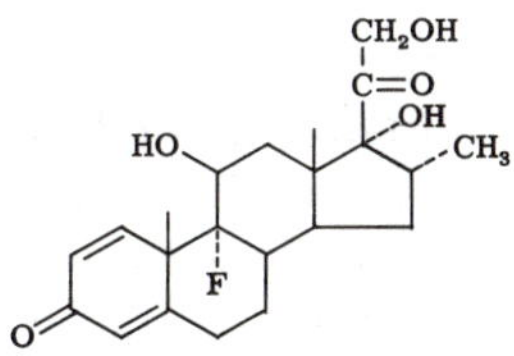

Δ^1-Dehydro-9α-fluoro-16α-methylcortisol (dexamethasone)

(XVIII)

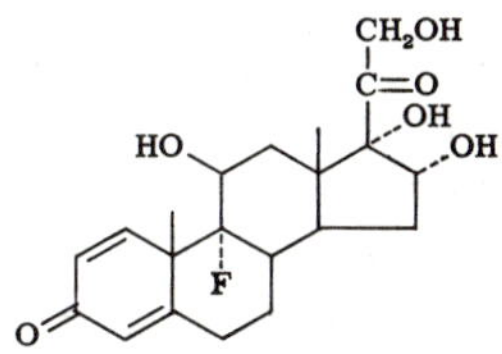

Δ^1-Dehydro-9α-fluoro-16α-hydroxycortisol (triamcinolone)

(XIX)

Fig. 5.14 *(Continued)*

(Fig. 5.14, XII, XIV, XIX). Glycogenic activity is also reduced, but to a considerably smaller extent. The antiinflammatory properties (in both rats and humans) of hydrocortisone and prednisolone, as well as their 9α-fluoro-derivatives, are increased by methylation at C-16 (Fig. 5.14, VI, X, XV, XVIII).

Conversion of 16,17-dihydroxycorticoids to their acetals or ketals enhances their glucocorticoid and antiinflammatory potencies as much as tenfold. The lower molecular weight derivatives (with acetaldehyde or acetone, for example) promote sodium excretion, while those of higher molecular weight may induce some salt retention (Fried and Borman, 1958).

6

Relaxin

As noted earlier (see Chapter 1, Section III,D), the name relaxin was applied, originally, to that substance in the blood of several rodent species which would induce pelvic relaxation in estrous (or estrogen-treated) guinea pigs. Subsequently, relaxin preparations were shown to evoke a number of other physiological responses. Although the physiological role, if any, of relaxin is unknown in animals other than guinea pigs and mice, the range of its biological properties, and its unique occurrence as an ovarian protein hormone, label relaxin as an agent of more than cursory interest.

I. Assay

The full range of biological effects attributable to a pure relaxin preparation has not yet been established. It seems clear, however, that pelvic relaxation in guinea pigs and mice and inhibition of spontaneous uterine activity in rats are intrinsic properties of the same chemical entity (or entities).

A. Pelvic Relaxation in Guinea Pigs

If an immature female guinea pig is "primed" with estrogen (1 μg estradiol/day for 4–7 days) and then given a subcutaneous or intramuscular injection of relaxin in aqueous solution, palpable relaxation of the symphysis pubis occurs in about 6 hours. Relaxation can best be detected by manual palpation, with the ischial crests and the symphysis pubis held between thumbs and forefingers and the two halves of the pelvis moved past each other. The response is a transient one; depending upon the amount of relaxin injected, the effect disappears in 12–24 hours.

In their original description of the assay procedure, Abramowitz *et al.* (1944) defined a "guinea pig unit" (GPU) as the amount of relaxin which would induce unmistakable relaxation in two-thirds of a group of twelve guinea pigs sensitized as described above. Subsequently, Frieden and Hisaw (1950) found greater specificity and a steeper log dose–response curve if the character of response displayed by each animal, as well as the fraction of animals which respond, are taken into account. Both assays require a subjective evaluation by the operator, therefore the samples are coded to keep their identities unknown until after the test is completed. With some experience, however, solutions whose concentrations differ by a factor of two to four may readily be distinguished when eight to twelve animals are used at each dose level. Figure 6.1 shows the log dose–response curve obtained with a concentrate of pregnant rabbit serum. The amount of relaxin required to produce a "total response" of 120 is approximately equivalent to the Abramowitz guinea pig unit. Using twenty animals at each dose, Steinetz *et al.* (1962) established 95% confidence limits of 79–112% for the assay.

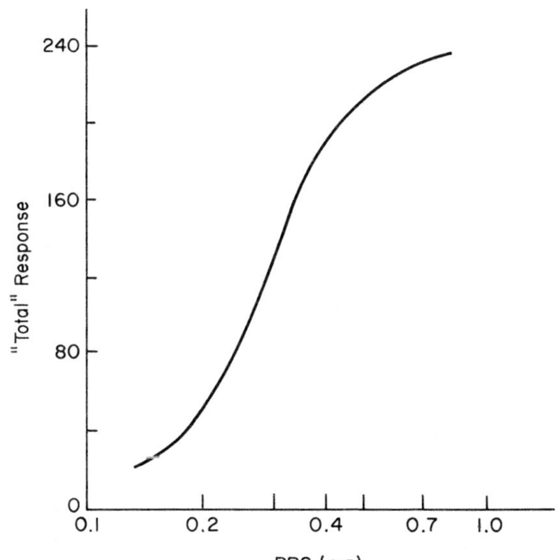

Fig. 6.1 *Assay of a pregnant rabbit serum (PRS) concentrate in estrogen-treated guinea pigs. Data of Frieden and Hisaw (1950).*

Guinea pigs used repeatedly (every other week) for relaxin assay, lose their sensitivity to the hormone. After 6–8 weeks, fewer than half the animals will respond to an amount of relaxin which originally relaxed all of them. Desensitization is probably due to the formation of anti-relaxin antibody.

B. PUBIC SEPARATION IN MICE

Hall and Newton (1947) discovered that relaxin would facilitate separation of the pubes in estrogen-treated mice. This finding led to the use of mice as assay animals. The response of mice to relaxin differs, in important respects, from that of guinea pigs; a longer period of estrogen pretreatment (7 days) is needed, and the maximum effect of relaxin is not observed until 24 hours after injection. Early studies of the effects of relaxin in mice suggested that another substance might be involved, since, while relatively crude preparations (2 GPU/mg) were very effective in mice, much larger doses (in GPU) of more active material (50–300 GPU/mg) were required to produce a comparable effect. The apparent paradox was resolved when it was found (Kliman and Greep, 1958) that the activity of purified relaxin preparations in mice was greatly enhanced by the use of a repository vehicle for relaxin administration. Apparently, the amount of time needed for relaxin to exert its effect in mice requires that its rapid destruction or elimination be avoided. In relatively inactive preparations this protection is presumably provided by other proteins. For the routine assay of purified relaxin preparations in mice, their solutions are diluted with the dye benzopurpurine 4B. Formation of a relaxin-dye complex prevents its rapid elimination.

When mice were first used for relaxin assay, x-rays were used to visualize the extent of pubic separation. This procedure was soon superseded by direct measurement of the length of the interpubic ligament after dissection to expose the symphysis pubis. The ligament was examined under a low power dissecting microscope equipped with a calibrated ocular micrometer. The length of the interpubic ligament in control estrogen-treated mice averaged 0.6 mm. Twenty-four hours after the injection of 1.0 GPU* of relaxin in 1% benzopurpurine 4B solution the ligament measured 2.5 mm. The response was linear with the logarithm of the dose over at least a fourfold range. The 95% confidence limits, using twenty animals per dose, were 86–116%.

C. INHIBITION OF UTERINE MOTILITY

Among the characteristic properties of relaxin-containing porcine ovarian extracts is the ability to abolish the spontaneous contractions of guinea pig

* Seven micrograms of a preparation which contained 150 GPU/mg.

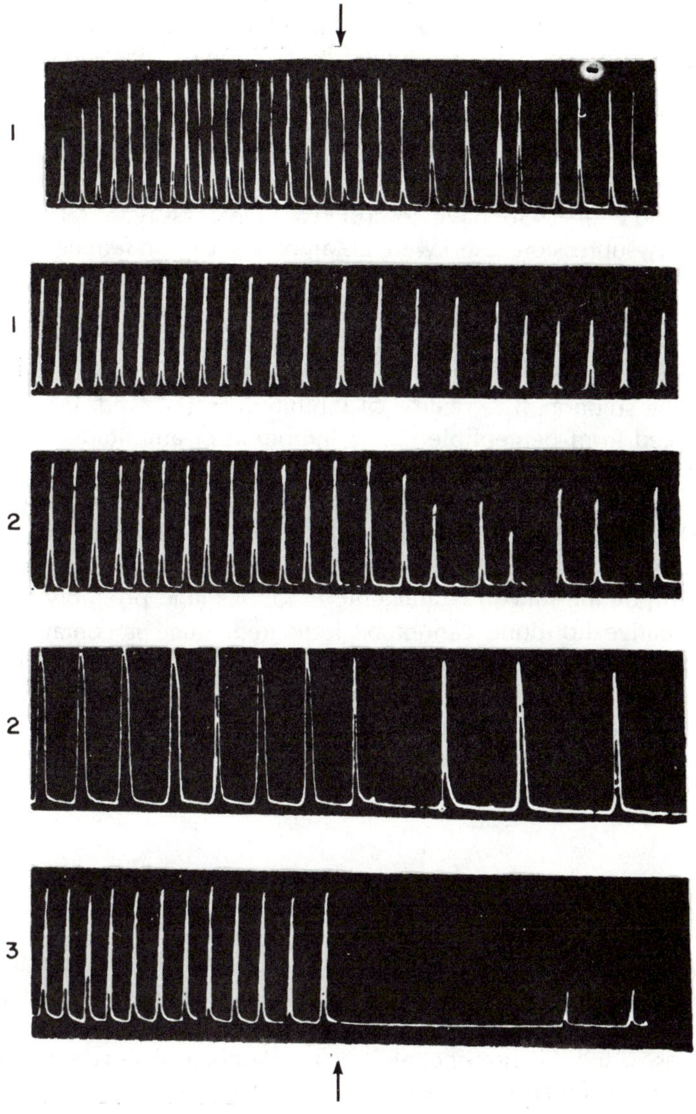

Fig. 6.2 *Inhibition of spontaneous contractions of rat uteri in vitro by relaxin. The numbers represent scores assigned to indicate the degree of inhibition. The arrows indicate the time of addition of relaxin in each experiment. Reproduced, with permission, from Steinetz et al. (1962).*

and rat uteri (Felton *et al.,* 1953; Sawyer *et al.,* 1953). For both kinds of animals, the ability of the samples tested to inhibit motility was proportional to their relaxin content, as determined by the guinea pig palpation assay, over a wide range of specific activities (Frieden and Hisaw, 1953). The close parallelism lends credence to the hypothesis that motility supression is an intrinsic property of relaxin. Similar effects of relaxin preparations on mouse uterine segments were described by Kroc *et al.* (1959).

Wiqvist and Paul (1958) have described a quantal assay for relaxin, based upon motility supression. Uteri were obtained from virgin female rats which had been ovariectomized, then given estradiol for 3 days to provide a uniform state of estrus. Each horn was divided transversely into two halves, which were suspended in aerated salt solution and arranged to record contractions. After a regular pattern had been established, the sample was added to the solution. The degree of inhibition was scored, using a scale which ranged from perceptible (25%) inhibition of amplitude (assigned a score of 1) to complete inhibition lasting 15 minutes or longer (scored as 3; Fig. 6.2). A plot of log dose vs. average score was linear over an eightfold range (0.01–0.08 GPU/ml). A similar assay using uteri obtained from mice in spontaneous estrus has been described (Kroc *et al.,* 1959).

Although porcine relaxin is antigenic in rabbits (and probably in guinea pigs), the native hormone cannot be iodinated, since it contains neither tyrosine nor histidine (*see* below). Sherwood *et al.* (1975) coupled relaxin with *N*-carboxytyrosine anhydride to form "polytyrosyl" relaxin, which retained biological activity. Using this material, a double-antibody radioimmunoassay for porcine relaxin was developed; it was reported to be sensitive to less than 1 ng of relaxin.

II. Occurrence

Relaxin has been found in the blood, ovaries, or placentas of a widely diversified group of mammals (Struck, 1967); among them are cats, cows, dogs, guinea pigs, horses, mice, pigs, rabbits, rats, sheep, and whales. In almost all cases, significant concentrations have been observed only during pregnancy. Some early reports (Pommerenke, 1934; Abramson *et al.,* 1937) suggested that relaxin is present in the blood of pregnant women, but this has not been confirmed. Using an immunofluorescent technique, Dallenbach and Dallenbach-Hellweg (1964) detected relaxin in human placentas, but Nagai (1966) was unable to observe any effect upon the symphyseal ligament of estrogen-treated mice when they were given an extract of 5 gm of human placenta. On the other hand, 50 mg of minced luteal tissue obtained from parturient women induced significant lengthening of the interpubic ligament.

There have been two reports of the occurrence of relaxin in nonmammalian sources. Steinetz (1959) found relaxin in an extract of rooster testes and in the ovaries of pregnant sharks. Mammalian testes are apparently free of relaxin.

Antiserum to porcine relaxin, prepared in rabbits, inhibited the action of rooster relaxin as well as porcine relaxin *in vivo* (mice); it also cross-reacted (Ouchterlony test) with mouse, rat, rooster, and whale relaxins. On the other hand, no cross-reaction could be seen with relaxin of pregnant rabbit serum, nor did anti-p-relaxin antibody cross-react with serum obtained from guinea pigs in late pregnancy but antibody-treated mice still responded to relaxin from this source (Cohen, 1963; Cohen and Steinetz, 1966). However, when a concentrate of pregnant rabbit serum was first treated with either acetic acid or urea, the antibody was inhibitory.

Little or no relaxin can be detected in the ovaries of nongravid sows, but relaxin appears in this organ early in pregnancy. The relaxin content increases rapidly thereafter, reaching a peak concentration of 250–500 GPU/gm of fresh tissue by the time the fetuses are 5–6 inches long, and remaining at this level until parturition. Ovaries obtained from pregnant sows are therefore the best source for the convenient preparation of relaxin in large quantity. For many physiological experiments, however, pregnant rabbit serum offers some advantage in reproducibility and convenience. The blood serum of rabbits exsanguinated late in pregnancy (25–30 days) invariably contains 10–25 GPU/ml of relaxin; a simple alcohol fractionation, followed by precipitation of the alcohol-soluble fraction with acetone, affords a stable powder with good relaxin activity.

III. Chemistry

Two peptides with relaxin activity have been isolated from porcine ovarian extracts (Sherwood and O'Byrne, 1974; Frieden *et al.*, 1974). Both are basic proteins, with isoelectric points in the range of 9.7–10.7. Each peptide contains 49–53 amino acid residues, with calculated molecular weights of 5600–6000; the molecular weights estimated from equilibrium sedimentation studies were 6300 (Sherwood and O'Byrne, 1974) and 6700 (Frieden *et al.*, 1974). Both peptides contain relatively large amounts of cysteine (6 residues per mole) and neither contains detectable quantities of histidine, proline, or tyrosine. Relaxin probably possesses an insulin-like structure, since after reduction and carboxymethylation two subunits of approximately equal size can be isolated.

As yet, little is known about the structural requirements for relaxin activity. Relaxin is inactivated by even mild reducing agents and by trypsin. Activity was retained after nitrous acid treatment; this suggests the dispensibility of at least some of its free amino groups. Esterification of the free carboxyl groups with methanol, however, destroys activity.

7

The Pancreatic Hormones

I. Insulin

A. ASSAY

1. *In Vivo Methods*

For standardization of insulin preparations, the induction of hypoglycemia in rabbits or of convulsions in mice by the intravenous or subcutaneous administration of its solutions have long been employed. Indeed, the "unit" of insulin activity was originally defined as the smallest amount of material which would reduce the blood sugar of a rabbit to 45 mg% within 4 hours of its injection. Approximately 0.04 mg of crystalline bovine insulin is effective. In mice, approximately 0.07 mg will produce convulsions in 50% of a group of twenty-four mice within 1.5 hours after injection.

Both the rabbit and mouse assays require relatively large quantities of insulin and are thus inadequate for the determination of physiological levels of the hormone. Much greater sensitivity to insulin can be achieved by an *in vivo* assay employing alloxan-diabetic, hypophysectomized, adrenomedullated rats maintained on glucose (Anderson and Long, 1948). In such animals, the intravenous administration of 1.0 mU (approximately 4×10^{-5} mg) of insulin will reduce the blood glucose to 50% of its initial value, and a significant change can be detected in response to 0.125 mU (5×10^{-6} mg). Even this improved sensitivity is, however, inadequate for most studies of insulin concentrations in physiological fluids.

2. *In Vitro Methods*

In 1940 Gemmill discovered that the addition of insulin to the suspending fluid increased the rate at which the isolated rat diaphragm removed glucose from the medium. This observation became the basis for successful attempts to measure the insulin content of blood and other fluids. As described by Randle (1956), the method involves the incubation of washed hemi-diaphragms from fasted rats in buffer containing 2.5 mg/ml glucose for 3 hours and then determining the remaining glucose in the incubation medium. The logarithm of the insulin concentration is linearly related to the cube root of glucose uptake, and as little as 0.125 mU (5×10^{-6} mg) insulin/ml can be detected.

Another tissue which has been widely employed is the rat epididymal fat pad. Haugaard and Marsh (1952) had observed that insulin increased the oxygen consumption of rat adipose tissue *in vitro*. Subsequently, it was discovered that the oxidation of glucose to CO_2 by adipose tissue was also sensitive to the action of insulin (Winegrad and Renold, 1958). A technique was devised for quantifying the response (Reynold *et al.*, 1960) based upon the incubation of glucose-1-^{14}C with rat epididymal tissue slices, and determining the amount converted to $^{14}CO_2$. With insulin present, radioactivity recovered as CO_2 was increased 40–400%, the lower figure being the average found when 10 μU (4×10^{-7} mg) insulin was added to each vessel. The log dose-response curve was linear over the range 3–500 μU ($1.2 - 20 \times 10^{-6}$ mg).

As indicated earlier, the most sensitive methods for insulin determination are immunological ones, especially those employing radioisotopically labeled compounds. It will be recalled that the first application of the radioimmunoassay technique to hormone analysis was the estimation of plasma insulin. In current practice antibody raised in guinea pigs by porcine insulin is used, since the properties of anti-porcine and anti-human insulin are nearly identical. Sensitivity to 0.1×10^{-6} mg/ml is claimed.

B. CHEMISTRY

Since the original elaboration of the structure of bovine insulin by Ryle *et al.*, in 1955, the structures of fifteen other insulins from vertebrate

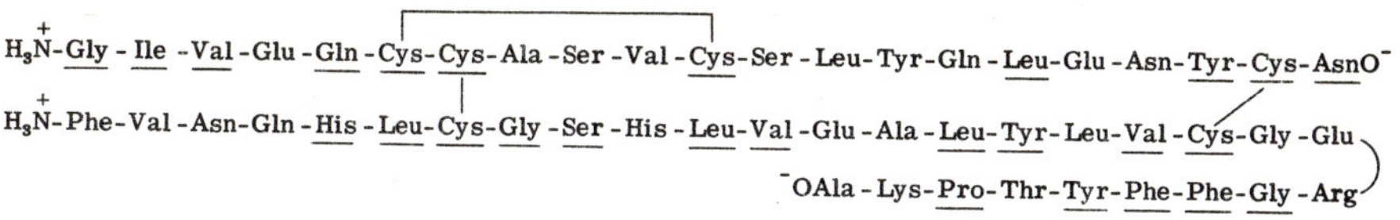

Fig. 7.1 *The amino acid sequence of bovine insulin. Invariant amino acids are underlined.*

species (or subspecies) have been determined. These include both terrestrial and pelagic mammals, the domestic chicken, and the North Sea cod. In addition, the compositions and partial structures of a number of other fish insulins (bonito, toadfish, anglerfish, and hagfish) are known.

A representation of the amino acid sequence of bovine insulin is shown in Fig. 7.1. Table 7.1 compares the sequences of seventeen insulins of known structure; bovine insulin is used as a "standard." Comparison of the known sequences indicates that 11 of 21 positions in the A-chain are invariant, being occupied in all insulins of known structure by the same amino acids; sixteen positions (of 30) in the B-chain share this property. Invariant positions are underlined in Fig. 7.1.

All mammalian (and chicken) insulins have a B-chain that consists of 30 amino acid residues. Insulins isolated from the islet tissue of some fish (bonito and toadfish) have only 29 amino acids in the B-chain, the C-terminal amino acids being lysine and serine, respectively. The B-chain of cod insulin consists, like mammalian insulin, of 30 residues; however, the C-terminus is lysine (corresponding to B^{29} of bovine insulin) and the full complement of 30 residues has apparently been achieved by adding methionine to the N-terminus. A second toadfish insulin has a B-chain indentical to that of cod insulin. Anglerfish insulin likewise displays a B-sequence displaced by one amino acid residue; in this instance valine is the N-terminal amino acid.

Two distinct insulins have been isolated from rat pancreas, and, as indicated above, toadfish islet tissue has also yielded two insulins. As Table 7.1 shows, the two rat insulins share the same A-chain but differ in the residue at B^{29}. Although complete structures of the toadfish insulins are not known, their A-chains differ by one residue (Ile replaces Lys, probably at A^{10}). Methionine is N-terminal for the B-chains of both toadfish insulins; one B-chain terminates in Ser at B^{29}, the other in the sequence Pro-Lys at $B^{29,30}$. Both rat isocoids have been detected in individual rat pancreases. All animals of this species thus appear to be homozygous with respect to two similar insulin-producing genes. Multiple insulins have also been found in bonito and flounder.

In general, differences between different mammalian insulins involve fewer than half a dozen residues, and the insulins of dog, pig, finback whale, and sperm whale are chemically, but not necessarily immunologically, identical. Guinea pig insulin provides a striking exception; as compared to

TABLE 7.1 Comparison of Insulin Sequences[a]

Species	A-chain										B-chain														
	4	8	9	10	12	13	14	15	17	18	0	1	2	3	4	10	13	14	17	20	21	22	27	29	30
Cow[b]	Glu	Ala	Ser	Val	Ser	Leu	Tyr	Gln	Glu	Asn	—	Phe	Val	Asn	Gln	His	Glu	Ala	Leu	Gly	Glu	Arg	Thr	Lys	Ala
Sheep, goat			Gly																						
Pig[c]		Thr		Ile																					
Whale (sei)				Thr																					
Horse		Thr	Gly	Ile																					
Elephant		Thr	Gly																						Thr
Human		Thr		Ile																					Thr
Rabbit		Thr		Ile																					Ser
Rat 1	Asp	Thr		Ile										Lys											Ser
Rat 2	Asp	Thr		Ile										Lys										Met	Ser
Chicken		His	Asn	Thr								Ala	Ala										Ser		
Guinea pig	Asp		Gly	Thr	Thr	Arg	His			Ser				Ser	Arg	Asn		Thr	Ser	Gln	Asp	Asp	Ile		Asp
Cod	Asp	His	Arg	Pro	Asp	Ile	Phe	Asp	Gln		Met	Ala	Pro	Pro			Asp				Asp		Asp		—

[a] *Only variable amino acid residues are shown.*
[b] *Bovine insulin is used as a "standard."*
[c] *Pig, dog, sperm whale, and fin whale are identical.*

bovine insulin, this molecule differs in seven residues in the A-chain and ten in the B-chain, including the carboxy terminus. Fish insulins are also very different from bovine insulin, but guinea pig and fish insulins are even more dissimilar. Dayhoff (1972) has suggested that the evolution of insulin has proceeded from a common primordial peptide (of unknown composition) along two divergent lines; one leads through chicken insulin to the various mammalian insulins (except guinea pig), the other leads to the various fish insulins.

Falkmer (1972) and De Martinez *et al.* (1973) looked for indications of the occurrence of insulin in the tissues of invertebrates. Acid alcohol extracts of tissues of starfish, sea squirts, whelks, octopus, and crabs significantly enhanced the synthesis of glycogen in mouse hemi-diaphragms; this effect was inhibited by antiserum to mammalian insulin. Oyster hepatopancreas, incubated with labeled leucine, produced a series of labeled proteins which had properties similar to both insulin and proinsulin.

C. STRUCTURE–ACTIVITY RELATIONSHIPS

With a single exception, all the mammalian insulins which have been studied possess the same intrinsic activity (24 IU/mg) when measured by the rabbit hypoglycemic method, the mouse convulsion test, or the fat pad assay. The exception, not surprisingly, is guinea pig insulin, which possesses about one-fourth the activity of bovine insulin in the mouse convulsion assay. When bovine and guinea pig insulins are compared with respect to their abilities to induce hypoglycemia in guinea pigs, however, their activities are the same.

Despite close similarities in primary structure, the various mammalian insulins can readily be distinguished immunologically. This distinction extends even to insulins from different species, which appear to possess the same primary structure, e.g., porcine and sperm whale insulins; des-alanine pork and des-threonine human insulins.

The comparative biochemistry of the fish insulins is more confusing. Bonito insulin, anglerfish insulin, and insulin from cod caught in North American waters are about as active (20–26 IU/mg) in the mouse convulsion and fat pad assays as bovine insulin. On the other hand, insulin from North Sea cod was reported to be only half as active as bovine insulin in the fat pad assay, and hagfish insulin was found to have only 7% (2 IU/mg) of the activity of bovine insulin in the rat epididymal fat pad assay. Humbel (1963) has reported a figure of 7.7 IU/mg for the activity of a purified toadfish insulin fraction, using the fat pad assay; the purified fraction was essentially homogeneous electrophoretically, although the possibility of partial inactivation of the product was not ruled out.*

* This explanation was preferred by Humbel.

Very soon after insulin was isolated, it was discovered that reduction of any of the disulfide bonds in insulin led to a complete loss of biological activity. Neither the free amino groups nor the free hydroxyl groups of insulin are essential; no loss in activity occurs on acetylation or O-sulfation of the molecule. Although the C-terminal alanine of the B-chain may be lost without damage, removal of the C-terminal asparagine of the A-chain leaves less than 5% of the activity. In contrast, both N-terminal sequences are expendable. Digestion of insulin with leucine aminopeptidase removes an N-terminal pentapeptide from the A-chain and an N-terminal hexapeptide from the B-chain; the residue, however, retains 45% of its original activity. Modification of the exposed tyrosyl residues (as by iodination) leads to progressive loss of activity.

Although it has proved possible to synthesize the two chains of insulin, systematic studies of the effects of replacing individual amino acids have, until recently, been hampered by the low yields which consistently accompanied earlier attempts to combine the A- and B-chains to form a complete insulin molecule. Katsoyannis and his co-workers, however, were able to obtain high yields of active insulin by allowing native A-chain tetrathiol to react with the S-sulfonated derivative of native B-chain. Although a large number of products are theoretically possible, the major product was insulin, isolated in 60–80% yields based on the amount of B-chain sulfonate used. It was concluded that the information neccessary for proper covalent bond formation to restore the unique structure of the hormone is built into the primary chain structure. (However, this conclusion is at variance with the inability to reoxidize reduced insulin with significant recovery of activity). Armed with this procedure, the Brookhaven group (Katsoyannis *et al.*, 1967) have successfully resynthesized insulin from a variety of synthetic and native A- and B-chains. The combination yields (again based on the amount of B-chain used) are summarized in Table 7.2. Also listed in Table 7.2 are the specific activities of the several products as determined by the mouse convulsion assay on the isolated insulin hydrochlorides. Although insulin yields varied, being lowest when both chains were synthetic in origin, the specific activities of all the product molecules were the same, within experimental error, as natural ruminant or human insulin.

Note that the insulin prepared from bovine A-chain and human B-chain represents a "hybrid" insulin which does not occur naturally in any species.

In order to examine the effects of modifications of the amino acid sequence upon the biological activity of insulin, modified A-chains have been prepared and recombination experiments attempted with native (bovine) B-chain (Weber *et al.*, 1967). These experiments showed that activity was recovered when Ser^{12} was replaced by Ala, Asn^{18} by Ala, Tyr^{19} by Phe, and Asn^{21} by Ala. Positions 12 and 18 had been known to be mutable, but all naturally-occurring insulins contain Tyr at A^{19} and Asn at A^{21}. On the

TABLE 7.2 Recombination of A- and B-Chains of Insulin

Chains used for recombination		Combination yield (%)	Specific activity (IU/mg)
A	B		
Sheep (synthetic)	Bovine (natural)	30–38	25
Bovine (natural)	Sheep (synthetic)	17–19	22
Sheep (synthetic)	Sheep (synthetic)	12–16	25
Porcine (natural)	Bovine (natural)	35–50	25
Human (synthetic)	Bovine (natural)	30–42	22
Bovine (natural)	Human (synthetic)	18–23	22
Human (synthetic)	Human (synthetic)	15–22	24

other hand, Weber was unable to recover significant activity when modifications (Leu for Val, Ala or Gly for Ile, and Ala for Gly) were introduced in the first three residues of the A-chain. This finding was somewhat unexpected, since the entire N-terminal heptapeptide sequence of the A-chain had been found to be at least partly dispensable.

D. PROINSULIN AND THE BIOSYNTHESIS OF INSULIN

The manner in which insulin is synthesized, and, in particular, the mechanisms which underly the formation of the single intrachain and the two interchain disulfide bridges, has excited the interest of biochemists and endocrinologists for many years. The failure of reduced A- and B-fragments to recombine spontaneously in significant yield suggested the possibility that the information necessary for the establishment of the unique configuration characteristic of native insulin resided in a larger precursor molecule, of which both the A- and B-chains were a part. Of interest in this connection are the results of some experiments performed by Givol *et al.* (1965), who observed a marked difference in behavior between reduced reoxidized ribonuclease, on the one hand, and insulin- and urea-denatured chymotrypsin, on the other, when acted upon by an enzyme from beef liver which catalyzed disulfide interchange. For ribonuclease the most stable form appears to be the native configuration, since the reduced, reoxidized (and still active) enzyme was not inactivated by the liver enzyme. In contrast, urea-unfolded chymotrypsin was rapidly inactivated by the enzyme. When the beef liver enzyme was introduced into a solution of insulin at pH 7.2 both the solubility and the peptide maps characteristic of native bovine insulin were quickly modified. It was concluded that native active configurations for both chymotrypsin and insulin were not the most favored ones; by analogy to the precursor–product relationship between chymotrypsinogen and chymotrypsin, it was concluded that insulin was synthesized from a larger precursor.

Efforts to isolate the presumptive precursor had been made in 1965 by Wang and Carpenter, who tried unsuccessfully to find in pancreatic extracts a molecule larger than insulin which contained the characteristic heptapeptide sequence: Gly-Phe-Phe-Tyr-Pro-Lys (found in insulin at B^{23-29}). In a paper which appeared almost simultaneously with Givol's, Humbel showed by comparison of the results of longterm and pulse-labeling techniques that the single proline residue in the A-chain was labeled at a rate intermediate between the rates of labeling of the two prolines at B^3 and B^{28}. He concluded that the single-chain precursor theory was excluded by his data (Humbel, 1965).

The discovery of proinsulin resulted from a careful study of an islet cell, insulin-producing pancreatic adenoma, which became available to D. F. Steiner and P. Oyer at the University of Chicago. Slices of the tumor were found to incorporate labeled amino acid into protein *in vitro*. When the labeled proteins were fractionated by gel filtration several peaks of radioac-

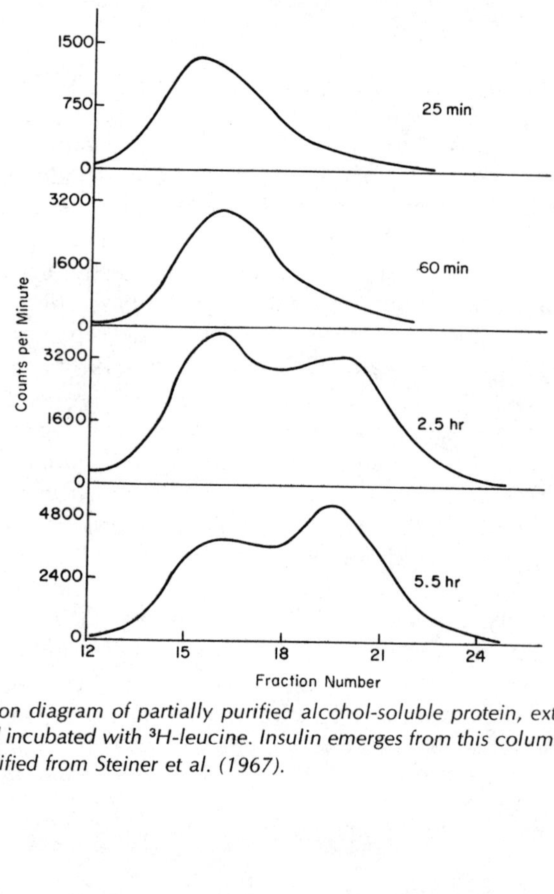

Fig. 7.2 *Elution diagram of partially purified alcohol-soluble protein, extracted from islet tumor slices, and incubated with ³H-leucine. Insulin emerges from this column with its peak at fraction 20. Modified from Steiner et al. (1967).*

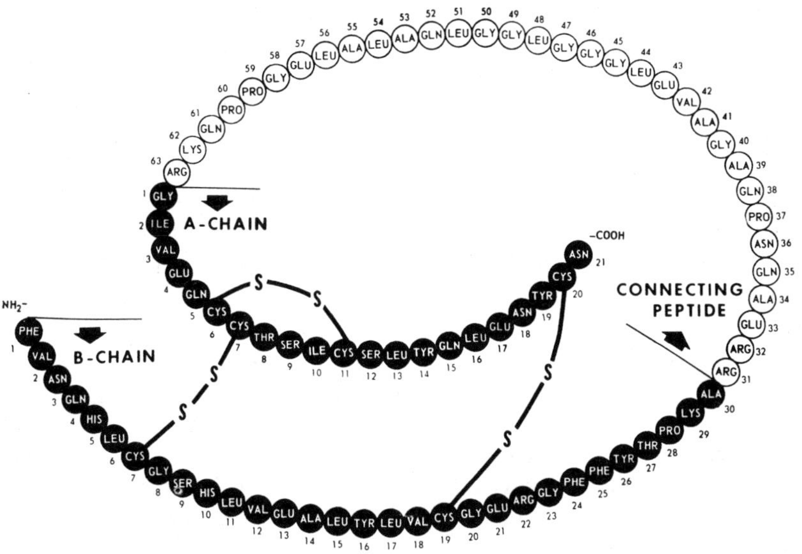

Fig. 7.3 *Representation of the proinsulin molecule (porcine). Reproduced, with permission, from Steiner et al. (1969).*

tive protein were found. One was insulin; another was a substance larger than insulin which was of high specific radioactivity and was bound tightly by anti-insulin serum. Insulin could not be separated from the unknown substance by any of the usual techniques of protein separation, but exposure to trypsin resulted in the rapid appearance of insulin while more prolonged digestion liberated the characteristic B^{23-29} heptapeptide. When the macromolecule was exposed to a reducing agent neither insulin subunit was released, indicating that each was linked covalently to the rest of the polypeptide. Finally, clear evidence of a precursor-product relationship for the unknown protein and insulin was obtained from experiments in which isolated rat islets were incubated for periods up to 5 hours with labeled phenylalanine (Fig. 7.2).

Structural studies have shown that the B-chain of insulin forms the amino-terminal end of the proinsulin molecule. This is followed by a 30-amino acid peptide segment (in bovine proinsulin) ending in arginine*; the latter is linked to the N-terminal glycine of A-chain. The sequences in the connecting peptides of both bovine and porcine proinsulins have been established. It is of some interest that two distinct proinsulins are formed by isolated rat islets, corresponding to the two insulins which are known to exist in this animal. Figure 7.3 represents a 3-dimensional view of porcine

* Porcine proinsulin includes a 33-amino acid connecting peptide.

proinsulin, together with the transformation caused by trypsin. The action of trypsin can also result in splitting the Lys-Ala bond at B^{29-30} to form desalanine insulin which is biologically fully active.

As noted above, when reduced insulin is reoxidized in air, the yield of insulin is only 1–2%, as determined by biological or immunoassay. Proinsulin, reduced in 8 *M* urea and allowed to reoxidize in air in slightly alkaline solution, recovers 60–70% of its original immunological activity. These results indicate that the conformation which leads to a biologically active insulin is thermodynamically favored for proinsulin, and that the penultimate step in insulin biosynthesis probably occurs spontaneously in the pancreas.

Proinsulin exhibits about 15–20% of the biological activity of an equivalent amount of insulin *in vivo.* Although it has not been possible to demonstrate significant transformation of circulating proinsulin to insulin, such a transformation, occurring within the confines of receptor cells, may account for this limited activity. Shaw and Chance (1968) studied the effects of pork proinsulin upon glucose metabolism in adipose tissue and in diaphragm *in vitro.* Like insulin, proinsulin enhanced the conversion of glucose-^{14}C to $^{14}CO_2$ and ^{14}C-fatty acids by rat epididymal fat pad and also stimulated the conversion of glucose to glycogen by rat diaphragm. However, since these actions could be opposed by pancreatic trypsin inhibitor, the activity of proinsulin in this instance appears to depend upon a proteolytic enzyme present in the target cell.

Evidence for a cod insulin precursor of a molecular weight about 10,000 and about thirty amino acids longer than insulin has been reported by Grant and Reid (1968).

II. Glucagon

A. ASSAY

Like insulin, glucagon can be measured using both *in vivo* and *in vitro* methods. *In vivo* methods are designed to measure its hyperglycemic effect in rats, rabbits, chickens, or cats; of these, the cat method originally devised by Staub and Behrens and subsequently modified by Smith and Robbins is recommended by Bromer and Behrens (1962). Fasted, hydrated cats (2.5–3 kg) are anesthetized with phenobarbital and a blood sample is taken. The glucagon solution is injected intravenously, and additional blood samples are taken at 8 minute intervals during the next 32 minutes. The assay may be repeated after 45 minutes. The injection of 0.1 μg/kg of crystalline glucagon will raise the blood sugar of the anesthetized cat by about 30 mg%; a dose twice as large resulted in an increase of 50 mg%.

Glucagon may be estimated *in vitro* by determining its effect upon glycogenolysis in rabbit liver slices. Glucagon is added in logarithmically spaced amounts (4×10^{-3} to 1.6×10^{2} μg/ml) to liver slices suspended in buffered saline. Changes in either glucose or inorganic phosphate may be followed.

Although the liver slice method described above is sensitive and economical of animals, time, and labor, it is subject to errors occasioned by nonspecific glycogenolytic factors; consequently, the response of relatively crude preparations does not parallel that of crystalline glucagon. Some of these problems are eliminated by a two-step assay in which phosphorylase in liver slices is first activated by glucagon and the tissue is then homogenized and centrifuged and the phosphorylase in the supernatant is incubated with freshly added glycogen. As compared to glucagon-free controls, the addition of 0.2–2.0 μg of glucagon will increase the amount of glucose formed by 10–65% (Unger *et al.*, 1959; 1961).

The action of glucagon upon phosphorylase is mediated by 3′,5′-AMP (cAMP), which is formed from ATP by adenyl cyclase. When washed membrane particles from rat liver are incubated with ^{14}C-ATP in the presence of glucagon, the formation of radioactive cAMP is much enhanced. Rat liver adenyl cyclase will respond vigorously to less than 0.1 μg/ml of glucagon (Fig. 7.4).

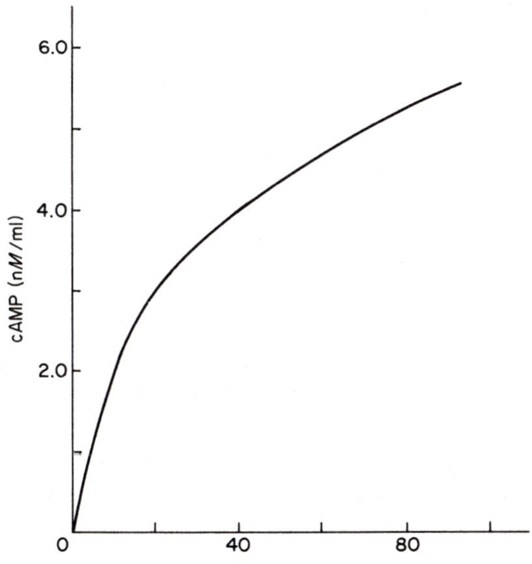

Fig. 7.4 *Formation of 3′,5′ cAMP in response to the addition of glucagon to a preparation of cat liver adenyl cyclase. Data of Makman and Sutherland (1964).*

A radioimmunoassay for glucagon, using a mixture of beef and pork glucagons as antigen for the production of rabbit anti-glucagon antibody has been described (Wright and Taylor, 1967). As in the insulin immunoassay, free and bound ^{131}I-labeled glucagon are separated by chromatoelectrophoresis. The method is reported to be sensitive to 10 pg of glucagon in 0.05 ml of solution.

B. CHEMISTRY

Although the existence of a pancreatic hyperglycemic factor was recognized as early as 1923, glucagon was not isolated in pure form until 1955 when Staub and his associates characterized crystalline glucagon as a low molecular weight polypeptide. Shortly thereafter, Bromer *et al.* (1957) established its amino acid sequence (Fig. 7.5).

Little is known concerning the comparative biochemistry of glucagon. The hormone has been isolated from bovine, porcine, and human pancreases. Human glucagon has the same amino acid sequence as bovine (and presumably porcine) glucagon (Thomsen *et al.*, 1972). The total synthesis of glucagon was accomplished by Wuensch (1967). The product was chromatographically and electrophoretically identical with the naturally occurring compound, but was only half as active when assayed in dogs.

A substance with many of the biological and immunological properties of glucagon (enteroglucagon) has been extracted from various regions (stomach, duodenum, jejunum, ileum, colon) of the gastrointestinal tracts of several kinds of animals (humans, dogs, pigs, rabbits). "Enteroglucagon" has not been extensively purified and almost nothing is known of its chemical properties. Like pancreatic glucagon, it is nondialyzable and is precipitated by 60% saturated ammonium sulfate. Although some have claimed that pancreatic and jejunal glucagon may be differentiated immunologically, the data are too fragmentary to warrant a firm conclusion.

1 2 3 4 5 6 7 8 9 10 11 12 13 14 15
H_2N-His-Ser-Gln-Gly-Thr-Phe-Thr-Ser-Asp-Tyr-Ser-Lys-Tyr-Leu-Asp-

16 17 18 19 20 21 22 23 24 25 26 27 28 29
Ser-Arg-Arg-Ala-Gln-Asp-Phe-Val-Gln-Trp-Leu-Met-Asn-ThrOH

Fig. 7.5 *Amino acid sequence of bovine and porcine glucagon. Dayhoff (1972, p. D-208).*

C. STRUCTURE–ACTIVITY RELATIONSHIPS

Among the earliest observations relating to the structural requirements for glucagon activity were those of Bromer (1964) that digestion with carboxypeptidase destroyed the hormone and that loss of activity, as measured in the anesthetized cat, could be correlated roughly with loss of Phe^{22}. However, the tricosapeptide, glucagon$^{1-23}$ synthesized by Wuensch and Wendelberger (1968), was found by Spiegel and Bitensky (1969) to be inactive in the hepatic adenyl cyclase assay. Spiegel and Bitensky also studied the action of cyanogen bromide on glucagon. The reaction product, which presumably consisted largely of glucagon$^{1-27}$, retained approximately 35% of the activity of unreacted glucagon, again determined by the adenyl cyclase assay. The difference was more than a quantitative one since the maximal response which could be obtained with the modified hormone was distinctly less than that produced by native glucagon.

Trypsin digestion also causes a rapid loss of glucagon activity. Three positions in the molecule should be susceptible to trypsin, including the bonds at Lys^{12}-Tyr^{13}, Arg^{17}-Arg^{18}, and Arg^{18}-Ala^{19}. As noted above, synthetic glucagon$^{1-23}$ was inactive; thus, any action of trypsin would be expected to be deleterious. Kakiuchi and Tomizawa (1964) purified an -SH dependent enzyme from liver which removed the N-terminal dipeptide His-Ser from glucagon; the product, glucagon$^{3-29}$, possessed an unspecified amount of activity.

The gastrointestinal hormone secretin is a 27-amino acid polypeptide. Twenty-one of the positions in secretin are occupied by amino acids which are identical with, or represent "conservative replacements" of amino acids in the same relative positions in glucagon. (A "conservative replacement" is one in which an amino acid has been replaced by one which is functionally similar, e.g., Glu for Asp, Arg for Lys, Leu for Phe, etc.). This close similarity is especially interesting in view of the common embryological origin of the pancreas and the duodenum. Despite these intriguing similarities, however, the two hormones do not share biological activities. Secretin, for example, is completely inactive in the adenyl cyclase assay; further, it has no effect upon the activity of native glucagon when added in amounts several times that of the glucagon present.

8

Parathyroid Hormones (PTH)

I. Assay

In his early studies of the parathyroid hormone, Collip (1925) used intact dogs as test objects. The dog assay is still the basis of the U.S. Pharmacopoeia standard of PTH activity; one USP unit is defined as one-hundredth of the amount which will raise the serum calcium of an adult dog by 1 mg% within 16–18 hours. For obvious reasons, this assay is too cumbersome for routine use in purification procedures. In the early 1950's, several laboratories succeeded in devising assays which were based upon the hypercalcemic response of parathyroidectomized rats to parathyroid preparations (Davies *et al.*, 1954; Munson, 1955; Rasmussen and Westall, 1957). In the assay devised by Munson, young (50–60-day-old) rats are placed on a low calcium diet for 4 days and then parathyroidectomized. Immediately after the operation, the unknown, or a standard PTH preparation, is injected and the serum calcium is determined 6 hours later. In untreated, parathyroidectomized rats, serum calcium is reduced from its normal value of 10.5 mg% to about 5 mg%; an adequate amount of parathyroid extract restores the calcium concentration to its preoperative value. Under these conditions, serum calcium concentrations are linear with the log of the PTH dose between 5 and 20 IU/animal (Fig. 8.1).

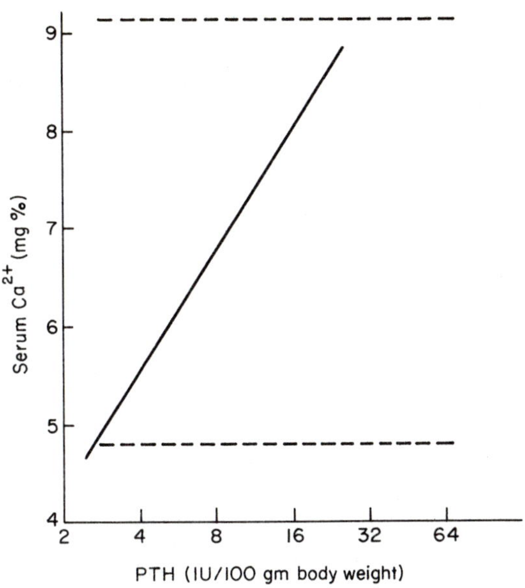

Fig. 8.1 *Elevation of serum Ca^{2+} in response to the injection of PTH in parathyroidectomized rats. The upper and lower broken lines represent the values for normal and untreated-parathyroidectomized animals, respectively.*

The rapidity of the hypercalcemic response in rats depends upon the stage of purification of PTH. Rasmussen found that the response to crude parathyroid extract persisted for 18 hours. As the extract was fractionated, the response was observed sooner (6 hours), and could no longer be observed after 14–16 hours. Aurbach (1959) noted that the addition of gelatin as a repository medium increased the activity of purified PTH, whereas no effect was evident with unfractionated parathyroid powder.

Parathyroidectomized mice are about 10 times as sensitive to PTH as are parathyroidectomized rats (Bethune *et al.*, 1967). Assays for PTH based upon its hypercalcemic effect in chicks (Parsons *et al.*, 1973) and in Japanese quail (Dacke and Kenny, 1973) have also been described. Birds are 2–4 times as sensitive to PTH as rats; in addition, the animals need not be parathyroidectomized and the time required is only 1 hour.

Parathyroid hormone also increases the circulating inorganic phosphate of the blood and increases urinary excretion of phosphate. Kenny and Munson (1959) have shown that the amount of inorganic phosphate excreted by rats during a 6-hour period following a PTH injection depends upon the amount of hormone given. The range for the "phosphaturic" assay in rats is 3–24 IU. A phosphaturic response to PTH can also be evoked in intact mice (Davies *et al.*, 1955). A collection period of 3½ hours was used, and a linear response was obtained with 0.1–3.0 IU of PTH.

Besides the effects upon serum calcium and urinary phosphate, a number of other indices of PTH action have been explored. Clark *et al.* (1960) injected $^{45}Ca^{2+}$ into rats; 45 days later they were placed on a Ca^{2+}-free diet for 5 days, then given PTH. Urine was collected during the ensuing 24 hours, and the total radioactive Ca^{2+} excreted was determined. In one set of experiments, the increase in labeled calcium, as compared to the control, was 15,000 CPM after 2 IU/100 gm and 74,500 CPM after 48 IU/100 gm. The response was linear with log dose between 2 and 32 IU/100 gm.

According to Zanelli *et al.* (1969) PTH will promote the dissolution of bone salt *in vitro*. When calvaria of young (6–9-day-old) mice were incubated in a tissue culture medium to which PTH had been added the Ca^{2+} content of the suspending fluid increased by 4–5 mg%. The response was sensitive to 0.02–1.0 IU/ml, and was thus about 100 times as sensitive as the Munson assay. The specificity and sensitivity of the assay was subsequently improved by Chu *et al.* (1971), who found that under the same conditions PTH inhibited the conversion of labeled citrate to $^{14}CO_2$.

Probably the most frequently used *in vitro* assay for PTH is the rat kidney adenyl cyclase assay. This enzyme catalyzes the reaction:

$$\text{Adenosine triphosphate} \rightarrow 3',5'\text{-adenosine monophosphate} + \text{pyrophosphate}$$

The enzyme is found in the plasma membrane of kidney and bone cells. For PTH assay a particulate fraction prepared from rat renal cortex is used as the enzyme source. The addition of as little as 0.14 IU of bovine PTH (b-PTH) causes a detectable increase in the rate of formation of the product (Fig. 8.2).

Parathyroid hormone has been found to be antigenic in both rabbits and guinea pigs; titers of 1:3000 may be developed in the serum of the latter species following the injection of purified (3000 IU/mg) b-PTH (Berson *et al.*, 1963). These antisera antagonized the biological effects of b-PTH and reacted with the purified radioiodinated hormone. A radioimmunoassay that utilizes ^{131}I-PTH (bovine) and depends upon electrophoresis to separate free and bound PTH was sensitive to 3 mU/ml (B/F = 1.0, compared to 2.5 in the absence of unlabeled PTH). When preparations ranging from 11–3000 IU/mg were compared immunologically, the ratio of biological to immunological activities varied by no more than a factor of two.

Although distinct immunological differences appear to exist, h-PTH, isolated from human parathyroids or from a parathyroid adenoma, cross reacts with anti-b-PTH antisera well enough to detect comparable con-

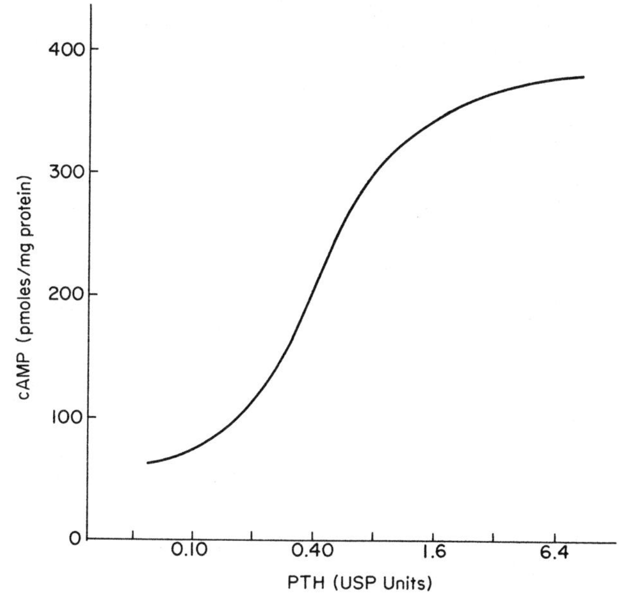

Fig. 8.2 *Activation of bovine renal adenyl cyclase by PTH in vitro. Data of Marcus and Aurbach (1969).*

centrations in human plasma. Using purified b-PTH as antigen, Tashjian *et al.* (1964) prepared an antiserum in rabbits, which he used in a complement fixation assay for PTH. The curves relating degree of hemolysis to PTH concentration were linear over the range 10–100 ng of hormone nitrogen (180–1800 mU).

II. Chemistry

An attempt to isolate parathyroid hormone was made by Collip as early as 1925; it has only been within the last decade, however, that efforts at isolation have met with success. In part, the difficulty of isolating PTH was due to the tenacity with which the hormone binds to other constituents, especially nucleic acids of parathyroid tissue. Extraction required the use of harsh reagents; until 1959, the most common solvent was dilute (0.2 *N*) HCl at elevated (70–100°) temperatures. Not surprisingly, this procedure was later shown to degrade native PTH, without, however, destroying all the biological activity. In 1959, Aurbach introduced the use of 70% phenol to disrupt the PTH–nucleic acid complex and obtained high yields of material which assayed 1500–4000 USP units/mg. A mixture of 8 *M* urea, 0.2 *M* HCl and 0.1 *M* cysteine has also been used; purification subsequently yielded fractions with activities of 3000 U/mg.

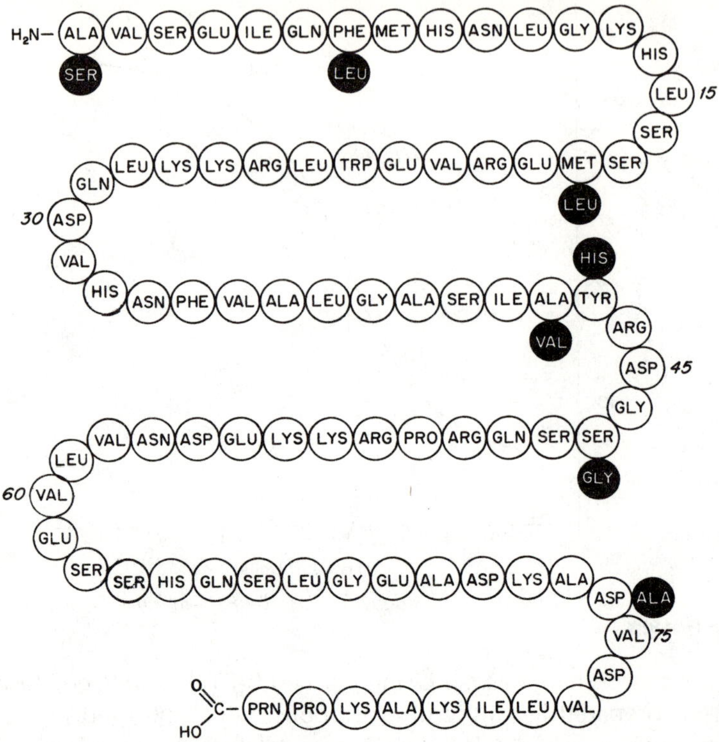

Fig. 8.3 *Amino acid sequences of bovine (open circles) and porcine (shaded circles) parathyroid hormones. Reproduced, with permission, from Potts et al. (1971).*

Purified, electrophoretically homogeneous bovine parathyroid hormone is a single chain polypeptide containing 84 amino acids (Fig. 8.3). Bovine parathyroids also contain two variants of the major form of PTH; both contain a threonine residue (absent in b-PTH) and one less valine residue. Figure 8.3 also shows the sequence of porcine PTH, isolated by Woodhead *et al.* (1971). p-PTH has serine as the N-terminal amino acid instead of alanine; in addition, 6 other amino acid substitutions occur. *In vivo,* b- and p-PTH have the same activities (2000–3000 U/mg); *in vitro* (adenyl cyclase assay), p-PTH is only about one-third as active as b-PTH.

Extracts of chicken parathyroids contain a hypercalcemic principle which has about the same molecular weight as b-PTH, as judged by gel filtration experiments (MacGregor *et al.,* 1972). Chicken PTH has been partially purified (600 U/mg by a modified mouse calvarium assay). In radioimmunoassays using anti-b-PTH antibody, the curve for chicken PTH is displaced two or three orders of magnitude to the right, as compared to pure b-PTH, indicating a low degree of cross reactivity.

O'Riordan *et al.* (1971) isolated small amounts of PTH from human parathyroid tissue. Its amino acid composition differs significantly from that of b-PTH (less Glu, Ile, Ser, Val; more Ala, Gly, Leu, Pro, Thr). Five of these substitutions appear among the 34 amino acids from the amino terminal end (Brewer *et al.,* 1972).

It has been known for a long time that PTH retains substantial biological and immunological activity upon fragmentation. Thus, from bovine parathyroid powder, extracted with hot hydrochloric acid, Rasmussen was able to isolate a number of calcium-mobilizing phosphaturic peptides with molecular weights ranging from 3800 to 5600. Their activities were all in the range of 750–1250 USP units/mg, i.e., from one-third to one-fourth the activity of "native" parathyroid hormone. When purified b-PTH was carefully hydrolyzed in dilute HCl, several fragments which retained activity *in vitro* and *in vivo* were formed. The smallest, as well as the most active, had an amino acid composition which corresponded to a 29-residue peptide from the amino terminal end of b-PTH (Keutmann *et al.,* 1972). Its activity was 650 U/mg. The occurrence of the 1–29 fragment corresponds to cleavage of the peptide bonds at either side of Asp^{30}. Other fragments resulting from the excision of other aspartyl residues (31–44; 46–55; 57–71; 77–84) have also been isolated; none of these were active.

The ability of PTH to sustain the loss of more than half the amino acids at the C-terminal end while retaining substantial biological activity does not extend to the N-terminal part of the molecule. Brief digestion with leucine aminopeptidase, sufficient to remove just three amino acids at the amino terminus, suffices to destroy activity completely. Trypsin, cyanogen bromide, performic acid, and acetic anhydride also inactivate. Some activity is left following treatment with tyrosinase, N-bromosuccinimide, and 2-hydroxy-5-nitrobenzyl bromide; the last two reagents are specific for Trp^{23}.

The structural requirements for PTH activity have also been studied by determining the activities of a series of synthetic peptides related to the native hormone. The data for nine such compounds are summarized in Table 8.1.

The purified b-PTH, assigned a value of 100 in Table 8.1 was calibrated against a Medical Research Council standard and was found to have 2500 U/mg *in vivo* and 3000 MRC U/mg *in vitro*. The regression lines for b-PTH^{1-34} were parallel to those obtained with b-PTH in both assays, but the slopes for the shorter peptides were distinctly lower. It is apparent from these data that the minimum polypeptide with PTH activity in the chick assay contains 28–34 amino acids in a sequence corresponding to the amino terminus of b-PTH.

TABLE 8.1 Biological Activities of Synthetic Peptides Related to Bovine PTH[a]

Peptide	Relative activity per mole of peptide	
	In vivo[b]	*In vitro*[c]
b-PTH	100	100
b-PTH^{1-34}	130	80
b-PTH^{2-34}	65	2
b-PTH^{3-34}	0.2	0.3
b-PTH^{1-26}	—	0.3
b-PTH^{1-27}	—	2
b-PTH^{1-28}	0.3	5
b-PTH^{1-12} + b-PTH^{13-34}	0.2	0.3

[a] *From Tregear et al., 1973.*
[b] *Chick hypercalcemic assay.*
[c] *Adenyl cyclase assay.*

III. The Nature of the Hormone in Circulation

The PTH molecule includes several antigenically distinguishable sites, as indicated by the fact that various fragments of the molecule interact to different extents with anti-PTH antibody. These facts have made it possible to distinguish several different immunoreactive components in glandular extracts, in the medium obtained after incubation of parathyroid explants, and in the general circulation. Plasma obtained from the thyroid veins of humans with normally active parathyroids contains mostly intact human PTH, but the principal immunoreactive component in the general circulation appears to be a C-terminal fragment with molecular weight about 7500 (Habener *et al.*, 1972). The same fragment, or one of similar size, comprises the main component identifiable in the plasma of hyperparathyroid patients; it is accompanied by native PTH and another, smaller (MW = 4500–5000) fragment (Canterbury and Reiss, 1972). Immediately after parathyroidectomy, the plasma concentration of native PTH increases, then rapidly decreases; after 30 minutes it is no longer detectable. One and one-half hours after the operation only the smallest fragment (MW = 4500–5000) remains. Since both PTH fragments are biologically inactive, estimates of plasma levels of active PTH by radioimmunoassay may be quite unreliable.

IV. Pro-PTH

The existence of a biosynthetic precursor of PTH (pro-PTH; calcemic fraction A) was demonstrated in 1972 (Kemper *et al.*, 1972), and its isolation and some of its properties reported shortly thereafter (Cohn *et al.*, 1972). Pro-PTH reacts with anti-PTH antibody, although higher concentrations (15–20 times that of PTH) are required, and is able to induce hypercalcemia in rats and bone resorption in the mouse calvarium assay. Amino acid analysis of purified pro-PTH indicates that it contains about 25 more amino acid residues than PTH; its molecular weight is therefore 12,100–12,500.

9

Calcitonin

I. Assay

The first method for quantitative estimation of the hypocalcemic principle of the thyroid gland was described by Hirsch, Voelkel, and Munson in 1964. Hirsch's assay was based on the fall in serum calcium during the first hour after injection of the hormone into rats maintained on a low calcium diet. As subsequently modified by Cooper *et al.* (1967), the assay was found to afford a linear log dose–response relationship between 0.015–0.060 MRC units of calcitonin.*

Larger doses of calcitonin not only cause a greater fall in serum calcium, but also prolong the period of hypocalcemia. Both variables have been combined into a single index for assay. Copp and Kuczerpa (1968) determined the area between the plasma calcium curves (determined at intervals during 6 hours) in treated and control animals. For young (36-day-old) rats, the response amounted to about 4 mg%-hours for about 0.010 MRC units (Fig. 9.1).

Older rats are less responsive to calcitonin. About five times as much hormone is required to produce a significant response in 77-day-old an-

* One MRC unit was defined as the hypocalcemic activity of 40 mg of an extract of hog thyroids prepared by the Medical Research Council, Mill Hill, London. 0.010–0.020 MRC units will lower the serum calcium by 1.5 mg% in young rats.

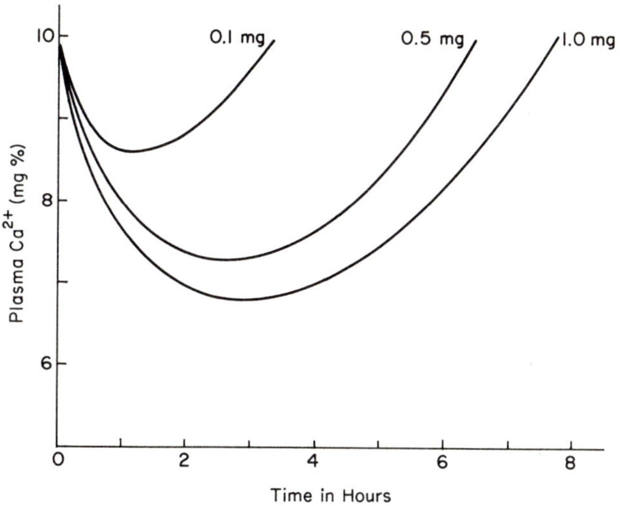

Fig. 9.1 *The effect of various quantities of calcitonin upon the magnitude and duration of the hypocalcemic response in 36-day old rats. Data of Copp and Kuczerpa (1968).*

imals; after 40 weeks rats are totally unresponsive (Fig. 9.2). It may be worth noting that only a slight diminution in PTH responsiveness occurs in older animals.

The hypocalcemic response in mice may also be used for the assay of calcitonin (Laljec *et al.,* 1967). Curiously, while mice and rats appeared to be equally sensitive to porcine calcitonin (p-calcitonin), extracts of human thyroids which were distinctly hypocalcemic in mice had no effect upon plasma calcium in rats.

Lequin *et al.* (1969) prepared antisera to calcitonin in rabbits. The antigen was a relatively crude (8 MRC units/mg) preparation of porcine calcitonin. A radioimmunoassay was developed with ^{131}I-labeled synthetic porcine calcitonin; a unique feature of the procedure was the use of dextran-coated charcoal to separate free from antibody-bound hormone. The small (MW 3600) calcitonin molecule was absorbed by dextran, while the larger antibody-hormone complex was excluded. Significant reduction of the B/F ratio was observed when the concentration of synthetic p-calcitonin was 20×10^{-11} *M*; this corresponds to 2×10^{-5} MRC units/ml.

Calcitonin from human thyroids cross reacts only slightly with rabbit anti-p-calcitonin antibody; the above assay therefore cannot be used for clinical purposes. A radioimmunoassay suitable for human calcitonin has been developed (Deftos, 1971), using either calcitonin isolated from a medullary thyroid carcinoma or a synthetic product. Deftos reported that concentrations of calcitonin, 0.01–0.1 μg/ml, may be detected by this method.

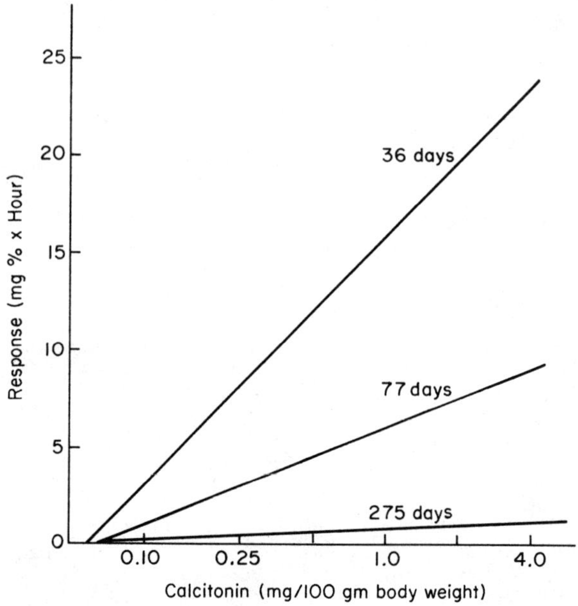

Fig. 9.2 *Effect of age upon the response of rats to calcitonin. Data of Copp and Kuczerpa (1968).*

II. Chemistry

The resolution of the problem of the chemical nature of calcitonin affords a striking example of the progress of protein chemistry since 1950. The existence of a hypocalcemic hormone produced by mammalian thyroids was first definitely established by Hirsch *et al.*, in 1963. By 1968, not only had the primary structure of porcine calcitonin been worked out (independently by three groups of investigators) but total syntheses had been reported by two of them. By 1970 the occurrence of calcitonins in a

		1				5					10				
Bovine	H_2N-	<u>Cys</u>-	Ser-	<u>Asn</u>-	<u>Leu</u>-	<u>Ser</u>-	<u>Thr</u>-	<u>Cys</u>-	Val-	<u>Leu</u>-	Ser-	Ala-	Tyr-	Trp-	Lys-
Ovine															
Porcine															-
Human			-Gly-						-Met-		-Gly-	Thr-		-Thr-	Gln-
Salmon											-Gly-	Lys-	Leu-	Ser-	Gln-

Fig. 9.3 *Amino acid sequences of bovine, ovine, porcine, human, and salmon calcitonins. Dayhoff (1972, pp. D-205 and D-206). The invariant amino acids are underlined.*

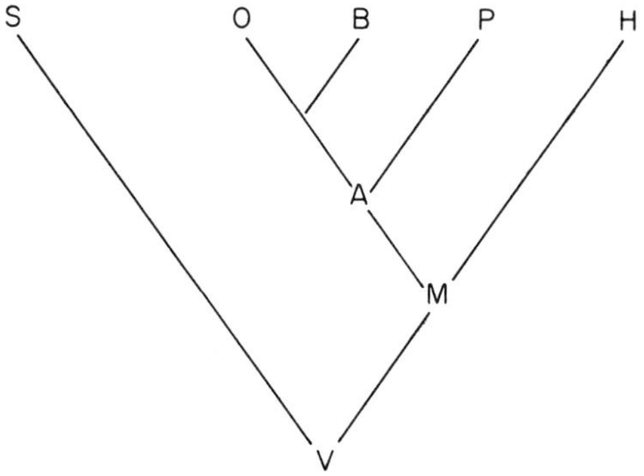

Fig. 9.4 *A possible evolutionary scheme for modern calcitonins. S, salmon; O, ovine; B, bovine; P, porcine; H, human; A, artiodactyl; M, common mammalian ancestor; V, vertebrate. Reproduced, with permission, from Staehlin, 1972.*

dozen or so vertebrate species had been established, and the sequences of two other mammalian (bovine, human) and one nonmammalian (salmon) calcitonins had been defined.

All of the calcitonins for which complete data are available are peptides with 32 amino acids. In Fig. 9.3 sequences of four mammalian and one nonmammalian vertebrate calcitonins are compared. Unlike the corticotropins, in which species differences are confined to a few amino acids, and to a restricted part of the molecule, some of the calcitonins display very marked differences in amino acid composition; the differences are distributed rather generally throughout the molecule. The three artiodactyl hormones (bovine, ovine, and porcine) are closely similar (1–3 residues). Human calcitonin differs from ovine calcitonin in 19 residues, whereas only 16 amino acids are replaced when human and salmon calcitonins are compared. Staehlin (1972) has suggested that all the calcitonins may have evolved from a common vertebrate ancestor (Fig. 9.4,V). Mutations may then have occurred to salmon calcitonin (Fig. 9.4,S) and to a common mammalian ancestor (Fig. 9.4,M). The latter, in turn, was presumably trans-

15 20 25 30

Asp-Leu-Asn-Asn-Tyr-His-Arg-Phe-Ser-Gly-Met-Gly-Phe-Gly-Pro-Glu-Thr-Pro(NH$_2$)

-Tyr-

Asn- -Phe-

-Phe- -Lys-Phe- -Thr- -Pro-Gln-Thr-Ala-Ile- -Val-Gly-Ala-

Glu- -His-Lys-Leu-Gln-Thr-Tyr-Pro-Arg-Thr-Asn-Thr- -Ser-Pro

Fig. 9.3 (*Continued*)

formed to human calcitonin (Fig. 9.4,H) and to a common artiodactyl calcitionin (Fig. 9.4A); minor modifications of the latter would lead to the calcitonins found in modern artiodactyls.

In addition to the major calcitonin component (s-CT-1) in salmon ultimobranchial glands, two active analogs have been isolated from the same source (Pless *et al.*, 1972). s-CT-2 is Asp^{15}, Phe^{22}, Ala^{29}, Val^{31}-s-CT-1, and s-CT-3 is Met^{8}-s-CT-2.

The sample of purified human calcitonin which is described in Fig. 9.3 was isolated from C-cell tumors of the thyroid. An active dimer of the molecule shown was also isolated from this source (Riniker *et al.*, 1968).

III. Biological Activity

Although the structures of only five calcitonins have been worked out in detail, calcitonin or calcitonin-like substances have been found in every vertebrate species which has been studied. The material available included ultimobranchial tissue from bony and cartilaginous fishes, reptiles, amphibians, and birds, the C-cell containing (parathyroid) regions of rabbits and dogs, and in the thyroids, parathyroids, and thymus glands of humans. Chicken ultimobranchial calcitonin appears to be somewhat larger (MW = 4000) than porcine calcitonin, as judged by gel filtration on Bio-Gel P-10.

Purified mammalian calcitonins (porcine, bovine, human) have activities in the range of 100–300 MRC units/mg. As noted earlier, a significant reduction in the serum calcium of young rats can be provoked by the injection of 0.010 MRC units of calcitonin; thus, only 0.03–0.10 μg of the hormone is required for a hypocalcemic response. The relative instability of some calcitonins at low concentrations may account for some of the reported spread in specific activities. Thus, one of the variants of salmon calcitonin (s-CT-3) has only 30% of the activity of the others, presumably because of the sensitivity of methionine to oxidation.

Purified calcitonin from salmon ultimobranchial glands is at least ten times as active as any of the mammalian calcitonins; its activity in rats was reported (Keutmann *et al.*, 1970) to be 2700 MRC units/mg. In mice, salmon calcitonin is relatively even more potent—one milligram was equivalent to 50,000 MRC units of porcine calcitonin. In general, nonmammalian calcitonins produce a longer lasting hypocalcemia than mammalian ones; in rabbits, the hypocalcemic effect of ultimobranchial calcitonin persists two to four times as long as an equivalent dose of porcine hormone (Fig. 9.5). Nonmammalian calcitonins also retain their activity longer when incubated with rat plasma.

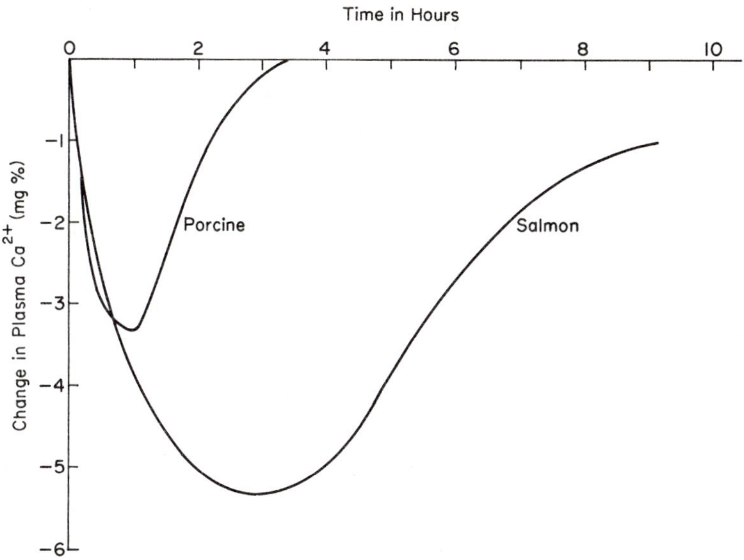

Fig. 9.5 *Comparison of the effects of equivalent doses (10 MRC units) of porcine and salmon calcitonins upon plasma* Ca^{2+} *in young rabbits.* (*From Copp, 1970.*)

Although rats have been the choice of most experimentors for studies of the biological actions of calcitonin, sensitivity of blood calcium to this hormone has been shown in mice, rabbits, frogs, fresh water eels, catfish, and properly prepared (parathyroidectomized) cockerels. Parsons and Reynolds (1968) have reported that preparations of porcine calcitonin which were equipotent in rats may evoke very different responses in mice, and similar effects were observed using ultimobranchial calcitonins from both chickens and salmon. Porcine calcitonin was active in both monkeys and humans. The concentration of calcium in the blood of sharks, killifish, and salmon were reported (Pang, 1971) to be insensitive to the administration of either mammalian or fish calcitonins, even though the ultimobranchial glands of some of these animals are rich sources of calcitonin.

A characteristic feature of calcitonin structure is the cyclic heptapeptide at the amino terminal end of the molecule (Fig. 9.3). The disulfide linkage apparently does not need to be intact for biological activity, since mercaptoethanol-reduced calcitonin was fully active (Brewer, 1969). However, if the reduced derivative was carboxymethylated, all activity disappeared. These facts suggest that the disulfide ring is restored (and necessary) *in vivo*.

The methionine residue at position 25 in porcine calcitonin may be oxidized to the sulfoxide or converted to the carboxymethyl sulfonium salt without damage to its biological properties; however, conversion to methionine sulfone resulted in an inactive peptide. In contrast, conversion of Met^8 in human calcitonin destroyed its hypocalcemic activity. Tyrosinase-oxidized and 2-hydroxy-5-nitrobenzyl calcitonin (the Trp residue is substituted) were both inactive, as was *N*-bromsuccinimide-treated calcitonin.

It was noted earlier that human calcitonin (h-calcitonin) does not react with antibody to p-calcitonin. Conversely, neither bovine, ovine, porcine, or salmon calcitonin will cross react with anti-human calcitonin antisera. Dogfish ultimobranchial calcitonin will crossreact with antibodies to salmon and porcine calcitonins but not with anti-h-calcitonin. Two lots of antiserum to h-calcitonin, collected in the same rabbit 8 and 17 months, respectively, after the first sensitizing injection reacted differently with peptide fragments obtained by proteolytic digestion of h-calcitonin; this fact has been used as evidence for the existence of several immunoreactive sites in the molecule (Dietrich and Rittel, 1970; Byfield *et al.*, 1972).

10

Hormones of the Anterior Pituitary

I. Growth Hormone

A. ASSAY

Three methods for the biological assay of growth hormone (GH) have gained wide acceptance: (a) the increase in weight of intact female rats that have stopped growing; (b) the increase in weight of immature hypophysectomized rats; and (c) measurement of the width of the tibial epiphyseal cartilage in hypophysectomized rats. In addition, the need for more sensitive procedures applicable to the concentration of growth hormone in blood and other fluids has sparked a large number of studies that have culminated in the development of a satisfactory radioimmunoassay. Weight gain in both adult and hypophysectomized rats is logarithmically related to the amount of growth hormone supplied, but the latter are at least five times more sensitive than the former. Thus, as little as 10 μg per day of porcine growth hormone will induce a sustained increase of 1.0 gm per day in the body weight of hypophysectomized rats. This effect can persist for as long as 90 days if growth hormone from a nonprimate source is used. (In contrast, rats become refractory to primate growth hormone after only 10 days).

Perhaps the most commonly used bioassay for GH is the tibia test [(c)

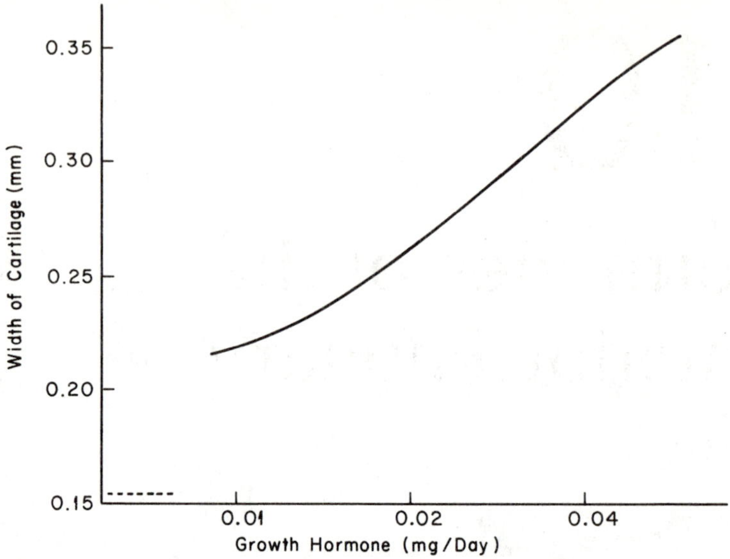

Fig. 10.1 *Epiphyseal cartilage (tibia) assay for growth hormone. The broken line represents the cartilage width in untreated animals. Data of Li et al. (1945).*

above]. This assay depends upon the fact that the epiphyseal cartilage of the long bones ceases to grow after hypophysectomy and that resumption of growth may be induced with GH. Young hypophysectomized rats are treated with GH for 4 days, the animal is killed on the fifth day, a tibia is removed, and the width of the epiphyseal cartilage, visualized by its resistance to silver staining, is measured. Figure 10.1, which represents data of Li *et al.* (1945), was obtained with purified bovine GH. Within limits of precision of the assay, dose–response curves of similar slope have been obtained with hormones isolated from pituitaries of sheep, hogs, whales, monkeys, and men.

Although the intact mouse is relatively insensitive to the actions of growth hormone, hypophysectomized mice respond with an increase in epiphyseal cartilage width. In the absence of thyroid hormone, the response is slow, 17 days being required for significant increases to occur. As a result, the use of the mouse as a test animal offers no advantage as far as sensitivity is concerned.

A number of specialized techniques have been applied to the assay of growth hormone. These include the increase of tail length in hypophysectomized rats, the rate of increase in blood urea in nephrectomized fed rats, the uptake of ^{35}S by tibial cartilage (hypophysectomized rat), and increase in the concentration of nonesterified fatty acids (NEFA) in dogs or humans.

While few of these procedures have gained general utility as routine assay tools, they may find application in special circumstances. Increase in NEFA in humans, for example, may be useful as a screening procedure to identify GH preparations which are active in man.

Most of the assay problems which arise during the isolation and characterization of growth hormone can satisfactorily, if somewhat laboriously and expensively, be met by one or another of the bioassays which have just been referred to. Even the most sensitive of these, however, are usually unsuited for the determination of growth hormone concentrations in blood or other body fluids. Inspired by the successful development of an immunoassay for insulin, attempts to devise a similar procedure applicable to GH were mounted in the late 1950's and early 1960's. In 1960, Reed and Bryan described a method for GH immunoassay, using hemagglutination as an end point. As little as 5×10^{-9} gm (5 ng) can be detected by this method.

Techniques for the radioimmunoassay of human growth hormone (h-GH) were described by several groups of workers soon thereafter (Utiger *et al.*, 1962; Glick *et al.*, 1963; Hunter and Greenwood, 1964). The various procedures differ principally in the means used to effect the separation of free and antibody-bound GH: precipitation with goat anti-rabbit serum antibody (Utiger); electrophoresis on paper (Glick); electrophoresis on cellulose acetate (Hunter). These methods permitted the semiquantitative estimation of GH concentrations (of the order of 0.2–100 ng/ml) in human plasma as well as in monkey plasma. It has been found, in fact, that inhibition curves using labeled h-GH and unlabeled monkey GH parallel those obtained with h-GH alone; while no cross-reaction could be demonstrated with bovine or porcine GH (b-GH or p-GH, respectively).

B. CHEMICAL COMPOSITION

The isolation of pure growth hormone from the pituitaries of domestic animals followed by only a few years the isolation of pure prolactin, and for much the same reason (i.e., its high concentration in pituitary tissue). Although the first isolation of purified bovine growth hormone (b-GH) included a reported yield of "only" 40 mg/kg of fresh glands (a quantity which is by no means small as these matters are usually reckoned), by 1954 recoveries of 2 gm/kg were routine.

Since 1955, growth hormone has been isolated from the pituitaries of eight other mammalian species. These include dogs, horses, humans, monkeys, pigs, rabbits, rats, and whales. In addition, substances with growth-promoting properties have been isolated from pituitaries of chickens and several kinds of fish. Although no purification was attempted, extracts of pituitaries of eleven kinds of primates (including gibbons, organutans, chimpanzees, and squirrel monkeys), bony fishes (paddlefish, sturgeon), cats, deer, bullfrogs, woodchucks, camels, lizards, anteaters, and sea lions displayed activity in the rat tibia test. Yields of GH have been fairly large in all species, ranging from 2–5 gm/kg of fresh glands.

Purified mammalian growth hormones contain from 1–3 IU/mg,* varying somewhat with the species of origin. In general, the most potent growth promoting substances have been isolated from human and rat pituitaries. As noted above, significant increases in the width of hypophysectomized rat epiphyseal cartilage can be demonstrated after giving 5 μg (0.015 IU) of GH over a 4-day-period. Another index of activity is the half-maximal tibial response, which requires a total of only 20–40 μg over a 4-day-period.

All the growth hormones which have been characterized are proteins; none have shown any evidence of the presence of nonamino acid components. Early studies of the molecular kinetic properties of b-GH had indicated that its molecular weight was close to 45,000 (Li *et al.*, 1945); this value was based on sedimentation behavior in the ultracentrifuge, as well as osmotic pressure measurements in 0.4 *M* $(NH_4)_2SO_4$ at pH 7.0. Subsequently, investigations of the properties of growth hormones of other species indicated that pig, sheep, and whale growth hormones were about the size of the b-GH molecule (40,000–48,000), while primate growth hormone was about half that size (25,000 and 21,500 for monkey and human hormones, respectively). It should be noted that because of the limited solubility of most growth hormones in salt-free solutions near pH 7 most of the molecular weight studies have been performed at low (3.6) or high (9.6) pH, usually in the presence of significant amounts of salt.

Although some early data by Li and Pedersen (1953) had suggested that b-GH undergoes a reversible dissociation to smaller molecules at pH 11.5, the 40,000 dalton figure for b-GH was not seriously challenged until 1963, when Andrews and Folley (1963) passed bovine, ovine, and porcine growth hormones through a column of Sephadex G-75 at pH 7.4. Under these conditions, all three hormones emerge from the column in narrow bands; the elution volumes corresponded to molecular weights of 20,000–22,000. Later, Andrews (1966) studied the gel filtration properties of a number of growth hormones as functions of concentration and pH. He found that the apparent molecular weights of all growth hormones were strongly concentration dependent, diminishing as the concentration decreased. He also showed that the molecular weights of all molecular species were lowest near pH 7.5, with some tendency apparent for all of them to aggregate at higher pH, and especially at lower pH. Estimates of the minimum molecular

* A unit of growth hormone activity has been defined (Li and Evans, 1948) as the daily dose that causes an increase of 40 to 60 gm in body weight over a 20-day period when given to plateaued female rats weighing 220 to 280 gm.

TABLE 10.1 Molecular Weights of Growth Hormones of Various Species[a]

	Species				
	Bovine	Ovine	Porcine	Monkey	Human
Molecular weight	26,000	24,000	22,500	21,000	20,500

[a] *From Andrews (1966).*

weights were made by extrapolation to infinite dilution at pH 7.5 (Table 10.1).

The estimates of monomeric molecular weights were subsequently verified by sedimentation velocity in glycine buffers of low ionic strength (Dellacha *et al.,* 1968) and in guanidine hydrochloride (Wilhelmi and Mills, 1968). Light scattering data at pH 9.5 and 11.5 yielded estimates of 24,700 and 16,500, respectively, for b-GH (Sonnenberg *et al.,* 1968). At pH 2.2–3.6 the sedimentation constant ($s_{20,w}$) of b-GH is approximately 2.3 S at low ionic strength and in the absence of neutral salts. Addition of even small amounts (0.06–0.10 *M*) of NaCl or KNO_3 increases $s_{20,w}$ to 3.0–4.2 S at the same pH. The striking tendency of b-GH to aggregate is indicated by the fact that b-GH will precipitate from its solution in glycine buffer if the NaCl concentration is increased to only 0.10 *M*.

Sodium dodecyl sulfate, an anionic detergent, will, like guanidine, depolymerize GH. In glycine-NaOH buffer (0.1 *M*, pH 9.4), $s_{20,w}$ for GH = 3.4 S. If 0.5% SDS is added, $s_{20,w}$ drops to 1.6 S. This corresponds to a decrease in molecular weight from 56,000 to 23,000; the latter figure probably includes some bound detergent.

Quite recently growth hormones from rat and rabbit pituitaries have been isolated. At pH 9.9 both these proteins sediment as single peaks with $s_{20,w}$ = 3.21 S, corresponding to molecular weights of approximately 45,000. Measurement of the osmotic pressure of solutions of rabbit GH in 6 *M* urea at pH 7.2 also pointed to a high figure (45,000) for the molecular weight. However, in 0.1 *M* glycine HCl, pH 3.55, the $s_{20,w}$ for rat GH was 2.24 S and that for the rabbit preparation was even lower, indicating that some dissociation had occurred. It seems likely therefore, that all (mammalian) somatotropins possess molecular weights in the range of 20,000 daltons; all but simian and human GH's exhibit a strong tendency toward aggregation, even in concentrated urea. The molecular weights of fish growth hormones also lie within this range. In view of the uncertainties introduced into molecular weights calculated from molecular kinetic properties of strongly aggregating substances, it would appear that the best estimates of the monomeric molecular weights of growth hormones would be those arrived at on the basis of amino acid composition—21,800 and 22,100 for ovine and human growth hormones, respectively.

Detailed sequence information is available for h-GH, o-GH, and b-GH (Niall *et al.*, 1973; Li *et al.*, 1973; Fernandez *et al.*, 1972), and approximate amino acid compositions are known for the growth hormones of five other species. These data are summarized in Fig. 10.2 and Table 10.2. Human and ovine GH's are single-chain peptides containing 191 amino acid residues, while the sequence proposed by Fernandez *et al.* for b-GH is 189 residues long. The sequences of o-GH and b-GH are identical except for two inversions, four replacements, and the deletion of two residues. Bovine GH displays microheterogeneity at position 126, sometimes occupied by Val and sometimes by Leu. Human GH differs from the ruminant growth hormones in approximately one-third of the amino acids present.

Major variations among different growth hormones occur in the number

TABLE 10.2 Amino Acid Composition of Mammalian Growth Hormones

	Residues/mole							
Amino acid	Cow[a]	Dog[b]	Pig[c]	Rabbit[c]	Rat[c]	Sheep[d]	Monkey[c]	Human[e]
Alanine	15	18	16–17	15	16	15	7	7
Arginine	13	13	12	13	12	13	11	11
Aspartic acid	16	17	15	15	14	16	21	20
Half-cystine	4	4	4	4	(4)[f]	4	6	4
Glutamic acid	24	25–26	24–25	24	25	24	27	27
Glycine	10	8	8	10	8	9	10	8
Histidine	3	3	3	3	3	3	3	3
Isoleucine	7	6	6	5	8	7	7	8
Leucine	25	26	24	24	22	27	23	26
Lysine	11	11	11	11	11	11	9	9
Methionine	4	3	3	3	3	4	3	3
Phenylalanine	13	13	12	11	12	13	13	13
Proline	6	8	7	7	7	6	10	8
Serine	12	15	14	13	13	13	17	18
Threonine	12	8–9	7	8	8	12	10	10
Tryptophan	1	(1)	1	1	1	1	1	1
Tyrosine	6	7	7	6	7	6	8	8
Valine	7	8	8	7	4	7	6	7
Total residues	189	194–196	182–184	180	178	191	192	191

[a] *Fernandez et al. (1972).*
[b] *Wilhelmi (1968).*
[c] *Wilhelmi and Mills (1968).*
[d] *Li et al. (1973).*
[e] *Niall et al. (1973).*
[f] *Data in parentheses uncertain.*

of polar amino acid residues (Table 10.2). Human and monkey GH's contain relatively more aspartic acid and serine, and relatively less arginine and lysine than bovine, ovine or porcine somatotropins. Wilhelmi has pointed out that the isoelectric points of growth hormones cluster in three groups, with the two primate hormones (4.9 and 5.2, respectively) being the lowest; dog, horse, pig, rabbit, and rat growth hormones have pI's between 5.9 and 6.3, while those of sheep and cattle are isoelectric at pH 6.8. In general these differences reflect corresponding differences in the relative proportions of dicarboxylic and basic amino acids.

Fellows *et al.* (1972) has called attention to a remarkable degree of homology between part of the growth hormone molecule (residues 39–78) and a number of other protein hormones, including pituitary and placental lactogens and the pituitary glycoprotein hormones. More than 60% of the residues in the corresponding sequences are either identical or the result of a single step gene mutation, supporting an earlier suggestion that the simple, as well as the glycoprotein hormones of the pituitary may have evolved from a common ancestral peptide.

Although the complete structures of other growth hormones are unknown, information concerning N- and C-terminal sequences is available. Most of the mammalian growth hormones which have been examined (canine, human, porcine, rabbit, rat, and cetacean) have Phe as the N-terminal amino acid. As shown in Fig. 10.2, sheep GH has Ala in this position. Bovine GH has consistently yielded equimolar amounts of Ala and Phe when examined by the Sanger procedure, in the proportion of one mole of each for 45,000 gm of protein. This was rationalized with earlier, larger molecular weight estimates by assuming the existence, in part of the molecule, of two chains, each with a free N-terminal amino acid. When the "true" molecular weight of b-GH was recognized to be 22,000, it was necessary to assume that even the best b-GH preparations consisted of two kinds of molecules, differing in their N-terminal amino acids and present in almost exactly equal amount. That individual animals are heterozygous for both allelic forms is indicated by the isolation of both forms of GH from single ox pituitaries.

More is known about C-terminal sequences. Bovine, human, porcine, canine, equine, and ovine hormones all have a tight loop of amino acids formed by a disulfide link between neighboring cysteine residues (Wilhelmi and Mills, 1968). The loop in animal somatotropins invariably contains one more amino acid than h-GH (Fig. 10.3).

C. COMPARATIVE BIOLOGICAL ACTIVITIES

Beginning in the late 1940's, attempts were made to apply b-GH preparations to the relief of hypopituitary function in man. Although occassional

		1									10										20					
(h-GH)		H_2N-Phe	Pro	Thr	Ile	Pro	Leu	Ser	Arg	Leu	Phe	Asp	Asn	Ala	Met	Leu	Arg	Ala	His	Arg	Leu	His	Gln	Leu	Ala	Phe
(b-GH)	H_2N-Ala			Ala	Met	Ser			Gly			Ala			Val				Gln	His						Ala
(o-GH)	H_2N-Ala			Ala	Met	Ser			Gly			Ala			Val				Gln	His						Ala
(h-PL)		H_2N-Val	Gln		Val								His				Gln				Ala					Ile

				30										40										50
(h-GH)	Asp	Thr	Tyr	Gln	Glu	Phe	Glu	Glu	Ala	Tyr	Ile	Pro	Lys	Glu	Gln	Lys	Tyr	Ser	Phe	Leu	Gln	Asn	Pro	Gln	Thr
(b-GH)			Phe	Lys					Arg	Thr			Glu	Pro	Gly		Arg			( )	Ile			Thr		Val
(o-GH)			Phe	Lys					Arg	Thr				Glu	Gly		Arg			( )	Ile			Thr		Val
(h-PL)									Thr					Asp							His	Asp	Ser		

									60										70					
(h-GH)	Ser	Leu	Cys	Phe	Ser	Glu	Ser	Ile	Pro	Thr	Pro	Ser	Asn	Arg	Glu	Glu	Thr	Gln	Gln	Lys	Ser	Asn	Leu	Gln	Leu
(b-GH)	Ala	Phe					Thr			Ala		Thr	Gly	Lys	Asn		Ala		Glu			Asp		Glu	
(o-GH)	Ala	Phe					Thr			Ala		Thr	Gly	Lys	Asn		Ala					Asp		Glu	
(h-PL)		Phe				Asp								Met										Glu	

					80										90										100
(h-GH)	Leu	Arg	Ile	Ser	Leu	Leu	Leu	Ile	Gln	Ser	Trp	Leu	Glu	Pro	Val	Gln	Phe	Leu	Arg	Ser	Val	Phe	Ala	Asn	Ser
(b-GH)									Ser	Glu			Glx		Gly	( )				( )			Thr		
(o-GH)													Gly		Leu				Ser	Arg			Thr	Asp	
(h-PL)									Glu							Arg					Met				Asn

```
                                     110                                          120
(h-GH)  -Leu-Val-Tyr-Gly-Ala-Ser-Asn-Ser-Asp-Val-Tyr-Asp-Leu-Leu-Lys-Asp-Leu-Glu-Glu-Gly-Ile-Gln-Thr-Leu-Met-
(b-GH)          -Phe-   -Thr-   -Asp-( )-Arg-       -Glu-Lys-                               -Leu-Ala-
(o-GH)          -Phe-   -Thr-   -Asp-( )-Arg-       -Glu-Lys-                               -Leu-Ala-
(h-PL)              -Asp-Thr-   -Asp-       -Asp-   -His-                   -Gln-           -Glu-

                    130                                     140                                     150
(h-GH)  -Gly-Arg-Leu-Glu-Asp-Gly-Ser-Pro-Arg-Thr-Gly-Gln-Ile-Phe-Lys-Gln-Thr-Tyr-Ser-Lys-Phe-Asp-Thr-Asn-Ser-
(b-GH)  -Arg-Glu-Val-               -Thr-       -Ala-       -Leu-               -Asp-               -Met-
(o-GH)  -Arg-Glu-               -Val-Thr-       -Ala-       -Leu-               -Asp-               -Met-
                                    -Arg-                   -Leu-

                                        160                                       170
(h-GH)  -His-Asn-Asp-Asp-Ala-Leu-Leu-Lys-Asn-Tyr-Gly-Leu-Leu-Tyr-Cys-Phe-Arg-Lys-Asp-Met-Asp-Lys-Val-Glu-Thr-
(b-GH)  -Arg-Ser-                                       -Ser-               -Asn-Leu-His-   -Thr-
(o-GH)  -Arg-Ser-                                       -Ser-                   -Leu-His-   -Thr-
(h-PL)          -His-

                    180                                     190
(h-GH)  -Phe-Leu-Arg-Ile-Val-Gln-Cys-Arg-( )-Ser-Val-Glu-Gly-Ser-Cys-Gly-PheOH
(b-GH)  -Tyr-       -Val-Met-Lys-       -Arg-Phe-Gly-   -Ala-       -Ala-   OH
(o-GH)  -Tyr-       -Val-Met-Lys-       -Arg-Phe-Gly-   -Ala-       -Ala-   OH
(h-PL)              -Met-               ( )                                 OH
```

Fig. 10.2 *Amino acid sequences of human, bovine, and ovine growth hormones and human placental lactogen (human chorionic somatomammotropin). The growth hormone sequences have been aligned to display maximum homology. Amino acid deletions are indicated by ( ). Source: h-GH, h-PL. Niall et al. (1973); b-GH, Fernandez et al. (1972); o-GH, Li et al. (1973).*

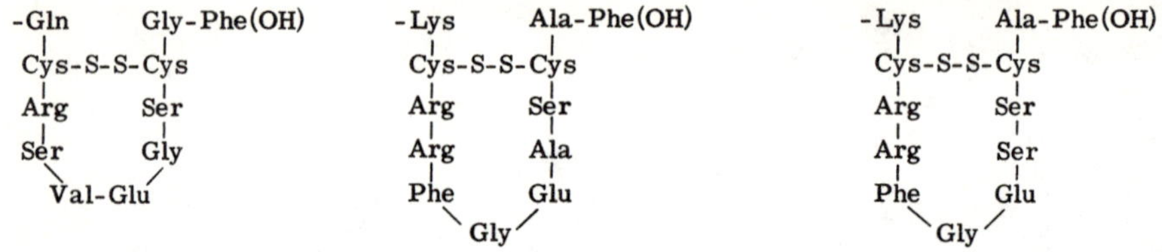

Human Bovine, ovine Canine, equine, porcine

Fig. 10.3 *C-terminal sequences of growth hormones. The amino acid compositions of the C-terminal dodecapeptides of canine and equine growth hormones are identical with that of porcine somatotropin, and the sequence of the last eight amino acids is known to be the same in the last two. Hence, it is assumed that the complete sequences are identical.*

hints of positive physiological effects were sometimes claimed, it could be stated unequivocally in 1959 that " . . . currently available preparations of (bovine) growth hormone have no anabolic protein action in man." (Knobil and Greep, 1959). This was all the more disappointing since experience with other hormones, especially insulin and ACTH, had encouraged the belief that other peptide hormones might be clinically useful.

Other evidence that the phenomenon of specificity in growth hormone action was not confined to bovine growth hormone also appeared early. In 1954, Wilhelmi (1955) showed that a substance isolated from the pituitaries of commercial fish (hake, pollack, cod) stimulated growth in hypophysectomized killifish, but was ineffective in the rat tibia test. In contrast, b-GH was even more active in fish than was fish GH. A little later it was shown that while monkeys, like men, do not respond to b-GH, extracts of monkey pituitaries, with growth-promoting properties in rats, would cause nitrogen retention in monkeys.

The results of some 15 years of research on phylogenetic specificity in growth hormone physiology are summarized in Table 10.3. The growth hormones of teleost fishes are active in fishes, but not in rats. (Lungfish pituitary extract is, however, active in the rat). Pituitary extracts from birds, reptiles, and amphibians have growth-promoting effects in rats, as do the pituitaries of all mammals which have been examined. Dogs are also generally responsive to mammalian growth hormones. Birds are not responsive to b-GH. Finally, primates respond exclusively to primate GH.

Guinea pigs are anomalous in their responses to GH. Hypophysectomized guinea pigs continue to grow at a rate which is indistinguishable from that of intact guinea pigs, and neither intact nor hypophysectomized guinea pigs are responsive to either bovine or primate (monkey) GH (Knobil and Greep, 1959). Neverless, the guinea pig pituitary contains GH (or a substance with similar properties), since its extracts have growth-promoting effects in the rat.

Another aspect of biological specificity related to GH is illustrated by the results of long term experiments of the effects of primate and other mammalian growth hormones in rats. If hypophysectomized rats are treated with monkey or human growth hormone, growth resumes, but ceases again after about 10 days. On the other hand, bovine or cetacean GH elicits a growth response in hypophysectomized rats which persists for at least 90 days (Li *et al.*, 1959). Rats which are refractory to one primate hormone (e.g., human) are also insensitive to the other (monkey), whereas ox or whale GH initiates growth promptly if administered after a course of primate hormone injections.

An elegant and sensitive method for the detection of biological "relatedness" among protein hormones is to determine the extent of immunological cross-reaction between antibodies to one kind of protein and a homologous protein of another species. Thus, rabbit anti-b-GH will precipitate not only with b-GH but also with o-GH; it will not, however, react with human GH. Antigen–antibody reactions can be visualized using classical precipitin methods; they may also be studied by allowing antigen and antibody to diffuse toward each other in agar; with this method an optimal concentration range is automatically provided. In the Ouchterlony modification of the agar diffusion test (Fig. 10.4) several antigens contained in reservoirs are placed in a circle around a central reservoir containing antibody. The appearance of precipitin lines indicates an antigen–antibody reaction,

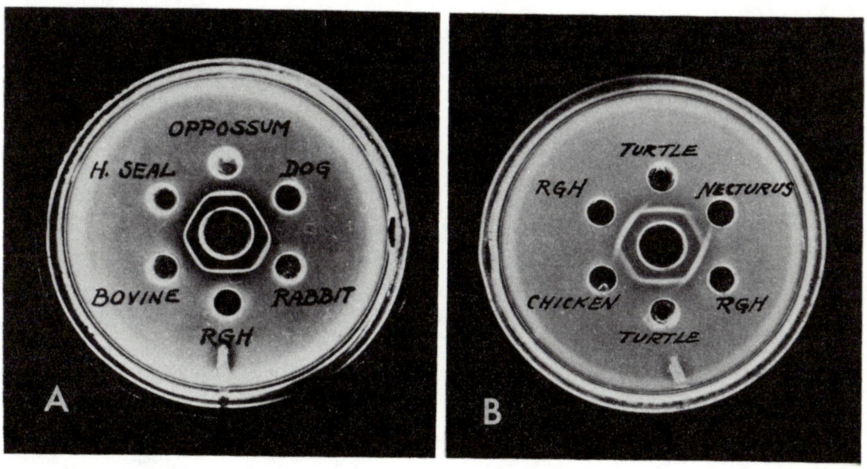

Fig. 10.4 *Ouchterlony plates showing precipitin reactions between anti-rat growth hormone (center well) and other mammalian and nonmammalian growth hormones (outer wells). The absence of spurs in plate A indicates qualitative identity of rat GH with other mammalian GH's. Spurs in plate B indicate only partial identity of rat, avian, amphibian, and reptilian GH's. The anti-rat GH antiserum was prepared in monkeys. Reproduced, with permission, from Hayashida (1969).*

TABLE 10.3 Phylogenetic Specificity of Growth Hormones[a]

Source of growth hormone	Tested in: Killifish	Frogs	Chickens	Cats	Dogs	Guinea pigs	Mice	Rats	Monkeys	Humans
Cod								−		
Hake	+							−		
Lungfish								+		
Mackerel								−		
Paddlefish								±		
Salmon								−		
Shad								−		
Sturgeon								±		
Bullfrog								+		
Lizard								+		
Turtle								±		
Chicken			+					+		
Anteater								+		
Camel								+		
Cat								+		
Cow	+	+	−	+	+	−	+	+	−	−
Deer								+		
Dog								+		

Guinea pig			?	+		
Horse				+		
Pig				+	−	
Rabbit				+		
Rat				+		
Sea lion				+		
Sheep	+	+		+		−
Whale				+		
Woodchuck				+		
Monkey	+		−	+	+	+
Man	+		−	+	+	+

[a] +, *Active;* −, *inactive;* ±, *activity uncertain.*

and the configuration of the intersecting lines for two different antigens can be interpreted in terms of their immunochemical similarity.

Another, somewhat more elaborate test of the degree of relatedness of two antigens to a third represents a variation of the procedure used for radioimmunoassay. Precipitation by antibody of radioisotope-labeled antigen is inhibited by the presence of another, cross-reacting antigen. A quantitative comparison of two antigens can be made by determining the amount of each required to inhibit precipitation of a third antigen by a preset amount (e.g., 50%).

Other techniques which have been used include the ability to induce anaphylactic reactions by injecting one kind of GH into guinea pigs which have been sensitized to another, and the ability of antiserum to one kind of hormone to diminish response to another *in vivo*.

Table 10.4 summarizes data from a number of sources on the ability of various kinds of growth hormones to cross-react with antisera to others. Of interest here is the fact that anti-b-GH interacts with sheep and deer GH (as well as with b-GH) whereas anti-rat GH serum reacts not only with growth hormones from other mammalian genera, but also with pituitary extracts from birds, reptiles, and amphibians. Using gel-diffusion techniques, reactions of identity could be observed between rat GH and the growth hormones of other mammals (Fig. 10.4); reactions with growth hormones of amphibians (necturus) and reptiles (turtles) were strong, but nonidentical. It

TABLE 10.4 Immunochemical Specificities of Growth Hormones

Source of growth hormone	Antibody to growth hormone, from[a]					
	Rats	Pigs	Sheep	Cows[b]	Monkeys	Humans
Chickens	+			−		
Camels				+		
Cows	+	+	+	+		+
Deer				+		
Horses		+		−		−
Rabbits	+	+		−		
Rats	+	+		−		
Sheep	+		+	+		−
Whales		+	−	−		−
Monkeys	−			−	+	+
Humans	−	−	−	−		+

[a] *Except for anti-pig growth hormone, the antisera were prepared in rabbits. Anti-pig growth hormone was prepared in guinea pigs.*

[b] *Growth hormones from bullfrogs, anteaters, woodchucks, guinea pigs, cats, sea lions, chameleons, and several kinds of fish did not cross-react with anti-bovine growth hormone.*

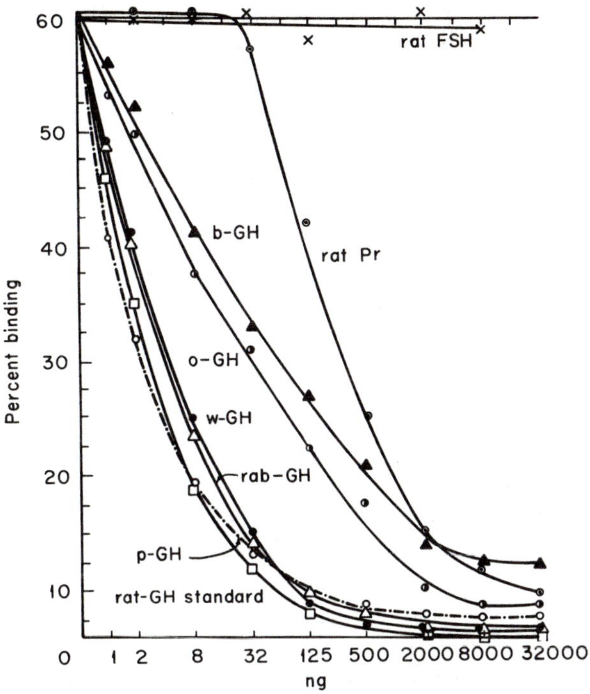

Fig. 10.5 *Cross-reactions of highly purified mammalian growth hormones [bovine (b-GH), ovine (o-GH); cetacean (w-GH) rabbit (rab-GH), porcine (p-GH)] with monkey anti-rat GH antiserum by means of a double antibody immunoassay. Data for rat prolactin (rat Pr) and rat FSH are also shown. Reproduced, with permission, from Hayashida (1969).*

would appear that rat growth hormone shares immunologically significant structural features with a wide variety of growth hormones.

Hayashida (1969) also used a radioimmunological approach to examine the effectiveness of various somatotropins to inhibit the interaction of rat GH and anti-rat GH antiserum. By this criterion, differences between the various mammalian hormones could readily be visualized. Figure 10.5 shows that only 4 ng of unlabeled rat GH was required to inhibit precipitation of ^{131}I-labeled rat GH (by monkey anti-rat GH serum) by 50%. Porcine GH was equally effective, while whale and rabbit growth hormones were less so; relatively large quantities of bovine and ovine hormones were required for inhibition. (Note that rat prolactin, in high concentration, was also effective, but that rat FSH was not; the interaction of prolactin with antiserum to GH could be accounted for by contamination with rat GH.)

The unique structural character of primate growth hormones is indicated by their failure to react with antisera to hormones other than those of primates. Tashjian *et al.* (1965) were able to establish an immunological hierarchy among primate growth hormones by studying their ability to react with anti-h-GH antibody; semiquantitative comparisons, based on complement fixation, were drawn. Three classes (suborders) of nonhuman primates were studied: growth hormones of the hominoideae (gibbons, chimpanzees, and orangutans) fixed more complement (when combined with anti-h-GH) than hormones of the cercopithecoideae (macaques, rhesus monkeys, and vervets); the single specimen of ceboideae (squirrel monkey) GH showed little cross-reaction except at relatively high antibody concentrations.

D. CHEMICAL MODIFICATION

Among the reagents which have been tested for their effects upon the biological activity of GH are iodine, performic acid, a number of reducing agents (including sulfite and dithiothreitol), and compounds which substitute amino groups. Selective acetylation of N-terminal amino groups can occur without loss of activity; however, if the ε-amino groups of lysine are attacked, activity is lost. Guanidinated b-GH is active, while succinylated GH is inactive. Much appears to depend upon the net charge on particular side chains.

Only one of the six tyrosine residues of b-GH may be iodinated without loss of activity. If more iodines are introduced, the loss of activity parallels their increase. Performic acid completely inactivates GH, either by oxidation of —S—S— bonds or by destruction of tryptophanyl residues.

In contrast with what happens to other protein hormones when treated with reducing agents, animal or human GH can be reduced without loss of activity. Sulfite, which cleaves the disulfide bond closest to the C-terminus, has essentially no effect upon either bovine or porcine GH, but does diminish the activity of human GH by 50–80%. However, when h-GH is reduced by mercaptoethanol or dithiothreitol nearly all of the activity is retained. Further, activity is retained when the reduced hormone is carbamidomethylated; however, the reaction of reduced GH with iodoacetic acid rather than iodoacetamide leads to essentially complete inactivation. Again, it appears that introduction of negatively charged centers into the molecule plays a deleterious role.

Some of the most interesting aspects of growth hormone chemistry derive from the results of studies of its fragmentation by proteolytic enzymes. It has long been known that proteolytic enzymes will release significant amounts of nonprotein (i.e., soluble in 5 or 10% trichloroacetic acid) material from growth hormones of various sources without affecting their growth-promoting activity. Thus, pepsin can convert about 40% of h-GH or 20% of b-GH to acid soluble material before the activity of either, as determined by the rat tibia test, begins to diminish. The sensitivities of the two hormones to trypsin is reversed, however; only 10% of the h-GH molecule can be removed by trypsin without loss of activity, while as much as 25% of b-GH can be removed by this means with the rest retaining essentially full activity. Leucine aminopeptidase will remove nearly one-fourth the amino acids at the amino terminal end of h-GH before growth-promoting activity begins to diminish (Li, 1956).

The results of these experiments assumed additional importance when it was reported that while native b-GH is devoid of activity in man, its tryptic, chymotryptic, or papain digestion products displayed some of the metabolic properties of primate GH. In a series of hypopituitary patients, Sonnenberg *et al.* (1968, 1969) found that the administration of trypsin-digested b-GH (t-BGH) to humans resulted in nitrogen and phosphorus retention, increased insulin resistance, and decreased tolerance to carbohydrate. Although these experiments were not consistently reproducible, they have provided encouragement for the suggestion that the characteristic physiological properties of somatropin reside in amino acid sequences which are common to hormones of several species. Moreover, the susceptibility of a particular species to native GH seems to be determined by other structural features in the molecule.

The nature of the "active sequences" have been clarified by experiments reported by Chillemi and Pecile (1971) and by Yamasaki *et al.* (1970, 1972). Chillemi and Pecile synthesized two peptides, corresponding to sequences 81–121 and 122–153 of h-GH; both were found to possess low, but significant, somatotropin activity in rats. Further, a mixture of 100 μg of each peptide was as effective as 400 μg of either ($\sim$12.5 μg of b-GH). The degree of homology between h-GH and the ruminant somatotropins in these two regions is very high (Fig. 10.2); there are only five "unacceptable" replacements in sequences of 42 and 32 amino acids, respectively. If the activity of somatotropin resides primarily in these regions of the native hormone, it might be expected that differences in species specificity would be reduced when the minimal peptides are compared.

Limited tryptic digestion was employed by Yamasaki *et al.* (1970) to isolate a b-GH fragment which retained nearly half the activity of the original somatotropin preparation and which also had metabolic activity in humans. The active fragment corresponded exactly in amino acid composition and sequence to residues 94–130 of b-GH and was homologous to residues 96–133 (with one deletion) of h-GH. Its resemblance to the active peptides synthesized by Chillemi and Pecile is obvious.

The larger h-GH fragment recovered by Yamasaki *et al.* from the tryptic digest, which apparently consisted of residues 1–93 and residues 131–191, linked by a disulfide bridge (53–164), had relatively little activity.

Additional evidence that the complete structure of h-GH is not required for activity came from an attempt, by Li and Yamashiro (1970) to synthesize h-GH. The attempt was only marginally successful, principally because it was based upon an incorrect structure for h-GH, first proposed by Li, Dixon, and Liu (1969). The compound actually synthesized differed from h-GH in several respects: (a) it contained only 188 amino acids instead of 191; (b) a 15-amino acid peptide sequence, which occupies residues 78–92 in h-GH, was erroneously placed at 17–31; (c) three amino acids Gln, Leu, and Arg, occupying positions 68, 93, and 94 in h-GH were omitted; and (d) a tripeptide sequence, Gly-Ser-Pro in h-GH (131–133) was replaced by Pro-Ser-Gly. Despite these significant differences, the synthetic "hormone" had about 10% of the activity of native h-GH by the rat tibia assay, and reacted with rabbit anti-h-GH antiserum. Note that the critical sequence described by Yamasaki *et al.* was present in the active synthetic product.

Frohman, Burek, and Stachura (1972) discovered that extracts of rat, dog, and human pituitaries as well as a GH-producing rat tumor contained, in addition to somatotropin, a much larger molecule which, like GH, reacts with homologous anti-GH antibody. While this substance, referred to as "large" growth hormone, accounted for only about 1% of the total immunoreactive GH of pituitary extracts, it accounted for 30–60% of the immunoprecipitable radioactivity of extracts of rat pituitaries incubated with radioactive leucine for periods up to 6 hours. However virtually none of the GH secreted into the medium during pituitary incubations (or into the blood *in vivo*) was large GH. Large growth hormone could be partially converted into GH by treatment with urea or guanidine hydrochloride, while digestion with trypsin failed to effect such a conversion. It was suggested that LGH consists of GH associated with another protein of much larger molecular weight, and that its role is related to the synthesis or release of GH (Stachura and Frohman, 1973). One of the possibilities mentioned was that it might represent a polysome composed of GH messenger RNA, ribosomes, and GH molecules in varying stages of completion; presumably enough of the latter contain the immunoreactive GH site to provide for the formation and precipitation of a complex with anti-GH antibody.

II. Adrenocorticotropin (ACTH)

A. ASSAY

1. In Vivo Methods

Early estimates of ACTH activity were based upon the ability of the hormone to increase the weight of the adrenal gland in either intact or hypophysectomized animals. These assays retain only historical interest, having been replaced for the most part by techniques which are faster or physiologically more significant. However, in 1957 Li *et al.* showed that adrenal weight increase in hypophysectomized rats was linear with the logarithm of the dose within a range of 1.5–22.5 μg of purified corticotropin per day (Fig. 2.1).

A major improvement in the speed and sensitivity of ACTH bioassays was introduced by the observation that stimulation by ACTH was accompanied by a rapid fall in adrenal ascorbic acid. An assay based upon depletion of adrenal ascorbic acid was developed by Sayers *et al.* (1948); subsequently, modifications were introduced by Thompson and Fisher (1953) and by Rerup (see Fisher, 1962). In hypophysectomized rats, adrenal ascorbic acid averages about 470 mg%. The subcutaneous administration of 0.1–3.0 μg of pure corticotropin/100 gm of body weight will reduce the ascorbic acid content by 20–150 mg% (i.e., to 450–320 mg%) in about one hour (Fig. 2.2). If the hormone is injected intravenously, the useful range is 0.01–0.1 μg per animal. Assays of various preparations using the subcutaneous route of administration appear to parallel more closely their clinical efficiency than do assays in which the intravenous route is employed.

The ACTH-stimulated adrenal gland discharges its ascorbic acid into the blood; an elevated ascorbic acid content can be detected in adrenal vein blood within minutes following an ACTH injection (Munson and Toepel, 1958). In 100-gm hypophysectomized rats, a significant increase can be seen following the injection of only 2×10^{-4} μg, and the log dose–response curve is approximately linear to 0.001 μg.

The injection of a number of substances other than ACTH (e.g., vasopressin) also results in the elevation of adrenal vein ascorbic acid. In an effort to improve the specificity of the response, Lipscomb and Nelson (1962) explored the effect of ACTH upon the concentration of blood corticosterone. In the unstimulated, hypophysectomized rat the rate of secretion of corticosterone, measured by a fluorescence technique, was 4.6 μg% per minute. Within a minute and a half of the systemic injection of 5×10^{-4} μg of ACTH, the rate of corticosterone secretion increased about fivefold. As little as 3×10^{-4} μg may be detected in this manner (Fig. 2.3).

2. *In Vitro Methods*

In 1953 it was found that when slices of adrenal glands from adult rats were incubated with ACTH, cortisol or a substance with similar spectroscopic properties was discharged into the medium (Saffran and Bayliss, 1953). The sensitivity of the method was rather low (0.03 μg being the minimum effective dose with 35 mg of adrenal gland slices) but it avoided some of the technical complexities (hypophysectomy, cannulation of the adrenal vein, etc.) of the *in vivo* methods. In some modifications of the *in vitro* method (Elliott *et al.*, 1954) the ability of corticoids to reduce tetrazolium chloride derivatives (a function of the α-ketol side chain) has replaced the estimation of steroid by UV absorption (a measure of the 3-keto-Δ^4-moiety in ring A).

The sensitivity of the *in vitro* assay for ACTH is increased manyfold if isolated adrenal cortical cells, obtained by brief digestion of quartered rat adrenals with trypsin, are incubated with corticotropin. A significant increase in the amount of corticosterone released into the medium during a 2-hour-period is obtained with ACTH concentrations of 1.5×10^{-5} μg.

Cohen *et al.* (1957) studied the responses of slices of functional adrenocortical tumors to ACTH *in vitro*. These tumors had originated spontaneously in irradiated animals and were easily maintained by transplantation. In the presence of ACTH, tumor slices readily secreted cortical hormones (mostly corticosterone), and a procedure for ACTH assay employing adrenal tumor slices and the essentials of the Saffran–Schally technique was devised (Cohen and Furth, 1959). A linear log dose–response relationship was obtained when 0.0025–0.03 μg ACTH was added to 100 mg slices (Fig. 2.4). This method was thus about one order of magnitude more sensitive than the rat adrenal slice method. Moreover, the fact that enough tissue (5–10 gm) for several assays could be obtained from a single animal was a distinct advantage.

Other proposed assays for ACTH include measurement of the corticosterone concentration of the adrenals of hypophysectomized rats (sensitivity range $2.5\text{–}20 \times 10^{-4}$ μg), the determination of urinary steroid excretion of ACTH-treated guinea pigs (0.25–10 μg), and the thymus involution assay in young rats (1.5–6 μg). A radioimmunoassay of ACTH, using ^{131}I-labeled corticotropin, has also been reported.

B. CHEMISTRY

Nearly 30 years ago two laboratories simultaneously described the preparation of active corticotropin preparations which, on the basis of electrophoretic and ultracentrifugal criteria, were said to be homogeneous proteins (Li *et al.*, 1943; Sayers *et al.*, 1943). Both preparations, from sheep and hog pituitaries, respectively, were reported to be proteins with molecular weight about 20,000, and both preparations were relatively inactive; daily doses of 0.10–0.2 mg were required to maintain adrenal weight in hypophysectomized rats.

In 1950, Payne, Raben, and Astwood found that acetic acid extracts of acetone-dried pituitary powder could be fractionated on cellulose (later,

1 5 10 15 20

H_2N-Ser-Tyr-Ser-Met-Glu-His-Phe-Arg-Trp-Gly-Lys-Pro-Val-Gly-Lys-Lys-Arg-Arg-Pro-Val-Lys-Val

			25					30					35				39
Bovine	-Tyr-	Pro-	Asn-	Gly-	Ala-	Glu-	Asp-	Glu-	Ser-	Ala-	Gln-	Ala-	Phe-	Pro-	Leu-	Glu-	PheOH
Ovine			-Asp-														
Procine									-Leu-		-Glu-						
Human											-Glu-						

Fig. 10.6 *Amino acid sequences of bovine, ovine, porcine, and human corticotropins. The sequence 1-24 is common to all four peptides. Invariant amino acids are underlined. Source: Li (1972).*

oxidized cellulose) to afford preparations which were 40–80 times as active as the earlier "pure" hormones. Within a relatively short time corticotropin preparations which were homogeneous by a variety of criteria were in hand. The criteria included countercurrent distribution (White, 1953; Bell, 1954), ion exchange chromatography (Dixon and Stack–Dunne, 1955), and electrophoresis and amino acid composition (Li and Dixon, 1956). The purified hormones from pig, sheep, and ox pituitaries had similar amino acid compositions and similar biological activities by the ascorbic acid depletion assay.

Purified corticotropins have now been isolated from pig, sheep, ox, and human pituitaries. All of these consist of a single peptide chain of 39 amino acids, and interspecies variations are confined to the amino acid residues in positions 25–32 (Fig. 10.6).

C. COMPARATIVE BIOLOGICAL ACTIVITIES

The international unit (IU) of corticotropin activity was originally established as being equivalent to 1.0 mg of a relatively crude ACTH preparation (La-1-A) prepared in 1946 by the Armour Laboratories. Subsequently, a second International Standard was made up and evaluated against the first; its activity (1.14 IU/mg) was defined in a way which preserved the constancy of the "unit" in biological terms. The biological activity of any corticotropin preparation (or analog) is evaluated by direct comparison with one or another standard preparation. Not surprisingly, the use of different assays sometimes leads to different relative activities for the same compound. Thus, purified pig corticotropin is approximately 100 times as active as the International Standard (La-1-A) by the adrenal ascorbic acid depletion assay, when both substances are injected subcutaneously, but only thirty times as active when both are given intravenously. Since the former correlates better with the clinical efficacy of the various corticotropins, adrenal ascorbic acid depletion following subcutaneous injection of the sample is the preferred index of activity.

TABLE 10.5 Biological Activities of Corticotropins from Various Animals[a]

Source	Activity (IU/mg)	
	In vivo	*In vitro*
Porcine	85	150
Bovine	140	140
Ovine	106	136
Human	133	131

[a] *Data from Li and Oelofson (1967).*

All of the naturally occurring corticotropins show similar adrenal-stimulating activity, both *in vivo* (ascorbic acid depletion or corticoid production) and *in vitro* (corticoid production) assays (Table 10.5).

Early reports suggested that ACTH isolated from human pituitaries possessed distinctly lower corticotropic activity (~26 IU/mg). However, Li and Oelofsen were able to isolate samples of α_h-ACTH with the activities shown in Table 10.5.*

D. STRUCTURE–ACTIVITY RELATIONSHIPS IN THE CORTICOTROPIN SERIES

Even before the isolation of pure α-ACTH, it was discovered that limited digestion of a corticotropin concentrate by pepsin did not diminish its biological activity. Brink *et al.* (1952) showed that such digests could be processed to yield preparations of high activity (reported to be 200–300 IU/mg) which could be distinguished from native, oxycellulose-purified ACTH when distributed in butanol–aqueous trichloroacetic acid systems. Bell *et al.* (1956) showed that pepsin digestion resulted in removal of eleven amino acids at the C-terminal end of the molecule; after defining the complete amino acid sequence of α_p-ACTH, Shepherd *et al.* (1956) concluded, on the basis of the lability of the Pro–Asp bond (24–25) to acid hydrolysis, that full corticotropin activity probably required no more than the peptide sequence corresponding to the first 24 amino acids from the N-terminus of porcine ACTH.

* C.H. Li (1959) suggested that the principal active corticotropin isolated from a particular animal species be designated α_x-corticotropin (x representing the species). Thus, α_p is porcine corticotropin, α_h is human corticotropin, etc. Other ACTH-active peptides derived from the same source are labeled β_x-, γ_x- . . . ω_x-corticotropin. A peptide with the amino acid sequence corresponding to part of a naturally occurring corticotropin is to be designated by a superscript indicating the sequence referred to. Thus, α_p^{1-27}-ACTH would represent a heptacosapeptide with an amino acid sequence identical with that of the first 27 amino acids (from the amino terminal end) of the principal porcine corticotropin.

This hypothesis was quickly verified. In 1956, Boissonas *et al.* reported that α^{1-20}-ACTH had some (2–3 IU/mg) corticotropic activity *in vitro*. Later, however, α^{1-19}-ACTH was synthesized in two laboratories; both reported activities of 20–30 IU/mg *in vitro* as well as *in vivo*. Finally, the tridecapeptide amide ($\alpha_{NH_2}{}^{1-23}$-ACTH) was found to have essentially full adrenocorticotropic activity (103 IU/mg) when assayed in rats using both ascorbic acid depletion and plasma corticosterone elevation as indices of ACTH action.

Table 10.6 summarizes available data relating to the biological activities of synthetic peptides with amino acid sequences resembling those in the N-terminal part of the ACTH molecule. The shortest peptide with significant corticotropic activity *in vivo* seems to be that corresponding to the N-terminal heptadecapeptide of ACTH (α^{1-17}-ACTH) or its amide, although Steelman and Guillemin (1959) once reported that α-MSH itself (*N*-acetyl α^{1-13}-ACTH) possessed low, but detectable, activity, and Hoffmann and Yajima (1962) found some activity in the α^{1-16}-ACTH amide. *In vivo,* the octa- and nonadecapeptide amides (α^{1-18}-ACTH amide and α^{1-19}-ACTH amide) are fully as active in the adrenal ascorbic acid test as native corticotropin. The nonadecapeptide free acid appears to be distinctly less active than its amide; it is possible that only part of the difference in activities of the eicosapeptide and its amide, originally attributed by Hofmann to the presence of inactive diastereomers in the former, may, in fact, be real. *In vitro,* full activity (equivalent to native ACTH) is reached only with the tricosapeptide.

The capacity to induce a maximum steroidogenic response [compared to

TABLE 10.6 Activities of ACTH Peptides[a]

Peptide	Sequence	Activity (IU/mg) *In vivo*	Activity (IU/mg) *In vitro*	Activity IU/μmole
α_s-ACTH	Ser-Tyr- · · · -Phe(OH)	106 (70–160)	136 (90–200)	480–620
$^{1-16}$-ACTH	Ser-Tyr- · · · -Lys(OH)	0.1	0.1	—
$^{1-17}$-ACTH	Ser-Tyr- · · · -Arg(OH)	5.4 (3.7–7.9)	5.2 (3.3–8.2)	10
$^{1-17}$-ACTH(NH_2)	Ser-Tyr- · · · -Arg(NH_2)	33 (26–42)	42 (30–59)	70–90
$^{1-18}$-ACTH(NH_2)	Ser-Tyr- · · · -Arg-Arg(NH_2)	133 (95–186)	33 (24–46)	75–300
$^{1-19}$-ACTH	Ser-Tyr- · · · -Arg-Pro(OH)	47 (29–77)	35 (23–55)	80–110
$^{1-19}$-ACTH(NH_2)	Ser-Tyr- · · · -Arg-Pro(NH_2)	147 (115–188)	52 (23–55)	120–340
$^{1-20}$-ACTH(NH_2)	Ser-Tyr- · · · -Pro-Val(NH_2)	111, 83	—	235
$^{1-23}$-ACTH(NH_2)	Ser-Tyr- · · · -Val-Tyr(NH_2)	103	91	260–290
$^{1-24}$-ACTH	Ser-Tyr- · · · -Tyr-Pro(OH)	106	110	320
$^{1-26}$-ACTH	Ser-Tyr- · · · -Asp-Gly(OH)	130 (80–210)	93 (70–125)	290–400

[a] *Boissonnas et al. (1956); Hofmann et al. (1961, 1962); Hofmann and Yajima (1962); Li and Oelofson (1967); Schwyzer and Kappeler (1963).*

porcine ACTH (p-ACTH)] in suspensions of adrenal cells is retained by α^{1-10}-ACTH, α^{4-10}-ACTH, and α^{5-24}-ACTH, although very high concentrations are required (Schwyzer *et al.*, 1971; Seelig and Sayers, 1973). In contrast, the response to α^{5-10}- or even α^{5-24}-ACTH is much more modest, while α^{11-24}-ACTH is not only completely inactive but possesses, in fact, the ability to inhibit p-ACTH-induced corticosterone synthesis when present in excess (Seelig *et al.*, 1971). These data suggest that the heptapeptide sequence:

Met-Glu-His-Phe-Arg-Trp-Gly (α^{4-10}-ACTH)

is required for activation of a (still hypothetical) cell receptor for ACTH, while the longer sequence (α^{11-24}) is capable of binding to the receptor without, however, being able to activate it.

One of the significant differences between the shorter peptides and native corticotropins revolves about their subcutaneous:intravenous potency ratios. As noted above, for native corticotropin this ratio is about 3.0. The shorter peptides, including the eicosapeptide and the tricosapeptide, exhibit ratios of 0.3, i.e., unlike native ACTH they are more effective when given intravenously.

Inasmuch as corticotropins isolated from pituitaries of various animals all display about the same biological activity, it seems clear that significant structural differences in the amino acids following Pro^{24} can occur without significant change in biological activity. On the other hand, relatively simple modifications within the sequence at the amino terminal end of the molecule have profound effects upon ACTH activity. A free amino group at the N-terminus appears to be essential; oxidation of the N-terminal serine with periodate, followed by reduction with borohydride (converting the seryl residue to a glycolyl residue) reduces activity *in vivo* fifty-to a hundredfold; *in vitro,* the reaction product retained about 10% of its original activity (Dixon, 1962; Boright *et al.*, 1962). If the periodate step is followed by a Cu^{2+}-catalyzed transamination with glutamate, which converts the glyoxyl residue to a glycyl residue, essentially full activity of the original molecule is retained. (Synthetic Gly^1-α^{1-23}-ACTH is also as active as α^{1-23}-ACTH.) If the N-terminal seryl residue is replaced by a "nonprotein" amino acid residue (β-alanyl, γ-aminobutyryl, or sarcosyl) the resulting peptide is found to be two to several times more active than the seryl peptide (Fujino *et al.*, 1970a). A characteristic feature of these compounds is prolongation of steroidogenic activity; it seems clear that the resistance of the "unnatural" peptide bond to plasma or tissue proteases is an important factor for the survival of the peptide. This conclusion is buttressed by the observation that Pro^1-α^{1-24}-ACTH and Lys^1-α^{1-24}-ACTH possess only about half the activity of α^{1-24}-ACTH. Finally, α^{2-23}-ACTH amide, from which the N-terminal seryl residue has been omitted completely, is also about half as active as the homologous tricosapeptide.

The amino groups of the lysine residues at 11, 15, 16, and 21 are essential for biological activity, as indicated by the fact that formylation of these groups results in an inactive product. α-b-ACTH, if methylated in acid methanol, loses most of its activity, but activity is restored by hydrolysis in weak alkali ($NaHCO_3$). This fact points to a free —COOH group at Glu^5 as being a prime determinant of corticotropic activity, since none of the other dicarboxylic amino acids (nor the C-terminal phenylalanine) can be needed; also, Gln^5-α^{1-19}-ACTH is only about one-third as active as α^{1-19}-ACTH.

When corticotropin is oxidized with hydrogen peroxide all of the (adrenal-stimulating) activity is lost. Since there is no cysteine in the molecule, the change in biological properties has been attributed to oxidation of the methionine residue (Met^4), first to methionine sulfoxide, which can be reversed by cysteine or thioglycollate, and then, irreversibly, to methionine sulfone. Other oxidizing agents which adversely affect the activity of ACTH are potassium persulfate, performic acid, and *N*-bromsuccinimide; the chemical nature of these reaction products have not been adequately characterized.

An interesting series of α^{1-23}-ACTH amide analogs have been synthesized by Geiger and his associates (1964). Phe^2-α^{1-23}-ACTH amide, in which the ring hydroxyl in residue 2 has been replaced by a hydrogen atom, retains about 65% of the activity of the original tricosapeptide. Ala^3-α^{1-23}-ACTH amide (Ala for Ser) is about half as active. Gln^5-β-3-pyrazolyl-Ala^6-α^{1-20}-ACTH amide has also been prepared synthetically; it turned out to be less active than α^{1-20}-ACTH amide, in both its corticotropic and melanotropic properties, but substantial activity of both kinds was retained.

On the other hand, Glu^5, Phe^9-α^{1-20}-ACTH amide possessed only 2–3% of the activity of the parent eicosapeptide (Hofmann *et al.*, 1970), and *0*-nitrophenylsulfenyl-Trp^9-p-ACTH, while retaining the ability to stimulate corticosterone production by rat adrenal cells, does so only if high (60 × p-ACTH) concentrations are used (Kumar *et al.*, 1972). Apparently, Trp^9 is rather more essential than His^6.

In view of the fact that oxidation of the Met^4 residues completely destroyed ACTH activity, it is interesting that substitution of Met^4 by some nonsulfur-containing amino acids (Leu, Ile) diminished, but did not obliterate corticotropic activity (Fujino *et al.*, 1970b). In hopes of obtaining a compound with corticotropic activity which would be more resistant to both peptidases and oxidizing agents, Boissonas *et al.* (1966) synthesized D-Ser^1, NLe^4-α^{1-25}-ACTH amide. This compound proved to be nearly six times as active as either α^{1-25}-ACTH amide or the native hormone, using the Sayers assay. *In vitro,* the differences were somewhat smaller (two- to threefold). It appears that most of the protection results from the presence of the residue of unnatural configuration, since D-Ser^{1}, Lys^{17,18}-α^{1-18}-ACTH amide and D-Ser^{1}, Orn^{17,18}-α^{1-24}-ACTH were also five to ten times as active as the parent peptides. All of these compounds display a marked prolongation of steroidogenic activity. They are also effective at very low dosage.

Some inactive corticotropin derivatives have been found to significantly enhance the activity of small amounts of native ACTH when tested on the steroidogenic function of adrenal or adrenal tumor slices *in vitro* (Cohen and Frieden, 1961, 1963). These products include persulfate-, performate-, and *N*-bromsuccinimide-oxidized ACTH. Sulfated or formylated ACTH were ineffective. It is probable that the potentiation was the result of competition by the inactive derivatives for enzymes which are responsible for inactivation of the native hormone.

III. The Glycoprotein Hormones

The two pituitary gonadotropins [follicle-stimulating hormone (FSH) and luteinizing hormone (LH)], pituitary thyrotropin (thyroid stimulating hormone, TSH), and chorionic gonadotropin (CG) are all glycoproteins containing from 7.5 to 25% carbohydrate in purified preparations. In every instance the link between the carbohydrate portion and the peptide chain is provided by an N-glycosidic linkage through the amide group of an asparagine or the hydroxyl group of a serine residue. Among the sugars frequently represented are fucose, galactosamine, glucosamine, mannose, and sialic acid.

In addition to their carbohydrate content, the glycoprotein hormones display some other unique similarities. Under the proper conditions, each one may be dissociated into two nonidentical peptide subunits; while the subunits are themselves devoid of significant biological activity, they can be recombined, activity being restored in the process. The individual subunits also display some remarkable similarities; one of the subunits isolated from ovine luteinizing hormone (o-LH) is identical with one prepared from either bovine luteinizing hormone (b-LH) or bovine TSH, and the low molecular weight subunit of human luteinizing hormone (h-LH) is identical with one from human FSH (h-FSH) and strikingly similar to one of the subunits of human chorionic gonadotropin (h-CG).

A. Pituitary Gonadotropins

1. *Assay*

Although a variety of methods have been used in the past for the assay of FSH (Gemzell and Roos, 1966), the most useful and reliable methods depend upon the increase in ovarian weight in either rats or mice. Small amounts of LH will synergize with FSH in promoting ovarian growth. Steelman and Pohley introduced the practice of giving a large dose of chorionic gonadotropin along with the sample being tested. This had two effects: (1) it augmented the response to small doses of FSH and (2) it eliminated interference by variable LH contamination.

In the Steelman–Pohley assay (1953), immature (21- and 22-day-old) rats are injected three times a day for 3 days with a mixture of FSH and h-CG. The total dose of h-CG is 20 IU. Seventy-two hours after the first injection, the animals are killed and the ovaries weighed. In untreated animals, or those receiving h-CG alone, the combined ovarian weight is about 30 mg; this increases to 60 mg when 1.0–1.5 IU* of FSH is given, along with h-CG, during the 3-day period. The log dose–response curve is linear from 0.5–4 IU.

Brown (1955) has described a similar procedure with immature mice, using 40 IU of h-CG as an augmentor. While a direct comparison of the two assays has not been made, data supplied by Schmidt–Elmendorf *et al.* (1962) suggested that the mouse assay is 2–10 times as sensitive as the rat assay.

For the determination of FSH in small quantities of blood and urine, a still more sensitive procedure is required. Midgley (1967) has described a radioimmunoassay for FSH using rabbit anti-h-FSH antiserum and ^{131}I-labeled h-FSH. Contaminating anti-LH antibody was removed by adsorption with h-CG. The "double-antibody" method was employed to precipitate the antigen–antibody complex. When applied to pituitary extracts and postmenopausal urine, the Midgley procedure correlated extremely well with bioassays of the same preparations using the Steelman–Pohley method.

Using h-FSH of high specific activity (12,000 IU/mg) as both antigen and standard, Wide *et al.* (1973) reported that they were able to detect concentrations of less than 10 ng/ml FSH in serum and urine by radioimmunoassay. Since they used only 0.10 ml serum, their method was sensitive to 0.1–1.0 ng of FSH. Cunningham and Hebert (1973) used polystyrene tubes to adsorb anti-FSH antibody, and reported binding of radioiodinated FSH which was inhibited by the simultaneous addition of 0.3–30 ng of unlabeled FSH.

For many years, LH assays generally followed a procedure originally described by Greep *et al.* in 1941. This assay depends upon the fact that LH will stimulate testosterone production by the testis; the androgen, in turn, acts upon the accessory sex tissues—in particular, the prostate—causing

* The proposed (1968) International Unit of FSH is defined in terms of the second International Reference Preparation, prepared from human menopausal urine (IRP-HMG). This material contains 8 IU of both FSH and LH per milligram. In comparison, NIH-FSH-S1 contains 26 IU/mg, (by the ovarian augmentation method) and NIH-LH-S1 contains 1500 IU/mg (by the ovarian ascorbic acid depletion assay).

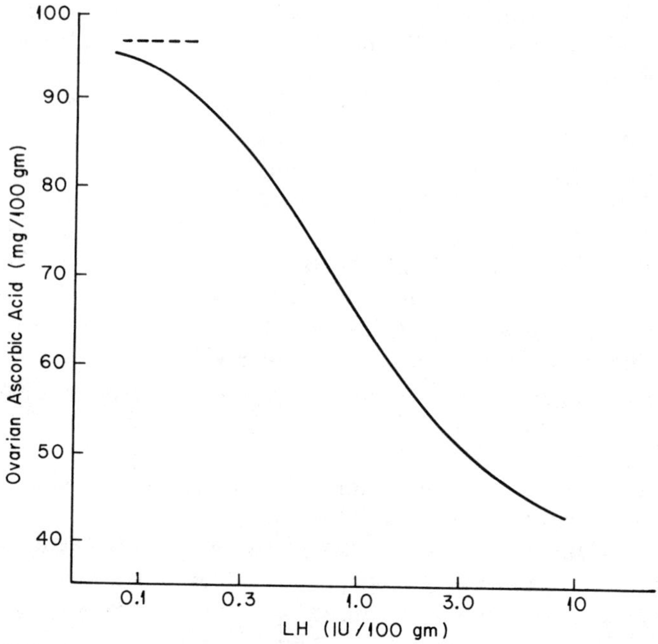

Fig. 10.7 *Ovarian ascorbic acid depletion assay for LH. Data of Parlow (1961).*

hypertrophy. In rats hypophysectomized at 21 days of age and used 2 weeks later, the weight of the ventral prostate increases from 7–8 mg to 25–30 mg following injections of LH over a 4-day period. The sensitivity of the assay is such that the amount of highly purified (homogeneous by many criteria) LH that is effective is from 0.5 to 5 μg.*

Like the rat adrenal, the rat ovary is rich in ascorbic acid; the luteinized ovary of the pseudopregnant rat contains about 1 mg ascorbic acid/gm of tissue. Parlow (1961) discovered that an early action of LH is to diminish the ascorbic acid content of the ovary. Within 4 hours, under the stimulus of an adequate amount of LH, the ascorbic acid content drops to 40% of its initial value.

In the ovarian ascorbic acid depletion (OAAD) test, as originally described by Parlow, immature female rats are brought into pseudopregnancy by the injection, first of a large dose of pregnant mare serum gonadotropin, followed by 25 IU of h-CG. About 7 (5–9) days after h-CG injection, the right ovary is removed and LH is administered intravenously. After 1 hour the left ovary is removed and its ascorbic acid content compared with that of the

* The International Unit of LH has also been defined in terms of the second IRP standard, which likewise contains 8 IU of LH/mg. NIH-LH-S1 is nearly 200 times (1500 IU/mg) as active in the ascorbic acid depletion test.

right ovary. The decrease in ascorbic acid content is roughly linear with the logarithm of the amount of LH over the range 0.15–3.7 IU (Fig. 10.7). Although the OAAD test is quite specific for LH, it is relatively useless for assays of LH in urine extracts because of their toxicity.

LH will also exhaust the ovary of its supply of cholesterol. Bell, Mukerji, and Loraine (1964) found that this phenomenon required far smaller quantities of LH than did a significant decrease of ascorbic acid. In animals made pseudopregnant by a combination of pregnant mare serum gonadotropin (PMS) and h-CG (see above) and injected with LH on the eleventh day of pseudopregnancy, approximately 0.5×10^{-9} mg $(0.2–0.7 \times 10^{-6}$ IU) of LH will reduce the cholesterol content of the heavily luteinized ovary from 1900 μg/100 mg to 1000 μg/100 mg within 5 hours. Cholesterol depletion is therefore at least a million times more sensitive as an indication of LH activity than is the OAAD or ventral prostate tests.

Despite its remarkable sensitivity, the cholesterol depletion assay has not found widespread use. This is due mostly to the biphasic nature of the response; while very small quantities of LH decrease ovarian cholesterol, larger quantities augment it, and still larger quantities diminish it again (Skosey and Goldstein, 1966). The complete dose–response curve for LH, therefore, shows two inflections, which makes its application subject to considerable uncertainty.

Since the ventral prostate weight assay represents a chronic physiological response to LH, while the ascorbic acid depletion assay measures an acute biochemical reaction, it is not surprising to find the relative activities of LH preparations from different sources differing according to the assay procedure used. Thus, NIH-LH-S1 (from sheep pituitary glands) has 50 times the LH activity of the second International Reference Preparation (IRP) when assayed by the ventral prostate method, but nearly 600 times the activity of the second IRP when both are assayed by the ovarian ascorbic acid depletion assay. Parlow (1968) has compared the relative potencies, using the two assays, of LH's from seven different sources; a fiftyfold difference in relative activity was encountered when comparing the LH activities of h-CG and o-LH by the two assays. It is significant that the circulatory half-life times for these two preparations were very different, being approximately 15 minutes for o-LH and nearly 5 hours for h-CG.

An assay for "total gonadotropic activity" that is particularly suitable for clinical studies, depends upon the synergistic effects of mixtures of LH and FSH upon the uterus of immature mice (Brown and Billewicz, 1962). A mixture of FSH and LH, similar to that found in human urine, affords greater stimulation of uterine growth than either does alone. With mixtures of NIH-FSH-S1 (about 25 IU/mg) and NIH-LH-S1 (about 50 IU/mg by ventral prostate assay) maximum uterine weight is achieved with a mixture consisting of 20% LH and 80% FSH. Under the conditions used by Brown and Billewicz

(22-day-old mice, 5 subcutaneous injections over a period of 3 days) maximal increase in uterine weight (approximately five- to sixfold increase over controls) was obtained with a total dose of 70–140 μg of mixed gonadotropins. This corresponds to 1.4–2.8 IU FSH and 0.7–1.4 IU LH.

Ovarian hyperemia, occurring within a few hours after sample administration, and detected by gross examination of the ovaries, has also been used as an index of gonadotropic activity, principally LH. Ellis (1961) has described a variation of this test which measures the accumulation of radioactivity in the ovaries 15 minutes after injection of radioiodinated serum albumin (and 2 hours after the hormone preparation was given). The method is sensitive to 0.5–2 μg NIH-LH-S1. However, large amounts of FSH interfere, and the method has not enjoyed wide use.

Radioimmunoassays for LH have been developed by Midgley (1966), by Odell *et al.* (1967a), and by Sand and Torjesen (1973) among others. All three assays take advantage of the fact that antisera to purified h-CG preparations will cross-react with pituitary LH. Both ^{131}I-labeled h-CG and ^{131}I-pituitary h-LH have been used as the radioactive substrate. For separation of bound from unbound hormone either the double-antibody precipitation or adsorption by dextran-coated charcoal are methods of choice. Radioimmunoassays for LH generally give parallel log dose–response curves for LH preparations of widely different specific activities, and good agreement has been reported between determinations of LH content by the ovarian ascorbic acid depletion method and by radioimmunoassay, but antibody-bound radioactive LH can be displaced by either TSH, FSH, or both.

Radioimmunoassays for LH are sensitive to 0.2–6.4 ng (0.3–9 mU) of human pituitary LH.

Reichert, Leidenberger, and Trowbridge (1973) have described a radiobioassay for LH which depends upon the ability of the particulate fraction of a rat testis homogenate to bind LH. The homogenate is first incubated with a nonradioactive LH solution, then with radioiodinated h-LH. The mixture is then centrifuged and the radioactivity of the supernatant solution determined. As the concentration of nonradioactive LH is increased, binding of iodinated LH diminishes, and more of it is found in the supernate. A linear relationship has been found between the log of the LH concentration and the unadsorbed radioactivity when the concentration of LH lies between 3 and 20 ng. Again, good correlation between the radioligand assay and various biological properties of LH preparations has been demonstrated.

Human chorionic gonadotropin closely resembles, in its biological properties, human pituitary LH. Its ready availability, compared to gonadotropin of pituitary origin, and its significance for the onset and progress of pregnancy, have encouraged the development of many procedures for its detection and quantitative estimation. Amphibians (frogs, toads) as well as mammals (cats, mice, and rabbits) have been used as assay animals. The earliest procedure, that of Aschheim and Zondek (1927), was based upon the development of ovarian hypermia in immature rats; this is rapid (4 hours) and sensitive, but being a quantal assay it is more suitable for clinical studies than for following the steps in a purification procedure. Human chorionic gonadotropin also causes an increase in ovarian weight in rats, but relatively large quantities are required. It will also stimulate the expulsion of sperm in frogs and toads; at one time this was a widely used procedure for pregnancy diagnosis. It is relatively insensitive, however, and the sensitivity varies with the season.

Methods based upon the secondary effects of h-CG are also numerous. These depend upon the fact that h-CG will induce the ovaries to secrete estrogen and the testes to secrete androgen. The hormone may then be detected by its effect upon other tissues of the reproductive tract. Thus, Delfs (1941) showed that the immature rat would respond to h-CG by an increase in uterine weight. The weight increase was linear with the dose over the range 0.25–1.0 IU of h-CG.*

Like LH, h-CG may be assayed by the increase in seminal vesicle or ventral prostate weights in male rats and by the ovarian ascorbic acid depletion test in females. In 21-day-old males, injections of 8–10 IU of h-CG, over a 3-day period, will more than double the prostatic weight. The response is linear between 2 and 5 IU (Loraine and Gaddum, 1950).

Chorionic gonadotropin was one of the first hormones to which immunoassay techniques were applied and is the only one for which agglutination (including hemagglutination) and complement fixation reactions have been used extensively. Both methods are sensitive to 0.5–5 IU of h-CG.

Techniques for the radioimmunoassay of h-CG differ little in principle from any of the similar assays which have been described for other protein hormones. Antiserum to h-CG is developed in rabbits; the quality of h-CG used as antigen has varied from 1,000 to 16,000 IU/mg with little apparent effect (Wilde *et al.*, 1967). Some improvement in specificity may be realized by adsorbing the antiserum with an extract of urine from hypophysectomized nonpregnant subjects. To separate antigen–antibody complexes from unbound antigen, both precipitation with anti-rabbit globulin serum and starch gel electrophoresis have been used; in addition, Thomas and Ferin (1968) have reported that satisfactory separation of the complex from unbound h-CG can be accomplished by adding dioxane to a concentration of 66%.

The sensitivity of the radioimmunoassay has been reported to be such that as little as 7×10^{-4} IU may be detected. On the assumption that "pure"

* An International Unit of h-CG was originally (1939) defined as the biological equivalent of 0.10 mg of a standard preparation. A more highly purified material serves as the current (second) International Standard; One IU is equal to 0.0013 mg of this preparation.

h-CG possesses an activity of approximately 20,000 IU/mg, this identity corresponds to 0.035 ng of protein. Other authors give 2 ng as the upper limit.

2. *Chemical Nature*

a. *Follicle-Stimulating Hormone.* Although pituitaries of several kinds of animals have been used for the preparation of FSH, most of the published work deals with the properties of ovine, equine, or human pituitary FSH. Ovine FSH preparations that appeared to be homogeneous by electrophoresis, immunoelectrophoresis, or ultracentrifugation have been produced in several laboratories (Roos and Gemzell, 1964; Papkoff *et al.*, 1967; Cahill *et al.*, 1968; Cahill and Hart, 1969; Sherwood *et al.*, 1970). Purified ovine FSH has an activity of 1300–5000 IU/mg (50–200 × NIH-FSH-S1) by the Steelman–Pohley augmentation assay. Equine FSH that showed only a single component upon disc electrophoresis and was also apparently homogeneous by sedimentation equilibrium (Nuti *et al.*, 1972) contained 1750–3100 IU/mg. Purified human pituitary FSH appears to be distinctly more active than either the ovine or equine hormones; values from 2600–11000 IU/mg have been reported.

Estimates of the molecular weights of FSH from nonhuman sources cluster about 30,000 as determined by sedimentation velocity or sedimentation equilibrium; dissociation into smaller units or pH-dependent aggregation were apparently responsible for earlier estimates which ranged from 16,000 to 39,000. [The monomeric unit of h-FSH was reported by various investigators to range from 31,000 to 48,600 (Ryan *et al.*, 1970; Saxena and Rathnam, 1971; Moffezoli *et al.*, 1972; Reichert and Lawson, 1973).] However, the structure of h-FSH proposed by Shome and Parlow (1974a,b) indicates a peptide molecular weight of 22,360; if the molecule contains 18% carbohydrate the total molecular weight can be reckoned to be 27,270.

As noted above, a unique property of the glycoprotein hormones lies in the fact that they can dissociate into inactive subunits; with FSH, dissociation occurs when the native hormone is exposed to 8 *M* urea at pH 7.5 or to 1 *M* propionic acid (Reichert, 1971; Amir, 1972; Parlow and Shome, 1974). When the dissociating agent is removed, activity is gradually (and incompletely) restored during prolonged incubation at 37°–40°.

The carbohydrate content of FSH preparations has been reported to be 14–25%, depending upon the species. Papkoff and Ekblad (1970) found that ovine FSH contained 13–14% carbohydrate, most of it associated with the smaller subunit. Equine FSH contains 25% carbohydrate (Nuti *et al.*, 1972), while human FSH was found to contain 18% (Papkoff, 1972). Hexose, hexosamine, fucose, and sialic acid were all present.

Recently, amino acid sequences for the two subunits of h-FSH have been proposed by Shome and Parlow (1974a,b). The structure of h-FSH-α is iden-

```
                                          10                                                        20
H2N(Asx-Ser)-Cys-Glu-Leu-Thr-Asn-Ile-Thr-Ile-Ala-Ile-Glu-Lys-Glu-Glu-Cys-Arg-Phe-Cys- Ile -Ser - Ile - Asn-
                              |                                                                         |
                             CHO                                                                       CHO

                          30                                 40
-Thr-Thr (Thr, Asx, Trp)-Glu-Thr-Cys-Ala-Gly -Tyr-Cys-Tyr-Thr-Arg-Asp-Leu-Val -Tyr-Lys-Asp-Pro-

                   50                           60
-Ala -Lys-Pro-Arg - Ile -Gln -Lys-Thr-Cys-Thr-Phe-Lys-Glu -Leu-Val -Tyr-Glu -Thr-Val -Arg-Val -Pro-

        70                                         80                                            90
-Gly -Cys-Ala -His -His -Ala -Asp-Ser -Leu-Tyr-Thr-Tyr-Pro-Val -Ala -Thr-Gln -Cys-His -Cys-Gly -Lys-

                                     100                                           110
-Cys-Asp-Ser -Asp-Ser -Thr-Asp-Cys-Thr-Val -Arg-Gly -Leu-Gly -Pro-Ser -Tyr-Cys-Ser -Phe-Gly -Glu -

        110
-Met-(Glx, Lys) OH
```

Fig. 10.8 *Amino acid sequence of h-FSH-β. Heterogeneity was observed at both the amino and carboxyl termini. Shome and Parlow (1974b).*

tical with that of h-LH-α (Fig. 10.9); the structure of h-FSH-β is shown in Fig. 10.8. The carbohydrate moieties are attached to asparagine residues 49 and 75 in the α-(smaller) subunit and to asparagine residues 7 and 24 in the β-(larger) subunit. The α-subunit contains 89 amino acid residues, while the β-subunit contains 111–115 residues. The variation in peptide size of the β-subunit is accounted for by heterogeneity at both the NH_2-terminal end (where the sequence Asx-Ser occurs in some molecules) and the COOH-terminal end (with a minor component ending in Glx and Lys). Recombination experiments have shown that it is the β-subunit of FSH which is hormone-specific; that is, α-subunits of other glycoprotein hormones can be recombined with FSH-β to give products with FSH activity. In radioimmunoassay systems developed for intact h-FSH, h-FSH-α is only weakly interactive, while h-FSH-β is strongly interactive. On the other hand, h-FSH-β shows only slight reactivity to anti-h-FSH-α antibody.

One of the characteristic features of FSH is its relatively high cysteine content (14 half cystines per mole). It is surprising, therefore, to find that neither mercaptoethanol nor cysteine inactivates FSH. It has been reported, however, that h-FSH is inactivated when it is alkylated with iodoacetamide. FSH is resistant to the actions of both trypsin and chymotrypsin; since LH is destroyed by these enzymes, a preparation relatively free of LH can be prepared by digestion of pituitary extracts with pancreatin. h-FSH is inactivated by both pronase and bacterial neuraminidase, as well as by ptyalin.

The picture which thus emerges suggests that the FSH molecule elaborated by the human pituitary is a rather asymmetric (f/f_0 = 1.49) but compact molecule composed of two noncovalently bonded subunits of approximately equal size. It has been suggested that the carbohydrate portion forms a protective envelope over the peptide chains, a conclusion suggested by the resistance of the native, fully sialylated molecule to various proteolytic enzymes.

Compared to FSH isolated directly from human pituitaries, human menopausal gonadotropin, which is also of pituitary origin (but isolated from urine) has distinctly lower biological activity (approximately 25–50 × NIH-FSH-S1) (Roos and Gemzell, 1965; Donini *et al.*, 1968). The purified product, characterized electrophoretically and in the ultracentrifuge, sedimented more slowly than did pituitary FSH ($s_{20,w}$ = 1.9 vs 2.9 S). Nonetheless, its behavior on DEAE-cellulose and on gel filtration was indistinguishable from that of pituitary FSH. Donini's preparation had a very high carbohydrate content (28.6%) and was especially high in sialic acid (8.6%). It seems likely that this material represents pituitary FSH which has been modified chemically during its passage through the body.

b. *Luteinizing Hormone (LH).* Purified LH has been isolated from bovine, equine, ovine, porcine, and human pituitaries. Purified animal LH is 2–6 times as active as the NIH standard preparation, assaying 3000–9000 IU/mg. Purified human LH, like human FSH, seems to be intrinsically more active than that from other kinds of pituitaries; its reported activity ranges up to 15,000 IU/mg (Peckham and Parlow, 1969).

Recent estimates of the molecular weights of LH, employing sedimentation, osmotic pressure, or exclusion chromatography techniques range from 26,000 to 30,000 (Amir, 1972), the lower figure being the molecular weight of h-LH. Although some early estimates of the carbohydrate content of ovine LH were as high as 36%, more recent data incline to a more modest 15–20% (Amir, 1972). Closset *et al.* (1972) reported that their h-LH preparation contained 16.0% carbohydrate, including relatively large amounts of galactose, glucosamine, mannose, and sialic acid and smaller quantities of fucose, glucose, and galactosamine (Table 10.7). These data are consistent with the fact that the amino acid content of h-LH accounts for approximately 86% of the total weight of the molecule (assumed molecular weight = 26,000). Courte *et al.* (1972) reported approximately the same amount of carbohy-

TABLE 10.7 Carbohydrate Content of Human Luteinizing Hormone (h-LH)

Constituent	Residues/mole[a]
Fucose	1.4
Galactose	3.3
Galactosamine	1.1
Glucose	1.0
Glucosamine	7.4
Mannose	7.3
Sialic acid	2.4

[a] *Based on a molecular weight of 26,000.*

drate (13.6%) in b-LH; interestingly, they found no sialic acid. Ovine LH also contains only traces of sialic acid and its biological activity is unaffected by neuraminidase. In contrast, purified h-LH retains only 12–16% of its original activity when treated with neuraminidase.

In 1967, Papkoff and Samy discovered that when ovine LH was subjected to countercurrent distribution in a mixture of aqueous ammonium sulfate, dichloroacetic acid, ethanol, and *n*-propanol it separated into two subunits of approximately the same size, but with different amino acid compositions. Subsequently, other kinds of LH, including those from rats, cattle, pigs, and humans have been shown to undergo a similar dissociation, which can also be accomplished by exposure to high concentrations of urea or guanidine hydrochloride, or to low pH. It has been established that all of these hormones consist of two noncovalently linked glycopeptides. By convention, the subunit of ovine LH with a low partition coefficient in the Papkoff–Samy system is referred to as LH-α, while that with the high partition coefficient is LH-β. This convention has been extended to LH subunits from other species as well. Neither subunit possesses significant LH activity, but the native active hormone is slowly reconstituted when neutral concentrated solutions of the two protomers are incubated (Papkoff and Samy, 1967; De La Llosa and Jutisz, 1969).

The isolation of LH protomers greatly simplified the task of obtaining detailed information concerning the structure of LH. To date, the complete amino acid sequences of both subunits of bovine, ovine, porcine, and human LHs have been established (Figs. 10.9 and 10.10). Bovine and ovine LH-α's are N-acylated 96-amino acid peptides, identical in sequence with oligosaccharides attached (by *N*-glycosidic linkage) to Asn residues 56 and 82. Porcine LH-α is shorter by 6 amino acid residues at the amino terminal end; in addition, 4 "conservative" amino acid replacements are found in the rest of the chain. Human LH-α is also shorter (by 7 amino acids) at the amino terminal end, compared to bovine or ovine LH-α; in addition, 22 amino acid replacements and one inversion (Cys^{88}-Ser^{89} in ovine, Ser^{81}-Cys^{82} in human) are evident when the two peptides are compared.

As shown in Fig. 10.10, bovine and ovine LH also share identical β-subunits, each with 119 amino acid residues (Maghuin–Register and Hennen, 1972). Porcine LH-β contains one more amino acid, while h-LH-β is only 115 amino acids long. Fifteen amino acid replacements (and one additional amino acid) distinguish p-LH-β from o-LH-β; there are 37 replacements in h-LH-β, in addition to two deletions and a dipeptide missing from the COOH terminus. The carbohydrate in all four LH-β's is linked to Asn^{13}; in h-LH-β, Asn^{30} also is part of a glycopeptide.

Ward *et al.* (1973) have established the position of the disulfide links in o-LH-β, as follows: Cys^{9}-Cys^{88}; Cys^{23}-Cys^{73}; Cys^{26}-Cys^{110}; Cys^{34}-Cys^{93}; Cys^{38}-Cys^{100}; Cys^{57}-Cys^{90}.

	10
Human	H_2N-Val-Gln-Asp-Cys-Pro-Glu-Cys-Thr-Leu-Gln-Glu-Asn-Pro-Phe-
Bovine, ovine	H_2N-Phe-Pro-Asp-Gly-Glu-Phe-Thr-Met- -Gly- -Lys- -Lys- -Lys-Tyr-
Porcine	H_2N-Thr-Met- -Gly- -Lys -Lys- -Lys-Tyr-

	20 30
Human	-Phe-Ser-Gln-Pro-Gly-Ala-Pro-Ile-Leu-Gln-Cys-Met-Gly-Cys-Cys-Phe-Ser-Arg-Ala-Tyr-Pro-
Bovine, ovine	-Lys- -Asp- -Tyr-
Porcine	-Lys-Leu- -Tyr-

	40 CHO 50
Human	-Thr-Pro-Leu-Arg-Ser-Lys-Lye-Thr-Met-Leu-Val-Gln-Lys-Asn-Val-Thr-Ser-Glu-Ser-Thr-Cys-
Bovine, ovine	-Ala- -Pro- -Ile- -Ala-
Porcine	-Ala- -Pro- -Ile- -Ala-

	60 70 CHO
Human	-Cys-Val-Ala-Lys-Ser-Tyr-Asn-Arg-Val-Thr-Val-Met-Gly-Gly-Phe-Lys-Val-Glu-Asn-His-Thr-
Bovine, ovine	-Ala-Phe-Thr-Lys-Ala- -Asn-Val-Arg-
Porcine	-Ala-Phe-Thr-Lys-Ala- -Asx-Ala-Arg- -Ser-

	80
Human	-Ala-Cys-His-Ser-Cys-Thr-Cys-Tyr-Tyr-His-Lys-SerOH
Bovine, ovine	-Glu- -OH
Porcine	-Glu- -Cys-His- -OH

Fig. 10.9 *Amino acid sequences of human, bovine, ovine, and porcine LH-α. The sequence of the bovine subunit was established by homology with b-TSH-α. Source: h-LH-α, Sairam et al. (1972); b-, o-LH-α, Dayhoff (1972, pp. D-198 and D-199); p-LH-α, Maghuin-Register et al. (1972).*

Leidenberger and Reichert (1973) found that vertebrate LH's could be segregated into four groups depending upon their abilities to displace h-LH from its combination with rat testicular homogenate (see Section III, A, 1). Monkey and human pituitary LH were comparable in effectiveness, followed, in order, by: (a) bovine, equine, ovine, and rat LH; (b) chicken and rabbit LH; and (c) canine and porcine LH. Human chorionic gonadotropin was nearly as effective as human LH in this comparison.

Donini *et al.* (1968) have described the isolation of an electrophoretically homogeneous LH from human menopausal urine (HMG; pergonal). The final product contained about 800 IU/mg (about half the activity of NIH-LH-S1). It was also a glycoprotein. It contained slightly more hexose than hexoseamine and a smaller amount of sialic acid (1.5%) than human pituitary LH. Estimates of the molecular weight (by gel filtration) gave a figure of 50,000 daltons.

B. CHORIONIC GONADOTROPIN

Early attempts to isolate h-CG from human pregnancy urine were made by Gurin *et al.* (1939, 1940), by Claesson *et al.* (1948), and by Zilliacus and

```
                                                  10                     CHO                                 20
                                                                          |
Human    H2N-Ser-Arg-Glu-Pro-Leu-Arg-Pro-Trp-Cys-His-Pro-Ile-Asn-Ala-Ile-Leu-( )-Ala-Val-Glu-Lys-Glx-Gly-Cys-
Ovine               -Gly-                -Leu-   -Gln-               -Thr-   ( )  -Ala-         -Glu-Ala-
Porcine             -Gly-                -Leu-   -Glx-               -Thr-  -Arg- -Ala-Glx-Asx   Ala-

                              CHO
                               |                                     40
Human    Pro-Val-Cys-Ile-Thr-Val-Asn-Thr-Thr-Ile-Cys-Ala-Gly-Tyr-Cys-Pro-Thr-Met-Arg-( )-Val-Leu-Gln-Ala-
Ovine                       -Phe-Thr-   -Ser-                       -Ser-  -Lys-Arg-   -Pro-Val-Ile-
Porcine                     -Phe-Thr-   -Ser-                       -Ser-      -Arg-   -Pro-Ala-Ala-

                 50                                  60
Human    Val-Leu-Pro-Pro-Leu-Pro-Gln-( )-Val-Cys-Thr-Tyr-Arg-Asp-Val-Arg-Phe-Glu-Ser-Ile-Arg-Leu-Pro-Gly-
Ovine               -Met-      -Arg-             -His-Glu-Leu-        -Ala-   -Val-
Porcine             -Val-   -Glx-Pro-            -Arg-Glu-Leu-Ile-    -Ala-   -Ser-

         70                                 80                                       90
Human    Cys-Pro-Arg-Gly-Val-Asp-Pro-Val-Val-Ser-Phe-Pro-Val-Ala-Leu-Ser-Cys-Arg-Cys-Gly-Pro-Cys-Arg-Arg-
Ovine       -Pro-           -Met-                                  -His-                      -Leu-
Porcine     -Pro-      -Asx-   -Thr-                               -His-                      -Leu-

                              100                                 110
Human    Ser-Thr-Ser-Asp-Cys-Gly-Gly-Pro-Lys-Asx-His-Pro-Leu-Thr-Cys-Asx-Glx-Pro-His (Ser, Lys, Gly)OH
Ovine       -Ser-Thr-           -Pro-Gly-Arg-Thr-Glx-   -Ala-       -His-  -Pro-Leu-Pro-Asp-Ile-LeuOH
Porcine     -Ser-Ser-           -Pro-Gly-Arg-Ala-Glx-   -Ala-       -Arg-  -Pro-Leu-Pro-Gly-Leu-LeuOH
```

Fig. 10.10 *Amino acid sequences of human, ovine, and porcine LH-β. Deletions are indicated by ( ). The amino terminal ends of o-LH-β and p-LH-β are acylated. Bovine LH-β is identical with o-LH-β except for residue 42 (Arg instead of Lys; Maghuin-Register and Dockier, 1971). Source: human, Shome and Parlow (1973); ovine, Ward et al. (1973); porcine, Maghuin-Register and Hennen (1972).*

Roos (1951). These early preparations contained 6000 to 8000 IU/mg; at least one of them was reported to be a crystalline material which was homogeneous upon extended Tiselius electrophoresis. More recently, however, preparations with activities of 12,000–20,000 IU/mg have been described (Got and Bourrillon, 1960; Van Hell *et al.*, 1966; Bell *et al.*, 1969; Bahl, 1969; Ashitaka *et al.*, 1970). Highly purified gonadotropins have also been isolated from the urine, plasma, and chorionic tissue of women with trophoblastic tumors (choriocarcinoma, hydatidiform mole, etc., Reisfield and Hertz, 1960; Wilde and Bagshawe, 1965; Pala *et al.*, 1973). Purified material obtained from molar tissue was less active (6500 IU/mg) than similar products from urine or plasma (20,000 IU/mg).

Although the biological activities reported for electrophoretically or immunoelectrophoretically homogeneous preparations show rather wide variations (8000–20,000 IU/mg), their chemical properties are remarkably similar. The most carefully characterized preparations [those of Got and Bourrillon (1960) and those of Bahl (1969)] were homogeneous by electrophoretic criteria, even though the biological activity appeared to be rather low. Graesslin *et al.* (1972) separated CM-Sephadex-purified h-CG into five components by isoelectric focusing. Their isoelectric points varied from 3.8 to 9.1 and their biological activities (by ovarian ascorbic acid depletion method) from 4600 to 18,500. Maximal activity coincided with a fraction with p*I* = 4.3; fractions with higher and lower isoelectric points were less active. The principal chemical difference appeared to be in the content of sialic acid, which varied from 2.9% (p*I* = 5.1) to 9.0% (p*I* = 3.8).

Estimates of the molecular weight of h-CG based on its sedimentation behavior range from 27,000 (in 0.1 *N* formic acid or 4 *M* guanidine hydrochloride) to 62,000. From its amino acid composition, the molecular weight of the peptide component may be calculated to be 25,400; since 25% of the molecule is carbohydrate, the weight of the complete molecule is about 34,000 daltons (see also Mori and Hollands, 1971).

Like the pituitary glycoprotein hormones, h-CG is dissociated into subunits by exposure to 8 *M* urea for relatively long periods (60 minutes at 37°; Swaminathan and Bahl, 1970). Separation of the subunits was accomplished by chromatography on DEAE-Sephadex. The two chains contain 92 and 147 amino acid residues, respectively (Fig. 10.11). The sequence of h-CG-α, as deduced by Bellisario *et al.* (1973) duplicates almost exactly that proposed by Sairam *et al.* (1972) for h-LH-α, except for the addition of three amino acids (Ala-Pro-Asx-) at the N-terminus, and the inversion of the Ser-Cys sequence at positions 81 and 82 in h-LH-α (84 and 85 in h-CG-α). h-CG-β and h-LH-β show considerably less homology; 18 amino acid replacements and two deletions appear when h-LH-β is compared with the first 117 residues of h-CG-β; the latter also contains 30 additional amino acids at the COOH terminus.

```
                                          10                                                         20
H2N-Ala-Pro-Asx-Val-Glx-Asx-Cys-Pro-Glx-Cys-Thr-Leu-Glx-Glx-Asx-Pro-Phe-Phe-Ser-Glx-Pro-Gly-Ala-Pro-Ile-Leu-Gln-

       30                                     40                                    50    CHO
                                                                                           |
Cys-Met-Gly-Cys-Cys-Phe-Ser-Arg-Ala-Tyr-Pro-Thr-Pro-Leu-Arg-Ser-Lys-Lys-Thr-Met-Leu-Val-Gln-Lys-Asn-Val-Thr-

                                                                                    CHO
              60                           70                                       |      80
Ser-Glx-Ser-Thr-Cys-Cys-Val-Ala-Lys-Ser-Tyr-Asn-Arg-Val-Thr-Val-Met-Gly-Gly-Phe-Lys-Val-Glx-Asn-His-Thr-Ala-

                      90
Cys-His-Cys-Ser-Thr-Cys-Tyr-Tyr-His-Lys-SerOH
```

(a)

```
                                               CHO
                                        10      |                                              20
H2N-Ser-Lys-Gln-Pro-Leu-Arg-Pro-Arg-Cys-Arg-Pro-Ile-Asn-Ala-Thr-Leu-Ala-Val-Glu-Lys-Glu-Gly-Cys-Pro-Val-Cys-Ile-

        CHO
         |                                   40                                         50
Thr-Val-Asn-Thr-Thr-Ile-Cys-Ala-Gly-Tyr-Cys-Pro-Thr-Met-Thr-Arg-Val-Leu-Gln-Gly-Val-Leu-Pro-Ala-Leu-Pro-Glx-

              60                                70                                              80
Leu-Val-Cys-Asn-Tyr-Arg-Asp-Val-Arg-Phe-Glu-Ser-Ile-Arg-Leu-Pro-Gly-Cys-Pro-Arg-Gly-Val-Asn-Pro-Val-Val-Ser-

                       90                                        100
Tyr-Ala-Val-Ala-Leu, Ser-Cys-Gln-Cys-Ala-Leu-Cys-Arg-(Arg)-Ser-Thr-Thr-Asp-Cys-Gly-Gly-Pro-Lys-Asp-His-Pro-Leu-

                                     CHO                                       CHO        CHO
   110                                |       120                               |    130   |
Thr-Cys-Asp-Asp-Pro-Arg-Phe-Gln-Asp-Ser-Ser-Ser-Lys-Ala-Pro-Pro-Pro-Ser-Leu-Pro-Ser-Pro-Ser-Arg-Leu-Pro-Gly-

              140
Pro-Pro-Asx-Thr-Pro-Ile-Leu-Pro-Gln-Ser-Leu-ProOH
```

(b)

Fig. 10.11 *Aminc acid sequences of* (a) *h-CG-α and* (b) *h-CG-β. Source: h-CG-α, Bellisario et al.* (1973); *h-CG-β, Carlsen et al.* (1973).

TABLE 10.8 Carbohydrate Content of Human Chorionic Gonadotropin (h-CG)[a]

Constituent	Residues/mole
Galactose	9
Mannose	9
Fucose	1
N-Acetylglucosamine	11
N-Acetylgalactosamine	3
Sialic acid	8

[a] *Bahl* (*1969*).

Human chorionic gonadotropin contains considerably more carbohydrate than either h-FSH or h-LH. Bahl's data for h-CG are summarized in Table 10.8. These data are in reasonable agreement with those of Schlumberger (1968); Mori and Hollands (1971) found considerably more galactose, mannose, and *N*-acetylglucosamine.

When h-CG is hydrolyzed by trypsin, a number of glycopeptides, with molecular weights in the range 3200–5100 are produced. Analysis of the carbohydrate units of the glycopeptides, using especially the information provided by the sequential application of specific glycosidases, led Bahl to postulate the presence of two oligosaccharide sequences in h-CG (Fig. 10.12).

There are 7 sites in h-CG where carbohydrate units are attached; two of these are in h-CG-α (Asn^{52}, Asn^{78}); of the other 5, all in h-CG-β, two are asparagines (Asn^{13} and Asn^{30}). The other three are serines 118, 129, and 131. Presumably the carbohydrate sequences are linked through either N-glycosidic or O-glycosidic bonds with amide or hydroxyl groups, respectively. It is not yet known whether the two large oligosaccharide sequences shown in Fig. 10.12 are attached to the same or to different chains. They account for most, but not all of the monosaccharides present, so smaller units must be attached to the other carbohydrate-binding sites.

As indicated in Fig. 10.8, 10.10, 10.11, the usual sequence around a carbohydrate-binding asparagine is -Asn-X-Thr or Asn-X-Ser. These in-

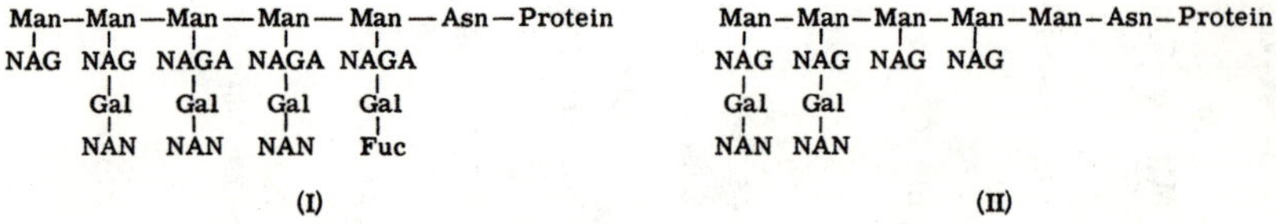

Fig. 10.12 *Proposed carbohydrate sequences in h-CG. Gal = galactose; Man = mannose; Fuc = fucose; NAGA = N-acetylglucosamine; NAG = N-acetylgalactosamine; NAN = N-acetylneuraminic acid.*

variant sequences have been suggested as the recognition sites for attachment of the oligosaccharides to asparagine.

The terminal glycosides of the carbohydrate units of h-CG are sialic acid (*N*-acetylneuraminic acid) residues, since h-CG may be desialyzed (by treatment with neuraminidase) without affecting the number of other sugar residues present. Desialyzed h-CG is essentially inactive *in vivo* (74 IU/mg vs 11,600 IU/mg) according to Mori and Hollands. However, asialo-h-CG retains full immunological activity, as well as being fully active in the radioligand-binding assay (Tsuruhara *et al.* 1972).

Chorionic gonadotropins are also found in the urine of other primates during pregnancy. Immunological comparisons, based upon the ability of antisera to subhuman primate hormones (or their subunits) to inhibit the biological activity of h-CG, indicated that gorilla and chimpanzee gonadotropins were much more similar to h-CG than is monkey gonadotropin (Hodgen *et al.*, 1973). This phylogenetic distinction was also supported by radioimmunoassay data; thus, while gorilla and chimpanzee CG preparations inhibited the combination of labeled h-CG-α or h-CG-β with their respective antibodies, monkey CG did not.

While gonadotropins from mammalian pituitaries are effective in stimulating gonadal (especially testicular) functions in lower vertebrates, the reverse seems not to be the rule. Thus, rat pituitary extracts significantly enhanced testis weight in chicks or turkey poults (values ranged from 60 to 200% over a 4-day period), but rat ovarian weights were not significantly increased when chicken or turkey pituitary extract was given to rats (Herrick *et al.*, 1962). Hartree and Cunningham (1969) were able to separate FSH and LH from acetone-dried chicken pituitaries; these preparations were only weakly active in mammals. In fishes and reptiles only a single gonadotropin with elements of both FSH and LH function seems to be present (Burzawa–Gerard and Fontaine, 1972). Its gonadotropic effects are demonstrable in lower vertebrates (*anolis,* chicks) but not in mammals. Ovine FSH was able to stimulate testicular growth, spermatogenesis, and steroidogenesis in male snakes (Licht, 1972).

C. THYROID-STIMULATING HORMONE

1. *Assay*

Early attempts to measure the concentration of pituitary thyroid stimulating hormone in tissue extracts or body fluids utilized changes in thyroid weight or in the histological development of thyroids of guinea pigs, rats, and chicks. In general methods which depend upon changes in thyroid histology are more sensitive and more reliable than gravimetric methods.

Both methods are at present mostly of archival value, having been replaced almost completely by methods which measure ^{32}P uptake, ^{131}I uptake, or ^{131}I depletion of thyroids of animals receiving the corresponding radioactive substrate.

Borell and Holmgren, in 1949, showed that the thyroids of TSH-treated guinea pigs accumulated ^{32}P more rapidly than did those of untreated animals. Others showed that the same results could be achieved more conveniently and economically using 1- or 2-day-old chicks. In the modification described by Pierce and Nyc (1956), 1-day-old white leghorn cockerels were given a single intracardial injection of TSH. Three hours later, each animal received $Na_2H^{32}PO_4$ subcutaneously and after another 3 hours the animals were killed and the thyroids counted after being cleaned of excess tissue. Seven to ten chicks were used at each dose level. Thyroid radioactivity was linear with the logarithm of the dose over the range 0.3–1.2 mU TSH.* Methods which depend upon ^{32}P uptake by thyroids of rats have also been described, but these offer no particular advantage compared to the chick method. The chick assay is at least ten times as sensitive as the guinea pig method.

Florsheim *et al.* (1957) have described an assay based upon the TSH-induced increase in radiophosphate uptake by beef thyroid slices *in vitro*. ^{32}P incorporation into phospholipid was increased by TSH, but labeling of either acid-soluble or protein-bound phosphorus was not affected. The response was linear with log TSH concentration (3–30 mU/ml) for incubation periods of 3 hours.

Thyroidal iodine uptake has been applied as an index of TSH activity in guinea pigs, rats, mice, chicks, and tadpoles. Again, the chick assay appears to be the most sensitive. Day-old chicks were given three injections of TSH at 24 hour intervals. Fifteen hours after the last injection radioactive iodine (as iodide) was injected; the thyroids were removed and counted 4 hours later. In untreated animals, approximately 10% of the ^{131}I injected appears in the thyroid. With a total dose of 12 mU of TSH, this figure was doubled, and increased to 43% with 60 mU (Postel, 1956).

One of the principal disadvantages of TSH assays based upon iodine uptake is the requirement for repeated injections, which perforce increases the amount of TSH required. Methods based upon the ability of TSH to stimulate discharge of stored ^{131}I are generally more sensitive. Guinea pigs, mice, and chicks have been used. Usually the animals were given thyroxine or a thyroid-supplemented diet to depress endogenous TSH production, and, in some cases, were kept on a low-iodine diet before the assay. Each

* The International Unit of TSH activity is defined as the activity of 13.5 mg of the International Reference TSH standard; the latter is a lactose-adulterated preparation of crude bovine TSH.

animal was given ^{131}I intraperitoneally and 1–3 days were allowed to elapse while the radioiodine level of the thyroid stabilized, and that of the plasma decreased to a low value. TSH was then administered and a short time later either thyroidal ^{131}I or plasma ^{131}I was determined. Either the decrease in thyroidal ^{131}I or the increase in plasma ^{131}I could be used as an index of TSH activity.

Adams and Purves (1955; 1957) used guinea pigs. The index of TSH activity was an increase in plasma ^{131}I 3 hours after intravenous injection of the hormone. The response was linear with the log of the dose from 0.1 to 0.6 mU TSH, plasma radioactivity having increased 50% after the injection of 0.4 mU. A useful feature of this procedure is that some proportionality between the amount of TSH given and the resulting response was retained for quantities of TSH as large as 15 mU, in response to which plasma radioactivity increased 500–600%.

McKenzie (1958) applied the Adams and Purves technique to the mouse and showed that its sensitivity was distinctly improved. Again, the increase in plasma ^{131}I 2 hours after the injection of TSH was linear with the log dose; the useful range was 0.05–0.45 mU. The magnitude of the increase was 100–200%. Both the guinea pig and the mouse assays have been adapted for the detection of the "long-acting thyroid stimulator" in blood.

A number of *in vitro* radiometric assays for TSH have been proposed. Bottari *et al.* (1963) used guinea pig thyroid slices, preincubated with ^{131}I. Sodium iodide was added to block additional accumulation of iodine and the radioactivity of the solution was measured. TSH was then added to the incubation, and after 2 hours the medium was again counted. The increase in radioactivity was proportional to the log dose between 0.1 and 2.0 mU. The method is slow, since overnight incubation with ^{131}I was required. Better results were obtained with goitrous thyroids taken from guinea pigs treated with methylthiouracil. Kirkham (1962) used potassium thiocyanate to stimulate discharge of ^{131}I after prolonged incubation with TSH. Kirkham's method is one of the most sensitive yet described for TSH; its working range is claimed to be from 0.007 to 0.030 mU TSH/ml.

Manley *et al.* (1969) have described an extremely sensitive assay based upon the decrease in the iodide space of guinea pig thyroid slices incubated in solutions of TSH. The thyroids were taken from guinea pigs treated with thiouracil. A dose–response curve with a working range of 0.0005–0.064 mU/ml of incubation medium was displayed. Using this assay, Bourke *et al.* (1969) were able to estimate TSH concentrations in sera of normal rats and obtain a clear difference between the response of these and thyroxin-treated animals.

A rare example of an assay for a mammalian pituitary hormone in a nonmammalian species is that devised by Friesen (1968) employing the carp.

The fish were given radioactive iodide and were allowed to equilibrate for several days. The administration of TSH induced release of thyroidal iodine into the surrounding water.

It has been known for more than 30 years that laboratory animals can develop antibodies to TSH in bovine pituitary extracts. Antibodies prepared against early crude TSH preparations showed extensive cross-reaction with other hormones. Purified TSH preparations from both bovine and human pituitaries became available about 1960; their accessibility led to the development of radioimmunoassays, especially for h-TSH. The subject has been reviewed in detail by Odell *et al.* (1967b). As usual, the assay depends upon the displacement, by unlabeled TSH, of ^{131}I-TSH from its combination with anti-TSH antibody. A plot of the fraction of radioactivity bound against the logarithm of TSH concentration was linear between 1.0 and 20 ng of human TSH and from 0.2 to 10 mU of bovine TSH. Lack of specificity in cross-reactions of h-TSH and anti-b-TSH militates against the use of b-TSH as an antigen for immunoassays of TSH in human plasma. Regression lines obtained (with anti-h-TSH antisera) for plasma of hypothyroid patients have the same slope as lines established for purified h-TSH.

2. *Chemical Properties*

Active thyrotropin preparations have been isolated from the pituitaries of all major classes of vertebrates, including fish (cod, carp, eels, mudfish), amphibians, birds, and a wide assortment of mammals. Although TSH isolated from the pituitaries of teleost fishes (cod, carp, eel) does not stimulate the thyroid glands of mammals, mammalian TSH will stimulate fish (trout, carp) thyroids; it has been reported, however, that trout do not respond to mammalian TSH at temperatures below 20°. TSH prepared from mudfish (*Protopterus annectens)* can be assayed in mice. The pituitaries of some fishes have TSH contents (measured in fish with a mammalian TSH standard) which may be ten- to twentyfold higher than those of mammalian pituitaries.

All of the TSH's which have been subjected to chemical characterization are glycoproteins with molecular weights in the range of 24,000–28,000. The compound that has received the most attention is bovine TSH. Almost all samples are polymorphic, containing two or more electrophoretically distinguishable, biologically active components. Although there have been occasional reports of b-TSH with activities of 60–80 IU/mg, Pierce's TSH, purified by chromatogrphy and countercurrent distribution (Liao *et al.*, 1969) as well as Condliffe's crystalline TSH (Condliffe and Jakoby, 1967) both assayed about 40 IU/mg. Specific activities of purified TSH's from other species range from 15 (sheep) to 70 (mouse tumor) IU/mg. If it is recalled that the sensitivity of *in vivo* assays range between 0.05 and 1.0 mU, it is easily calculated that the amount of purified TSH necessary for a physiological response is of the order of 1–20 ng.

The behavior of bovine TSH in the analytical ultracentrifuge seems to be that expected for a concentration-dependent aggregating system. Sedimentation analysis (Shome *et al.*, 1968) gave $s_{20,w} = 2.76$ S and a calculated molecular weight of 28,000 when the data were extrapolated to infinitely dilute solutions. At higher concentrations estimates of the molecular weight ranged up to 41,000. In 6 *M* guanidine hydrochloride, equilibrium sedimentation of both native and reduced, carboxymethylated TSH indicated that the molecular weight was between 24,000 and 26,500. A similar range of values was calculated from amino acid analysis.

In 1970, Liao and Pierce found that if TSH was incubated with 1 *M* propionic acid, it could subsequently be separated into two subunits, designated as b-TSH-α and b-TSH-β. Neither of the subunits had thyrotropic activity, but dissociation was readily reversible with restoration of biological activity. Each subunit consists of a single peptide chain: b-TSH-α has 96 amino acids and b-TSH-β has 112 (Fig. 10.8 and 10.13). Despite its shorter sequence, TSH-α emerges from a Sephadex G-100 column before TSH-β, probably because a difference in carbohydrate content leads to distinctly different Stokes radii. Liao's data (Liao and Pierce, 1970) indicate that whereas the carbohydrate content of bovine TSH-α is approximately 17%, that of b-TSH-β is only about 9%. TSH-α contains two separate carbohydrate chains, attached at Asn^{56} and Asn^{82}, while TSH-β contains only one (at Asn^{23}). Pierce has noted that heterogeneity of chemical composition occurs in both subunits. Thus, some molecules of b-TSH-β contain an additional methionine residue at the COOH terminus: similarly, some molecules of b-TSH-α do not have the Phe-Pro dipeptide at the amino terminal end, but begin instead with Asn.

As indicated in Fig. 10.8 the sequence of bovine TSH-α is identical with that of bovine (or ovine) LH-α. Considerable homology also exists between the β-subunits of TSH and LH; allowing for some differences in chain length, the half-cystines of b-TSH-β and o-LH-β can be aligned exactly and about half the total number of residues are either identical or represent conservative (one base change) substitutions.

Sairam and Li (1973a,b) separated TSH from human pituitaries into α- and β-subunits by countercurrent distribution and, aided by evidence of considerable homology with known peptides, were able to establish their amino acid sequences. Human TSH-α is identical, at least insofar as its peptide sequence is concerned, with h-LH-α (Fig. 10.8). Figure 10.13 includes a comparison of the sequence of h-TSH-β with that of b-TSH-β. Only 12 residue positions, including the C-terminal methionine, are different.

Active TSH preparations have also been isolated from sheep, hog, whale, and eel pituitaries, and from a TSH-producing, transplantable, mouse pitu-

10 20
Human H_2N-Phe-Cys-Ile-Pro-Thr-Glu-Tyr-Met-Thr-His-Ile-Glu-Arg-Arg-Glu-Cys-Ala-Tyr-Cys-Leu-Thr-Ile-
Bovine -Met- -Val- -Lys-

CHO 30 40
Human -Asn-Thr-Thr-Ile-Cys-Ala-Gly-Tyr-Cys-Met-Thr-Arg-Asp-Ile-Asx-Gly-Lys-Leu-Phe-Leu-Pro-Lys-
Bovine -Val- -Asx-Val-

50 60
Human -Tyr-Ala-Leu-Ser-Gln-Asp-Val-Cys-Thr-Tyr-Arg-Asp-Phe-Ile-Tyr-Arg-Thr-Val-Glu-Ile-Pro-Gly-
Bovine -Met- -Lys- -Ala-

70 80
Human -Cys-Pro-Leu-His-Val-Ala-Pro-Tyr-Phe-Ser-Tyr-Pro-Val-Ala-Leu-Ser-Cys-Lys-Cys-Gly-Lys-Cys-
Bovine -Arg- -Thr- -Ile-

90 100 110
Human -Asx-Thr-Asx-Tyr-Ser-Asx-Cys-Ile-His-Glu-Ala-Ile-Lys-Thr-Asn-Tyr-Cys-Thr-Lys-Pro-Gln-Lys-
Bovine

Human -Ser-TyrOH
Bovine -MetOH

Fig. 10.13 *Amino acid sequences of h-TSH-β and b-TSH-β. The amino acid sequences of h-TSH-α and b-TSH-α are identical with those of h-LH-α and b-LH-α, respectively. Source: h-TSH-β, Sairam and Li (1973b); b-TSH-β, Liao and Pierce (1971).*

itary tumor. Only tentative comparisons of chemical properties could be made among these various products, since they satisfied only minimal criteria of homogeneity. All of the samples were rich in proline and in hydroxyamino acids. Nonpolar aliphatic amino acids were relatively uncommon. It may be noted that both bovine and human TSH's have 22 half-cystine residues per mole, porcine TSH has about 16, sheep and mouse tumor TSH have about eight, and eel TSH only four. Most of the carbohydrate in b-TSH can be accounted for by fucose, mannose, glucosamine, and galactosamine (Howard and Pierce, 1969); human TSH has been reported to contain one mole of sialic acid, which can be removed without loss of activity.

In view of the similarity in amino acid composition between bovine and human TSH, it is surprising that antisera to these proteins show relatively little cross-reaction. To neutralize the biological activity of h-TSH, ten to one hundred times as much anti-b-TSH as anti-h-TSH was required, and anti-h-TSH did not inhibit b-TSH at all (Levy *et al.*, 1962; Utiger *et al.*, 1963). Wherry *et al.* (1970) have reported that monkey TSH reacts strongly with anti-h-TSH serum. In experiments in which graded amounts of unlabeled TSH were used to inhibit the binding of ^{131}I-h-TSH to rabbit anti-h-TSH, the curve obtained with monkey plasma (presumably containing monkey TSH) was superimposable over that obtained with h-TSH.

One unusual feature of TSH is its relative instability when purified. Lyophilized samples which assayed 20 IU/mg or more were found to lose nearly 50% of their activity after storage for several months, but it is possible to store frozen solutions of TSH for long periods without loss of activity.

D. RECOMBINATION AND HYBRIDIZATION AMONG THE GLYCOPROTEIN HORMONE SUBUNITS

The isolated subunits of FSH, LH, h-CG and TSH are virtually devoid of significant biological activity. Papkoff *et al.* (1971), by appropriate purification procedures, were able to reduce the residual activity of LH-α and LH-β to 1–2% of that found in the native hormone. The responses obtained by Pierce (1971) to 5–10 mU equivalents of TSH-α or TSH-β were indistinguishable from those of controls in the chick assay. The gonadotropic activity of h-CG-β was only 150–300 IU/mg (compared to 15,000 IU/mg for native h-CG); the fact that anti-h-CG antiserum, which does not bind h-CG-β, inhibits residual h-CG-β activity suggests that the subunit may have been contaminated with some native or reconstituted hormone (Rayford *et al.*, 1972).

Recombination of the homologous α- and β-subunits of the glycoprotein hormones can be accomplished in a variety of ways. The simplest is to mix subunits in 1:1 mole ratio in phosphate buffer, pH 7.0, 0.1 ionic strength, and allow them to react for 24 hours at 23°. Under these conditions, restoration of LH activity ranged from 20–144% in a series of 14 experiments (Papkoff *et al.*, 1973), with recovery usually 50–60%. Recombination of propionic acid-treated h-FSH restored somewhat more than one-third the original activity (Reichert, 1971), while recombination of h-CG subunits resulted in recovery of nearly 60% of the activity of the starting product (14,600 IU/mg) (Donini *et al.*, 1973). Similarly a mixture of TSH-α and TSH-β in buffer (pH 9.5) recovered about 50% of the calculated activity after standing 16 hours at 37°.

The discovery that b-LH-α and b-TSH-α share a common chemical identity raised the question of the possible functional identity of these two proteins. In fact, recombination studies using b-TSH-α and b-LH-β or b-LH-α and b-TSH-β indicated that the two α-subunits were interchangeable in respect to restoration of hormonal function. In each instance, the specificity of the response, (i.e., whether the recombinant possessed LH or TSH activity) was a function of the kind of β-subunit used. Thus, LH-α plus TSH-β had TSH activity, while TSH-α plus LH-β displayed only LH activity.

The α-subunit of h-CG is also interchangeable with TSH-α or LH-α in restoring activity when combined with isolated β-subunits of various kinds. Thus, h-CG-α plus b-LH-β was actually more active in the ovarian ascorbic

TABLE 10.9 Activities of Glycoprotein Hormone Subunit Combinations[a]

	Activity[c,d]		
Combination[b]	FSH	LH–CG	TSH
b-TSH-α		−	−
b-TSH-β			−
b-LH-α		−	−
b-LH-β		−	
h-CG-α		−	
h-CG-β		±	
b-TSH-α + b-TSH-β	(−)	(−)	+
b-TSH-α + b-LH-β		±	
b-TSH-α + h-CG-β		+	
b-TSH-β + b-LH-α			+
b-LH-α + b-LH-β	(−)	+	(−)
b-LH-α + h-CG-α		−	
b-LH-α + h-CG-β		+	
b-LH-α + h-FSH-β	+		
b-LH-β + h-CG-α		+	
b-LH-β + h-CG-β		−	
b-LH-β + h-FSH-α,β	−		
h-CG-α + h-CG-β	(−)	+	(−)
h-CG-α + h-FSH-α,β	+	−	
h-CG-β + h-FSH-α,β	±	+	
h-FSH-α + h-FSH-β	+	(−)	(−)

[a] *Data from Pierce, 1971; Pierce et al. (1971a).*
[b] *Abbreviations: b-TSH, bovine thyroid stimulating hormone; b-LH, bovine luteinizing hormone; h-CG, human chorionic gonadotropin; h-FSH, human follicle-stimulating hormone.*
[c] *Assay methods: FSH, Parlow method; LH, CG, ovarian ascorbic acid depletion; TSH, uptake of ^{32}P by chick thyroids.*
[d] *Key: − = near 0 activity; (−) $<10\%$ of native hormone; ± = 10–25%; + $>50\%$.*

acid depletion test than was reconstituted b-LH, while b-LH-α plus h-CG-β was indistinguishable from reconstituted h-CG (Pierce *et al.*, 1971a). A combination of h-CG-α plus b-TSH-β had good TSH activity, whereas b-TSH-α plus h-CG-β had no TSH activity.

Table 10.9 summarizes the results of a variety of recombination experiments.

It is clear from the above that: (a) the α-subunits of these glycoprotein hormones bear a close chemical relationship and can substitute more or less freely for each other, and (b) the biological determinant in each instance is a role conferred exclusively on the β-subunit.

It should be noted that failure of gonadotropin assays to distinguish between the various α-subunits is confined to acute assays in which the target organ is the ovary. Parlow *et al.* (1972) compared the activity of recombinations involving bovine LH-β or h-CG-β subunits in the ovarian ascorbic acid depletion assay with the effects of the same recombinations upon rat ventral prostate weights. In these experiments, clear differences attributable to the source of the α-subunit were observed. The "index of discrimination" (the ratio of the response in the ventral prostate to that in the OAAD assay) ranged from 0.9 (for b-LH-α plus b-LH-β) to 66.2 (for h-CG-α plus h-CG-β). With a given β-subunit (either b-LH or h-CG) the index of discrimination increased in the order b-LH-α < b-TSH-α < h-CG-α. Parlow concluded that recombinants containing h-CG-α possessed longer circulating lifetimes than those which included α-subunits from TSH or LH—a difference which would be much more apparent in the more prolonged response measured by ventral prostate weight increase. Some of these differences may be due to the carbohydrate components of the several subunits, as well as to slight differences in peptide sequence.

Studies of the behavior of the individual subunits and hybrid recombinations of b-LH, h-CG, and b-TSH by immunodiffusion and radioimmunoassay indicate that while the β-subunits of these hormones are also the principal determinants of immunological identity, the α-subunits retain some of their immunological uniqueness in combination with their complementary subunits. Thus, anti-b-LH antiserum reacts with intact b-LH or (less strongly) with b-LH-β, but not with b-TSH, while anti-b-LH-α or anti-b-TSH-α reacts with either b-LH or b-TSH, but not with their β-subunits (Pierce, 1971). On the other hand, little cross-reaction occurred between either h-CG-α or b-LH-α and anti-h-CG, as measured by their ability to displace ^{131}I-labeled h-CG from its combination with anti-h-CG. Inhibition of ^{131}I-h-CG-α interaction with anti-h-CG-α antibody was observed with native b-CG, and with an h-CG-α-b-LH-β hybrid, but not with reconstituted b-LH (Vaitukaitis *et al.*, 1972). It would appear that in some instances, the conformations necessary for expression of biological activity are not the same as those required for an immunological response.

IV. Prolactin

A. ASSAY

In an earlier section, the variety of physiological actions which prolactin (Pr, luteotropic hormone, LtH) exerts in mammals and birds was reviewed. Many of these have been used for assays; methods have been developed which are based upon (1) proliferation of the "crop sac" of pigeons or doves; (2) initiation of milk secretion in pseudopregnant rabbits; and (3) induction of decidual responses in the uterine horns of hypophysectomized rats or mice. Most of the research on isolation, purification, and properties of prolactin has been monitored by assays employing the crop sac method.*

For the crop sac assay, either juvenile (2–3 months) or adult pigeons may be used. Injection of 10–15 IU prolactin over a 4-day-period increases crop gland weight approximately 100%. The response (weight of the blotted gland) is linear with the log of the dose to 80–100 IU. Improvement of the assay, particularly reflected in increased sensitivity, has resulted from the use of older animals, increasing the number (but not the frequency) of injections, and by local, instead of systemic injection of the sample. When prolactin is injected directly into the skin over the crop, a circular region of proliferation can be defined, the diameter of which is proportional to the amount of hormone injected. In the assay modification described by Grosvenor and Turner (1958), a readily detectable response (diameter of proliferation ~1.0 cm) was achieved with a total dose of 0.010 IU given over a 4-day-period, and a linear response was obtained over a thirtyfold range of the amount of hormone injected. Some improvement in index of precision has also been achieved by determining the dry weight of the gland rather than weighing it when wet.

Both bovine and ovine prolactins are antigenic in guinea pigs. However, anti-prolactin sera cross-react with growth hormone, and development of a satisfactory assay for prolactin, which would be applicable to human serum, has been hampered by the apparent immunological indentity between human prolactin and growth hormone; while for immunoassays of prolactin in laboratory animals a supply of the homologous hormone is needed. Kwa and Verhofstad (1967) isolated rat prolactin from transplants of pituitary tumors and were able to prepare an antiserum to rat prolactin (r-Pr) in rabbits. A radioimmunoassay for rat prolactin was subsequently developed, using cellulose acetate electrophoresis to separate free and bound radioiodinated prolactin. In their hands the percent of ^{131}I-Pr bound was linear with the logarithm of the amount of prolactin bound over a hundredfold range (2.5–250 ng), and parallel curves were obtained for tumor prolactin, rat pituitary extract, and serum from tumor-bearing rats. A later, more sensitive modification increased the sensitivity to 0.05 ng r-Pr.

A useful *in vitro* assay for prolactin was devised by Shiu, Kelley, and Friesen (1973), based upon the observation that a fraction prepared from homogenates of mammary glands of pregnant rabbits primed with placental lactogen and hydrocortisone would specifically bind prolactin. The tissue fraction appeared to consist principally of membrane fragments. The procedure used was essentially the same as that devised by Reichert for LH assay using a testicular homogenate (see Section III, A, 1), i.e., competition

* An International Unit of Prolactin was established (in 1938) as the activity of 0.10 mg of a standard preparation. A second International Standard is now available; it has been shown to contain 22 IU/mg.

between unlabeled and ^{131}I-labeled prolactin for prolactin binding sites. Under suitable conditions, the addition of 10–1000 ng of prolactin/ml decreased the ratio of bound: free ^{131}I-prolactin from 3 : 1–1 : 3.

B. CHEMISTRY

Preparations of bovine and ovine prolactins (b-Pr and o-Pr) which satisfied minimal electrophoretic, ultracentrifugal, and solubility criteria for homogeneity were isolated by Li (1945) and by White (1942) more than 30 years ago; indeed, the crystallization of bovine prolactin was reported as early as 1937. These preparations were about three times as active in the pigeon crop assay as the first International Standard (i.e., 30–35 IU/mg). Although improved methods of isolation and purification were subsequently devised, essentially no improvement has been achieved as far as biological activity is concerned during the intervening decades. It seems clear, in fact, that early prolactin preparations represented the pure hormone, in contrast to the experience with ACTH and the gonadotropins.

That prolactin was the first pituitary hormone to be obtained in pure form is due mostly to the high prolactin content of the pituitaries of domestic animals. From one kilogram of sheep glands, Li (1957) collected 2 gm of prolactin which assayed 35 IU/mg; the final product represented nearly 80% of the total activity of the original pituitary homogenate.

Prolactin was characterized, in some early studies, as a protein of molecular weight 22,000–32,000, with an isoelectric point of 5.6–5.7. Bovine and ovine prolactins are indistinguishable in terms of their molecular-kinetic properties; their solubilities, however, are quite different, sheep prolactin being considerably more soluble at pH 2.25.

Cole and Li (1955) subjected 35 IU/mg sheep prolactin to countercurrent distribution in 2-butanol/0.35% dichloroacetic acid; after 100 transfers only a single symmetrical peak was seen. Nevertheless, 6 bands were detected on starch gel, and three of these (quantitatively the most important) were separated by chromatographing the mixture on DEAE-cellulose. All three fractions were active; they were shown to differ largely in their state of aggregation. Pure monomeric prolactin, with a molecular weight estimated to be about 23,000, was isolated after further chromatography. It gave a single band on starch gel and a single N-terminal amino acid (Thr) in the ratio of one mole/23,000 gm.

The complete amino acid sequence of ovine prolactin is shown in Fig. 10.14. The molecular weight calculated from the structure shown turns out to be 22,570, which agrees very well with the best earlier estimate of 22,720. There is no reason, therefore, to suppose that the molecule contains any nonamino acid components.

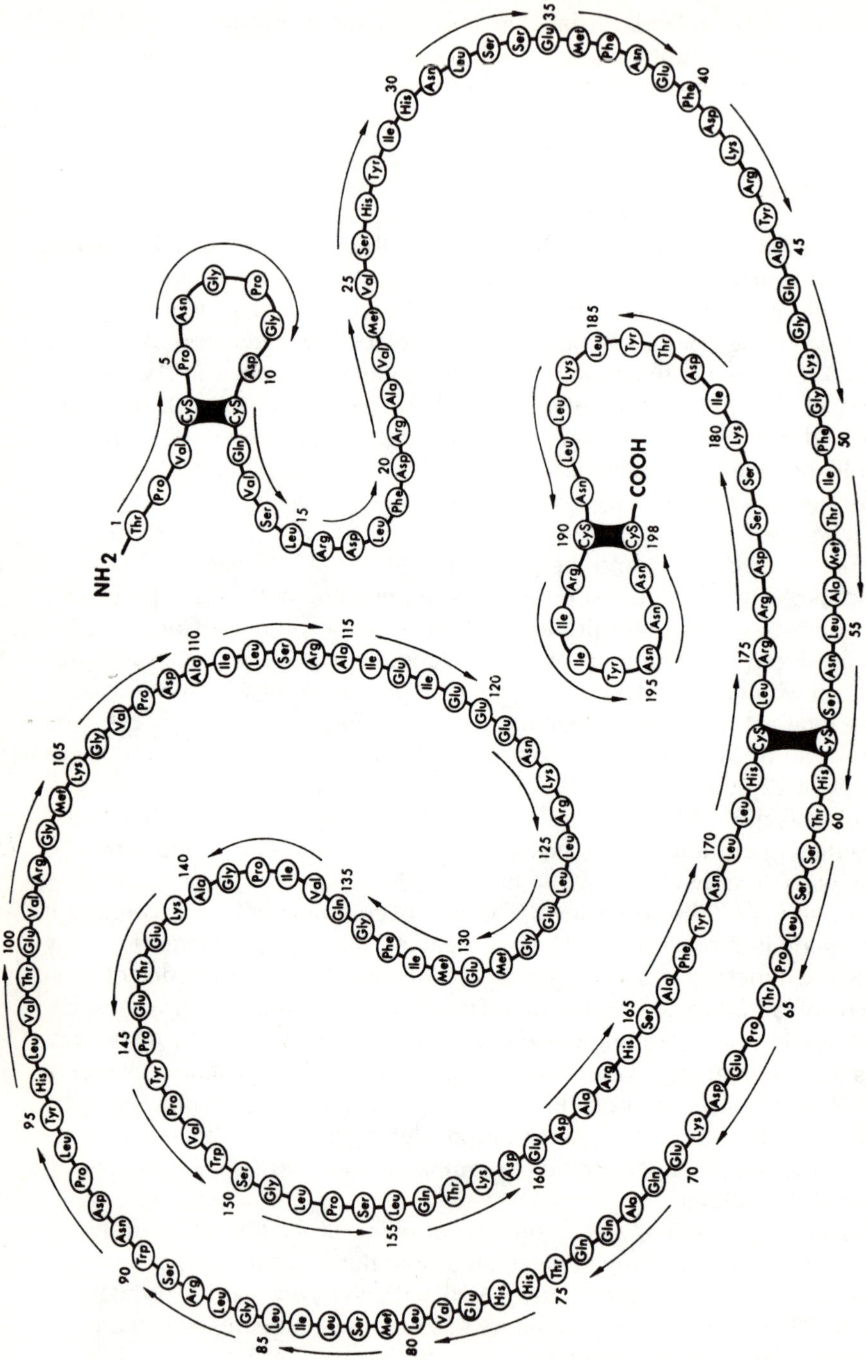

Fig. 10.14 *Amino acid sequence of ovine prolactin. Reproduced, with permission, from Li et al. (1970).*

Like the nonprimate somatotropins, o-Pr contains a tight disulfide-linked loop of nine amino acids at the carboxy terminus. In contrast to the growth hormones, however, one of the residues forming the loop in o-Pr is a C-terminal cysteine. In consequence, reaction with carboxypeptidase does not liberate free amino acids until the native protein has been reduced and alkylated.

Prolactin is a remarkably stable molecule. When a 1% solution is heated to 100° for 20 minutes, the biological activity is unaffected. Urea will dissociate oligomeric prolactin into smaller (monomeric) units; the original properties, including its activity, are restored upon removal of the urea. Complete iodination (7 moles/mole), reduction with thioglycollate, esterification, and acetylation destroy activity, as does extensive oxidation with performic acid. If the action of performate is restricted to the N-terminal threonine residue, activity is unaffected.

One unusual feature of prolactin chemistry appeared from studies of its susceptibility to chymotrypsin. After extensive digestion of o-Pr with chymotrypsin (50% of protein was converted to trichloroacetic acid-soluble material) Sluyser and Li (1964) isolated a fragment which possessed about half the specific prolactin activity of the original protein. This material was clearly different from o-Pr; Ala and Leu were found as N-terminal amino acids and carboxypeptidase liberated Leu and Phe from it. Nevertheless, it sedimented in the ultracentrifuge at nearly the same rate as native prolactin and had the same distribution coefficient in a butanol/dichloroacetic acid/water system.

Prolactin has been isolated from bovine, porcine, rat, and mouse pituitaries, in addition to sheep pituitaries. The molecular weights of the five mammalian hormones are not greatly different. Seavey and Lewis (1971) concluded from peptide mapping studies that b-Pr differed from o-Pr in but two respects: residue 107 in b-Pr is Ala instead of Val, and a histidine at residue 164 in o-Pr is missing in b-Pr. Porcine prolactin has 14 cysteines (instead of 6) and Ala as the N-terminal amino acid. Rat prolactin appears to be about 5 amino acid residues shorter than sheep prolactin, with the same number of half-cystine residues. The specific activities of purified prolactins from these species ranged from 28 to 50 IU/mg. Although the dose–response curves for rat and sheep prolactins parallel each other nicely when compared by the intradermal pigeon crop assay, discrepancies were noted when the same compounds were administered systemically.

Kwa *et al.* (1967) isolated prolactin from a transplantable, estrogen-dependent rat pituitary tumor. This substance was similar in many respects, including its immunological properties, to rat pituitary prolactin.

While the separation of prolactin from other pituitary hormones, including growth hormone, is a relatively easy matter when pituitaries of domestic animals are used, the separation of h-Pr from h-GH proved to be an intractable problem for a long time. Preparations of either growth hormone or prolactin from human (or monkey) pituitaries always contained both activities, although their ratios often showed wide variation. Consequently, an unequivocal conclusion concerning their identity (or nonidentity) was not possible. However, several kinds of evidence argued for the "separation of properties" hypothesis.

Fresh cultures of human fetal pituitaries secrete both prolactin and growth hormone into the medium. As the cultures age, however, the output of growth hormone steadily decreases, while that of prolactin increases. After 33 days, prolactin activity had increased five- to tenfold, while that of somatotropin decreased by 90%. Further, antiserum prepared using the culture fluid as antigen inhibited prolactin in human serum as well as that from the culture medium, while neither was inhibited by anti-GH antibody.

Other evidence suggesting that h-Pr and h-GH are separate hormones came from W. R. Lyons' laboratory. Lyons compared the epiphyseal cartilage effects and the lactogenic indices (milk secretion in hypophysectomized rats) of 50 human pituitary fractions known to possess somatotropin activity. The mammotropin : somatotropin ratios varied over a hundredfold range; further, the crop-stimulating activities were unrelated to these ratios (Lyons, 1969).

In 1971, two laboratories reported the separation of h-Pr from h-GH. Guyda and Friesen (1971) used affinity chromatography (chromatography of pituitary extracts on a column of sepharose which had been coupled to anti-h-Pr antibody*) for the separation. Lewis *et al.* (1971) chromatographed somatotropin-containing human pituitary fractions on DEAE-cellulose with an ammonium bicarbonate gradient. Prolactin emerged just before growth hormone. The two proteins could be distinguished electrophoretically, h-Pr migrating slightly more slowly than h-GH at pH 9.5, and slightly more rapidly at pH 4.5. Human prolactin contained 22–31 IU/mg prolactin activity by pigeon crop assay and 0.40 IU/mg somatotropic activity (purified h-GH contains 2.6 IU of somatotropic activity per milligram). Its molecular weight was about 22,000 and its N-terminal amino acid was Leu. The amino acid sequence is known for the first 40 residues from the amino terminal end (Niall *et al.*, 1973).

C. COMPARATIVE BIOLOGY

Nicoll and Nichols (1971) extracted pituitaries of four classes of tetrapods (mammals, birds, reptiles, and amphibians) and subjected the extracts to electrophoresis at pH 9.5. Fractions of similar or identical mobilities were

* The anti-h-Pr antibody was produced by injecting sheep with fluid obtained by incubation of human pituitary tissue *in vitro,* and was purified by chromatography on a Sepharose–h-PL (human placental lactogen) column.

assayed for crop-stimulating activity. In all cases, prolactin activity was associated with a discrete, rapidly moving band of protein. Activity was greatest in mammals and amphibia, lowest in birds.

Prolactin has been implicated in a greater variety of responses in fishes than any other hormone—from nest-building and resistance to thermal stress to pigmentation and the movement of ions across gill membranes. Prolactin isolated from tetrapod pituitaries will induce all of these effects, but the extent to which extracts of fish pituitaries will produce the responses to prolactin typically shown by birds and mammals is not so clear. Crop-stimulating activity has been found only in the pituitaries of lungfishes and in two of eight species of teleost fishes examined (Nicoll and Bern, 1968). Stimulation of mammary gland secretion is a property reserved, apparently, to tetrapod prolactins, while luteotropic activity is confined to mammals. Fluorescein-labeled anti-*o*-Pr antibody has been found to localize in specific cells of pituitaries of *Fundulus heteroclitus*.

V. Placental Lactogens

In 1962 Josimovich and MacLaren discovered that a protein isolated from human placentas at term showed significant immunological cross-reaction with rabbit anti-h-GH antibody. When tested in hypophysectomized rats, this preparation showed only modest tibial activity, but was active in the pigeon crop assay and in stimulating milk production in pseudopregnant rabbits. This substance has been called human placental lactogen (h-PL) or human chorionic somatomammotropin (h-CS). It has also been isolated from retroplacental plasma. Methods for its purification have been described by Friesen (1965) and by Florini *et al.* (1966). The prolactin-like activity of h-PL varies with the assay used; h-PL shares with h-GH the characteristic of low crop stimulating activity and high activity in the rabbit lactogenic test. Forsyth (1969) compared the crop-stimulating and lactogenic activities of four different preparations against the same ovine prolactin standard; the preparations contained 22–25 IU/mg of lactogenic activity, but only 1.4–4.2 IU/mg of crop-stimulating activity.

Purified h-PL is a single-chain polypeptide, containing, like h-GH, 191 amino acid residues. Its molecular weight is therefore approximately 22,000. Like growth hormone, it shows some tendency to aggregate in aqueous solution. When subjected to electrophoresis on starch gel at pH 8.6, it moves somewhat more rapidly than h-GH.

The complete amino acid sequence of h-PL was elucidated by Li, Dixon, and Chung (1971), and later verified, with some minor corrections, by Niall (1971). The h-PL sequence may be compared to that of h-GH in Fig. 10.2. It may be seen that there is a high degree of homology between the two structures, 165 of the 191 residues being identical and many of the others being "highly acceptable" or "acceptable" changes. Thus an 86% degree of homology exists between the two molecules; this suggests they may have a common origin in a primordial polypeptide.

The limited information available also indicates a considerable degree of homology (92%) between h-Pr and the first 50 amino acids (from the N-terminus) of o-Pr. There apparently has been an efficient conservation of prolactin sequence between lower orders of mammals and humans, while divergence is much more marked between growth hormones of the same species. Niall has speculated that the gene duplication which resulted in the emergence of h-PL may be a comparatively recent one, and that nonprimate mammals may lack a placental lactogen. Thus far, the only animal, other than man, in which a placental lactogen has been found is the monkey (Vinik *et al.*, 1973). Monkey placental lactogen possesses somatotropic activity (tibia test in hypophysectomized rats) and is more closely related immunologically to h-GH than to h-PL.

11

Melanocyte-Stimulating Hormone (MSH)

I. Assay

Although the effect of pituitary extracts upon the chromatophores (including melanophores) of various kinds of animals has been known for half a century, methods for the assay of MSH capable of semi-quantitative application have been developed only within the past 30 years. In 1944, Landgrebe and Waring developed a procedure for assessing the effects of pituitary preparations upon the web melanophores of light-adapted *Xenopus*. MSH-containing extracts were injected into the dorsal lymph sac, and the appearance of the melanophores was evaluated microscopically and recorded at intervals during the next 2–3 hours. The melanophore index (MI) was estimated on a scale of 1 to 5, the extremes being fully contracted (punctate) and fully expanded (stellate) melanocytes, respectively. The peak melanophore index, averaged for a group of eight to ten animals, was found to be linear with the log of the amount of hormone injected. Significant responses (MI = 2–4) resulted when 0.25–2.5 μg equivalents of the International Posterior Pituitary Standard powder were injected. Landgrebe and Waring proposed that the unit of MSH activity be defined as the amount contained in 0.5 mg of Posterior Pituitary Standard. Their assay was therefore sensitive to 0.0005–0.005 IU. (The MSH contents of the last three Posterior Pituitary Standards have been found to be the same within 10%.)

Although pituitary extracts are effective at relatively high dilutions, intact toads will darken in response to substances of nonpituitary origin as well, presumably because of the release of MSH from the animal's own pituitary. Hypophysectomy improves both the specificity and sensitivity of the assay.

The observation (Wright, 1948) that isolated pieces of frog skin would pale when immersed in Ringer solution and would darken perceptibly if pituitary extract was added to the surrounding fluid led Frieden *et al.* (1948) to devise a method for photometric estimation of the change in melanophore expansion. Pieces of skin from the legs and thighs of *Rana* were clamped in a holder so that the light transmission of a circumscribed area could be determined. Paling was accompanied by a decrease in light absorption, while the addition of pituitary extracts caused a rapid increase in absorbance. For the assay, the washed skin was immersed in a solution of the unknown and the change (increase) in absorbance recorded (in optical density units) as Δ_1. The unknown was then replaced by a standard pituitary extract, sufficiently concentrated to effect maximal darkening; the resulting change in absorbance (from the original baseline) was recorded as Δ_2. A

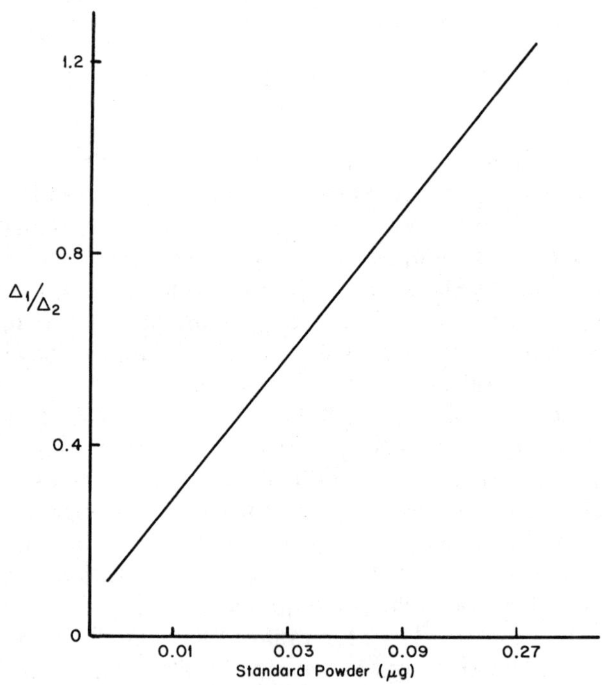

Fig. 11.1 *Photometric assay of MSH. Data of Frieden et al. (1948).*

plot of Δ_1/Δ_2 as a function of the logarithm of the MSH concentration was found to be linear over a thirtyfold concentration range. The midpoint of the regression line ($\Delta_1/\Delta_2 = 0.5$) coincided with a concentration of approximately 0.02 μg equivalents/ml of posterior lobe powder, corresponding to 4×10^{-5} IU/ml (Fig. 11.1).

Shizume, Lerner, and Fitzpatrick (1954) modified the photometric assay so that changes in skin reflectance coincident with melanophore expansion were measured. They also compared the responses of unknown and standard; as in the original procedure the ratio of the two responses was linear with the logarithm of the MSH concentration. The useful range was $1–16 \times 10^{-5}$ IU/ml. Although no direct comparison seems to have been made, the two *in vitro* assays appear to be comparable in both sensitivity and precision. It has been found that if skins of hypophysectomized *Xenopus* were used in the reflectance assay, the sensitivity was about doubled.

II. Chemistry

It was noted earlier that the intermediate hypophyseal lobe hormone (MSH) occurs in two forms, α and β. α-MSH has been isolated from pituitaries of cattle, pigs, horses, sheep, and monkeys. All of these animals secrete the same acetylated tridecapeptide:

Ac-Ser-Tyr-Ser-Met-Glu-His-Phe-Arg-Trp-Gly-Lys-Pro-Val (NH_2)

β-MSH is a larger molecule; in cattle, pigs, horses, sheep, and monkeys an 18-amino acid peptide is elaborated:

Bovine, ovine: Asp-Ser-Gly-Pro-Tyr-Lys-Met-Glu-His-Phe-Arg-Trp-Gly-Ser-Pro-Pro-Lys-Asp (b-β-MSH)
Pig: Glu^2-b-β-MSH
Horse: Glu^2-, Arg^{16}-b-β MSH
Monkey: Glu^2-, Arg^6-b-β-MSH

Human β-MSH is four residues longer at the amino terminal end:

Ala-Glu-Lys-Lys-Asp-Glu-Gly-Pro-Tyr-Arg-Met-Glu-His-Phe-Arg-Trp-Gly-Ser-Pro-Pro-Lys-Asp

Native α-MSH has an activity of 2×10^{10} (Shizume) Units/gm;* it is thus

* Most of the assay data which have been recorded for MSH preparations have been obtained using Shizume's assay, and activities have been expressed in terms of Shizume's laboratory standard. Fortunately, a correlation with the International Standard has been provided (Landgebe and Waring, 1962). One-half milligram of the International Standard is equivalent to 0.53 mg of Shizume's preparation; since the latter defined a "unit" of MSH activity as the effect produced by 0.04 μg of his preparation, 1 IU (0.5 mg of Internation Standard) is equivalent to 1.33×10^4 Shizume units. I shall continue the practice generally used, of reporting MSH activities in 'Shizume' units.

about 750 times as active as standard posterior lobe powder. Since its molecular weight is approximately 2000, it is apparent that *in vitro* α-MSH is active at a concentration of 2×10^{-11} *M*. β-MSH is distinctly less active than is α-MSH; estimates of the activity of native α-MSH range from 2×10^9 U/gm (ox, horse, monkey) to 5×10^9 U/gm (pig). The MSH activity of the docosapeptide from human pituitaries (human β-MSH) is apparently not known with assurance.

III. Comparative Pharmacology

The combination of relative simplicity of assay and relative accessibility has made the correlation of structure and biological activity in MSH analogs an attractive subject; as a result a great deal of effort has been expended in studying the biological activity of peptides related to MSH. The simplest compound possessing detectable MSH activity *in vitro* is the tetrapeptide, His-Phe-Arg-Trp (all L-), which was reported to have an activity of 4×10^4 U/gm.* On a weight basis this is 1/500,000 the activity of α-MSH; nevertheless, significant activity is displayed at 10^{-6} *M*. This sequence of four amino acids seems to be absolutely essential for MSH function, since neither the N-terminal octapeptide of α-MSH (which lacks the Trp residue) nor its C-terminal heptapeptide (in which His^6 is lacking) shows any activity at all. The pentapeptide, His-Phe-Arg-Trp-Gly, possesses about the same activity as the tetrapeptide; beyond this, addition of amino acids at either end (in the order found in α-MSH) increases activity greatly. Maximum activity is attained with the tridecapeptide (α-MSH); thereafter, activity falls precipitously to about one-hundredth the activity of the native hormone (e.g., the N-terminal hexadecapeptide of ACTH) and remains essentially constant (on a molar basis) with the addition of as many as 25 amino acids to the C-terminus (i.e., ACTH itself).

As isolated from pituitary tissue, the N-terminal amino group of α-MSH is acetylated; removal of the acetyl group diminishes the activity about tenfold. While acetylation or formylation of its amino groups (Ser^1, Lys^{11}) does not diminish (indeed, may enhance) activity, use of bulkier substituents (carbobenzoxy, tosyl) lowers activity, possibly by interfering with approach of the MSH molecule to receptor sites.

Some structure-activity relationships in a limited series of MSH fragments, analogs, and homologs, are summarized in Table 11.1.

It has been known for at least 35 years (Stehle, 1938) that treatment with alkali potentiates the MSH activity of pituitary extracts. Smaller quantities of peptide are required for darkening, either *in vitro* or *in vivo,* using alkali-

* Note that this sequence is found in all native MSH's.

TABLE 11.1 Structure-Activity Relationships in Compounds Related to α-MSH[a,b]

Compound[c]	MSH Activity (U/gm)	Compound	MSH Activity (U/gm)
α^{1-13}-MSH	2×10^{10}	Gly^{5}-α^{5-10}-MSH	2×10^{5}
Desacetyl-α^{1-13}-MSH	10^{8}	α^{6-9}-MSH	10^{4}
Desacetyl-α^{1-8}-MSH	0	Orn^{8}-α^{6-10}-MSH	3×10^{4}
α^{1-10}-MSH	4×10^{6}	Citrulline^{8}-α^{6-10}-MSH	Inhibitory
Desacetyl-α^{1-10}-MSH	3×10^{6}	α^{6-13}-MSH	8×10^{6}
Gln^{5}-α^{3-10}-MSH	7×10^{5}	F-Lys^{11}-α^{6-13}-MSH	8×10^{6}
α^{3-13}-MSH	10^{9}	α^{7-13}-MSH	0
Acetyl-α^{3-13}-MSH	5×10^{9}	α-AIB^{4},Gln^{5},F-Lys^{11}-α^{1-13}-MSH	2×10^{8}
α^{4-8}-MSH	0	(D)Trp^{9}-α^{6-10}-MSH	5×10^{4}
α^{4-10}-MSH	1.4×10^{6}	(D)Arg^{8}-α^{6-10}-MSH	10^{4}
Gln^{5}-α^{4-10}-MSH	2.8×10^{5}	(D)Phe^{7}-α^{6-10}-MSH	3×10^{5}
α^{5-10}-MSH	2×10^{5}	(D)His^{6}-α^{6-10}-MSH	Inhibitory
		α^{6-10}-MSH [all(D)]	Inhibitory

[a] *α-MSH: Ac-Ser-Tyr-Ser-Met-Glu-His-Phe-Arg-Trp-Gly-Lys-Pro-Val(NH$_2$).* (residues numbered 1–13 above the sequence)
[b] *Source: Hofmann (1962); Lande and Lerner (1967).*
[c] *F, formyl; AIB, aminoisobutyryl.*

treated material; in addition, the duration of the darkening response is much prolonged (Lerner, 1965). In 1963, Lee and Buettner–Janusch suggested that partial racemization of amino acid residues in the MSH molecule was responsible for this phenomenon. This suggestion, quickly reinforced by supporting evidence, stimulated interest in the biological activity of peptides containing amino acids of unnatural configuration. Hano *et al.* (1964), Koida *et al.* (1966), Yajima *et al.* (1966), and others have studied the behavior of synthetic analogs of the minimal pentapeptide, His-Phe-Arg-Trp-Gly, in which one or more of the amino acid residues (except glycine) have been replaced by their corresponding enantiomorphs. In general, it appears that responsibility for potentiation by alkali is chiefly, if not exclusively within the province of residues 2(Phe) and 4(Trp). Thus (L)His-(D)Phe-(L)Arg-(L)Trp-Gly and (L)His-(L)Phe-(L)Arg-(D)Try-Gly were both distinctly more active (three to one hundred fiftyfold) than the all (L) form *in vitro*. On the other hand, replacement of the other amino acids (His,Arg) by their unnatural isomers resulted in dimunution of activity (e.g., both (D)His-(L)Phe-(L)Arg-(L)Trp-Gly and (L)His-(L)Phe-(D)Arg-(L)Trp-Gly were both essentially inert). The all (D) pentapeptide, (D)His-(D)Phe-(D)Arg-(D)Trp-Gly, not only failed to disperse contracted melanophores of frog skin *in vitro* but prevented or reversed dispersion induced by either the all (L) pentapeptide or α-MSH. This property was shared to some extent by the (D)His and the (D)Arg analogs.

All of these data refer to effects upon isolated skins, using either *R. pi-*

piens or *R. nicromaculata*. The limited data that deal with the effects of diastereoisomeric peptides *in vivo* (Kastin *et al.*, 1965) reveal a similar, but not identical, set of relationships.

The stereochemical specificity of the melanocyte response indicates that it is possible to dissociate structural features which are recognized by a hypothetical melanophore receptor site and those which are responsible for melanin granule dispersion. Enhancement and prolongation of activity by (D)Phe- or (D)Trp-containing compounds is quite plausibly referable to slower rates of degradation, both intra- and extracellularly.

12

The Hormones of the Posterior Pituitary (Neurohypophysis)

I. Assay

As noted earlier mammalian posterior lobe extracts exert four principal actions in vertebrates: (1) a pressor effect; (2) an antidiuretic effect; (3) contraction of smooth muscle; and (4) milk ejection. Oxytocin and its physiological analogs may be detected by their effects on the rat uterus, blood pressure changes in anesthetized chickens, and changes in fluid pressure in rabbit mammary glands.

A. RAT UTERUS

A single horn of the uterus of a diestrous rat is suspended in modified Ringer's solution and aerated with 95% O_2/5% CO_2; the temperature is maintained at 32°–36°. One end of the uterus is fixed and the other is attached to the writing lever of a kymograph under a fixed load (1.25–1.3 gm). The addition of oxytocin to the bath fluid is followed by a contraction of the uterus. If care is taken to remain within the range of submaximal contractions, the intensity (amplitude) of the response is linear with the logarithm of the oxytocin concentration. The useful range is typically 0.04–0.08 IU/20 ml. Synthetic oxytocin has an activity of 500 IU/mg; hence a measureable response is induced by 0.004–0.008 μg/ml.

A useful discriminatory property of the rat uterus preparation results from the fact that while the activity of most octapeptides in the assay is potentiated by magnesium ion, oxytocin itself is unaffected. This property has been exploited by Munsick and by Sawyer in their studies of the comparative pharmacology of pituitary extracts.

B. AVIAN BLOOD PRESSURE

White leghorn chickens are anesthetized with sodium barbital and the blood pressure recorded via the ischiadic artery. The injection of oxytocin results in a reduction in blood pressure which is proportional to the logarithm of the dose within a relatively narrow range (0.2–0.4 μg, equivalent to 0.1–0.2 IU of oxytocin). Unknowns and standard preparations are injected at intervals of 3–5 minutes, and a suitably prepared animal may constitute a stable assay subject for as long as 6–12 hours. Occasionally birds may develop a tolerance to ocytocin, but sensitivity can usually be restored by discontinuing assays for one hour or more. Interference by contaminants (e.g., vasopressin) is not serious unless the vasopressin : oxytocin ratio is 2.5 or greater.

C. RABBIT MAMMARY GLAND

This appears to be the most sensitive, if not the most convenient, method for oxytocin assay. A lactating, anesthetized rabbit weighing about 2 kg is used. One of the ducts in the animal's nipple is cannulated and connected to a sensitive manometer. Oxytocin samples are injected intravenously; typically, the preparation responds to 1 mU (0.002 μg) of oxytocin by an increase of 16 mm H_2O in fluid pressure. Again, the index of discrimination is high; if the dose is reduced to 0.001 μg the increase is reduced by 75%.

Vasopressin can be measured by its effect on blood pressure in mammals, as well as by its antidiuretic properties in mammals and amphibians.

D. PRESSOR ACTIVITY

Rats, cats, and dogs have been used, but rats are preferred for reasons of convenience and economy. Rats weighing 400 gm or more are anesthetized with urethane, pithed, and the carotid artery is cannulated to record blood pressure; samples for assay are injected via the femoral vein. Significant pressor responses, amounting to 30–40 mm Hg, can be elicited with 0.006–0.008 IU of vasopressin. Since the pure hormone has a potency of

600 IU/mg, these figures correspond to 1–1.3 × 10^{-5} mg of vasopressin. Within this range, the log dose–response curve is nearly linear.

E. ANTIDIURETIC ACTIVITY

Rats are given water by stomach tube and the urine output is recorded at 10-minute intervals. If the output is at least 1.5 ml/10 minutes, the animals may be used. Vasopressin is administered subcutaneously or via the jugular vein. A significant diminution in urine volume may be obtained with as little as 12.5 microunits of vasopressin/100 g of body weight (rat); with doses between 50 and 200 μU/100 gm (8–30 × 10^{-5} μg) a graded response is obtained. Ethanol, by suppressing the secretion of endogenous antidiuretic hormone (ADH), improves the reliability of the assay.

Neurohypophyseal extracts also occasion a variety of other pharmacological responses in birds and amphibians, including oxytocic responses in avian and amphibian oviducts and increase of water transport across amphibian bladders (Munsick *et al.*, 1960). Since the relative effectiveness of different pituitary substances is different for each pharmacological end point, not only the pure hormones, but mixtures can be characterized, using a battery of tests. Sawyer and his colleagues have made elegant use of the comparative pharmacology of extracts of avian pituitaries to establish their composition; it was, in fact, by the use of such a pharmacological profile that the existence of vasotocin in chicken pituitaries was established.

Antibodies to both oxytocin and vasopressin, either free or conjugated with serum albumin or polylysine, can be raised in rabbits and sheep. This has permitted the development of radioimmunoassays for both compounds. Because of the relatively small size of the antigen, a wider choice for separation of free and antibody-bound peptide is available to the analyst. The radioimmunoassay for oxytocin covers the range 0.01–10 ng/ml, while that for either lysine or arginine vasopressin is useful for concentrations between 10–1000 ng/ml (Chard, 1973).

II. Chemistry

All of the neurohypophyseal hormones, including oxytocin, vasopressin, and their analogs are nonapeptides, possessing, as characteristic features, a hexapeptide ring bridged by a disulfide bond and a tripeptide "tail" (Fig. 12.1). All the known hormones possess similar structures, with variations in amino acid residues occurring at positions 3, 4, and 8. The structure of bovine oxytocin was established in 1953 by the Cornell group led by du Vigneaud and independently by Tuppy and Michl (1953).

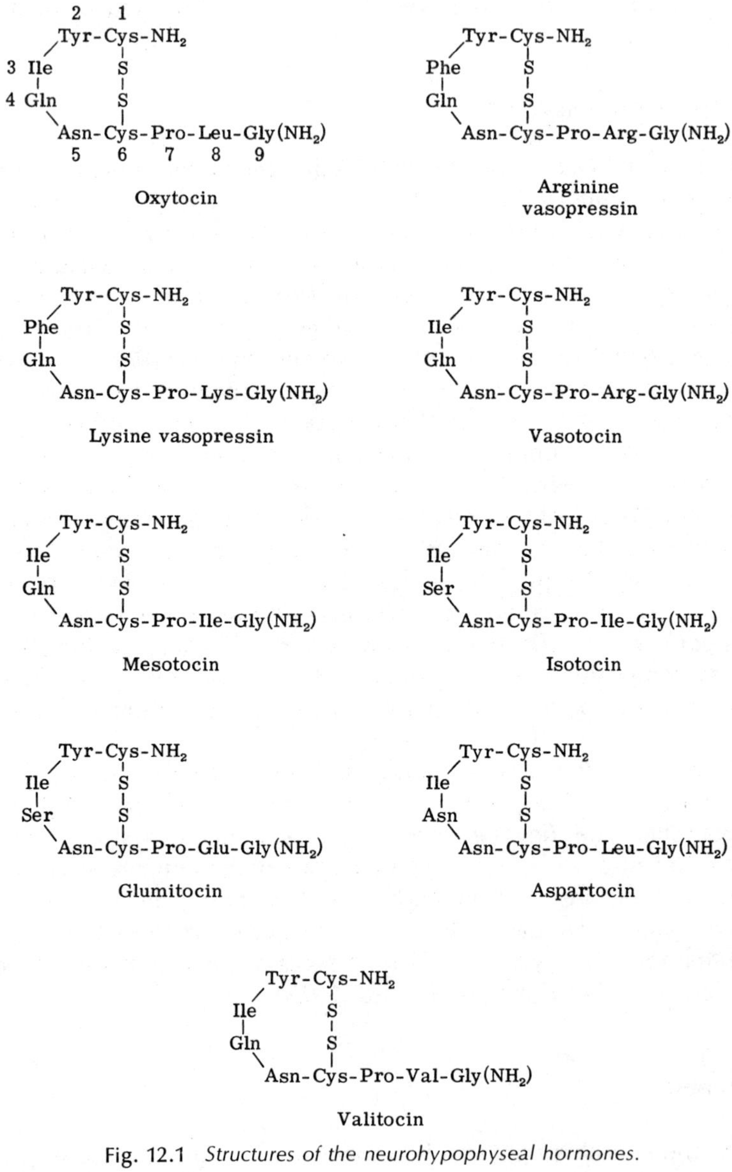

Fig. 12.1 *Structures of the neurohypophyseal hormones.*

In addition to being present in the pituitaries of all mammalian species examined thus far, oxytocin has been found in the pituitaries of birds, amphibians, reptiles, teleost fishes, lungfishes, and the ratfish, a cartilagenous fish.

Two vasopressins occur in mammals: arginine vasopressin (Phe^3,Arg^8-

oxytocin) and lysine vasopressin (Phe^3,Lys^8-oxytocin). Arginine vasopressin is more ubiquitous, appearing in rats, dogs, sheep, cattle, camels, monkeys, and man. It has also been found in a marsupial (opossum) and in a monotrene (the spiny anteater). Lysine vasopressin is confined to the pituitaries of domestic pigs and certain of its relatives, including the hippopotamus. Peccaries and wart hogs, inhabitants of semiarid regions, have retained the capacity to produce both vasopressins; examination of individual peccary pituitaries has shown that some animals produce one, some the other, while in still others, both hormones were found.

About 30 years ago Heller (1941) observed that extracts of pigeon pituitaries were much more active in stimulating water uptake by intact frogs than could be accounted for by any reasonable combination of oxytocin and vasopressin. A similar conclusion was reached by Munsick *et al.* in 1960, on the basis of assays of chicken pituitaries. In addition to ocytocin, these extracts were shown to contain a substance which was pharmacologically and chromatographically indistinguishable from Arg^8-oxytocin (arginine vasotocin), synthesized by Katsoyannis and du Vigneaud 2 years earlier (1958). Arginine vasotocin has been found in the pituitaries of every important nonmammalian group of animals except the elasmobranchs and is the only active peptide to be found in cyclostomes. Sawyer has suggested that arginine vasotocin is probably ancestral to all other neurohypophyseal hormones.

Five other analogs of oxytocin (or vasotocin) have been found in various orders of vertebrates. Mesotocin (Ile^8-oxytocin), as well as oxytocin, occurs in amphibians and reptiles. Isotocin (Ser^4,Ile^8-oxytocin) is found in bony fishes (Whittlestone, 1969). Variants of oxytocin seem to be more numerous among the cartilaginous fishes (sharks, dogfish, rays, and ratfish); glumitocin (Ser^4, Glu^8-oxytocin), aspartocin (Asn^4-oxytocin), and valitocin (Val^8-oxytocin) have been found in this group of animals. Unlike the other nonmammalian vertebrates, the pituitaries of cartilaginous fishes contain only small amounts of vasotocin (Acher *et al.*, 1972).

Several attempts have been made to work out reasonable schemes for the evolution of these hormones. Because of its ubiquitous occurrence, arginine vasotocin is assumed to be the ancestral nonapeptide. Six of the nine residues are invariant in all known oxytocic and pressor hormones. Consideration of possible mutations (single amino acid changes) leads to a scheme such as outlined in Fig. 12.2. Since cartilaginous and bony fishes arose from a common ancestor and diverged about 450,000,000 years ago, Acher *et al.* (1972) have suggested that arginine vasotocin has a minimum "age" of 500,000,000 years; mesotocin, 400,000,000; isotocin, 300,000,000; and aspartocin, glumitocin, and valitocin less than 180,000,000 years.

The occurrence of oxytocin in birds, amphibians, and reptiles indicates

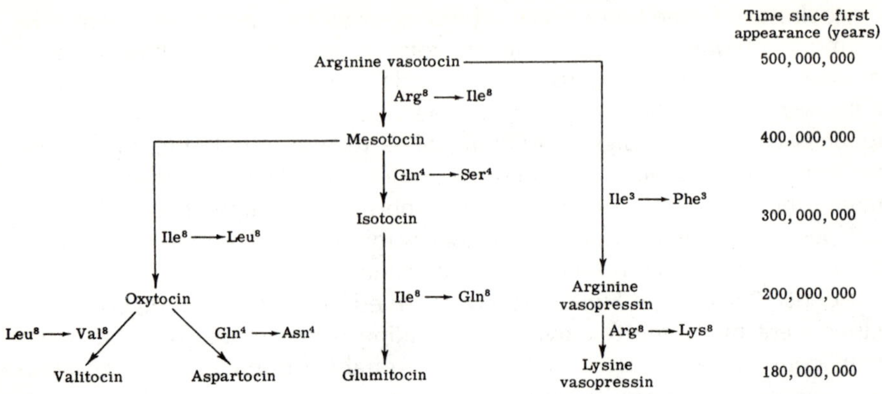

Fig. 12.2 *Hypothetical evolution of the neurohypophyseal hormones. Modified from Acher et al. (1972).*

that this hormone appeared at least 200,000,000 years ago; depending upon the significance of its presence in bony and cartilaginous fishes it could be much older.

III. Comparative Pharmacology

The synthetic genius of du Vigneaud, Boissonas, and others has made it possible to produce a large number of compounds which represent slight to major modifications of the structures of the naturally occurring neurohypophyseal hormones. As a result, a great deal is now known about the relationship between their chemical structures and physiological activities. Tables 12.1 and 12.2 include data concerning the comparative activities, in six bioassays, of 55 analogs of oxytocin or vasopressin.* The reference standard (the International Unit, IU) is defined as the activity of 0.5 mg of a sample of posterior lobe powder prepared expressly for the purpose. The current (1970) standard is the third in use since the first reference standard was prepared in 1926.

Nearly all the modifications which have been introduced into the oxytocin or vasopressin molecules have the effect of reducing or abolishing activity, whether measured *in vivo* or *in vitro*. Exceptions are 1-desaminooxytocin, which is significantly more active than oxytocin itself in both the rat uterus and avian depressor assays, and Ile^3 vasopressin (vasotocin), which has many times the frog bladder permeability activity of va-

* A summary of the activities of 115 analogs of oxytocin and vasopressin has been compiled by Schwartz and Livingston (1964). Note that estimates of analog activities, as reported by different authors, are frequently very different.

TABLE 12.1 Comparative Biological Activities of Oxytocin Analogs[a]

Compound	Activity (IU/mg)					
	Rat oxytocic	Avian depressor	Milk ejection	Rat pressor	Rat antidiuretic	Bladder permeability
Oxytocin (O)	450	450	450	5	5	360
1-Desamino O	685	733	400	1.1	15	75
1-*N*-Leucyl O	23	3			0.3	
1-Desamino-Phe^{2} O	25	61		0.04		
1-Desamino-Abu^{4} O[b]	95	180	270		0	0
Ala^{1,6} O (desthio O)	0	0				
Phe^{2} O	30	60	60	0.4	0.5	18
allo-Ile^{3} O	25	22	125	0.2	0.05	
Leu^{3} O	45		100			
N-Leu^{3} O	2–10	10–20		<1	<1	
Phe^{3} O (oxypressin)	16	45	90	3	18	<20
Val^{3} O	60		210			
Abu^{4} O	70	110	225	0.1	0.25	
Ala^{4} O	36	65	240	0	0	
β-Ala^{4} O	0.1	0.4	0.5	<0.1		
Asn^{4} O (aspartocin)	108	202	300	0.1	<0.1	
Glu^{4} O	1.5	0.5	11	0	0	
Gly^{4} O	5.5	2.8	17			
Ser^{4} O	195	230	255	<0.1	<0.1	
Asn^{4},Gln^{5} O	0.4	0.3		0.1		
Ser^{4},Ile^{8} O (isotocin)	150	320	300	<0.1	<1	
Ala^{5} O	0.25	0.25	1	0	0	
Ala^{8} O	141	135	208			
Gln^{8} O	58		256	34	5.9	1270
Gly^{8} O	16	7	46			
Ile^{8} O (mesotocin)	290	500	330		1	800
Val^{8} O (valitocin)	200	280	310			
Gly^{9} O (9-deamido O)	1.3	0.2	1.2	0		
9-Decarboxamide O	7	0	4	0	0	
(D)Cys^{1} O	2	0.2	0.4		0	
(D)Tyr^{2} O	6	34	34			
(D)Cys^{6} O	<0.1	0	0			
(D)Pro^{7} O	13	0	3.9			
(D)Leu^{8} O	20	20	50	0	0	
All (D) O	0	0				

[a] *Principal references: Schwartz and Livingston (1964); Sawyer (1966a,b); Jost and Rudinger (1969).*

[b] *Abu, α-aminobutyryl.*

TABLE 12.2 Comparative Biological Activities of Vasopressin Analogs[a]

	Activity (IU/mg)					
Compound[b]	Rat oxytocic	Avian depressor	Milk ejection	Rat pressor	Rat anti-diuretic	Bladder perme-ability
Vasopressin (VP)	15	55	65	400	430	70
Ala^{1,6} VP (desthio VP)		10		33	<0.1	
Phe^{2} VP	0.1	1	3	70	20	<6
Ile^{3} VP (vasotocin)	95	250	180	220	225	30,000
Ile^{3},Thr^{4} VP	200	830		105	280	
Ile^{3},Citr^{8} VP	80	120			4	800
Ile^{3},Orn^{8} VP	40	90	95	100		
Thr^{4} VP	19	320		105	230	
Citr^{8} VP	13		70	40	40	<5
His^{8} VP	7	5	20	2		<10
Leu^{8} VP (oxypressin)	16	30	90	3	30	20
Orn^{8} VP	10	20	50	360	90	
Lys^{8} VP (lysine vasopressin)	5	45	45	250	225	<20
1-*N*-Acetyl Lys^{8} VP		Inhibitory	0.1	Inhibitory		
1-Desamino, Lys^{8} VP	10	60	30	125	300	
Phe^{2},Lys^{8} VP	0.1	1	3	70	20	<6
Ile^{3},Lys^{8} VP	80	210	180	130	25	1,500
Abu^{4},Lys^{8} VP	1.5	15		10	710	
Ala^{4},Lys^{8} VP	0.5	2.2		1.6	30	
Asn^{4},Lys^{8} VP	3	25		55	25	
Ser^{4},Lys^{8} VP	0.9	10		3.3	70	
Thr^{4},Lys^{8} VP	13	265		50	155	

[a] *Principal references: Schwartz and Livingston (1964); Sawyer (1966a,b); Manning et al. (1973).*

[b] *Abu: α-aminobutyryl; Citr: citrulline.*

sopressin. However, acylation of the amino terminal nitrogen (1-*N*-leucyl oxytocin) severely reduces oxytocin activity, and 1-*N*-acetyl lysine vasopressin has been reported to inhibit vasopressin activity. Even such modest changes as replacing isoleucine by leucine (Leu^{3}-oxytocin), or leucine by isoleucine or valine (Ile^{8}-oxytocin, Val^{8}-oxytocin) result in compounds possessing reduced activity. The amino acids in positions 2, 4, 5, and 6 all share a common sensitivity to alteration; data concerning the effect of modifying residue 7 (Pro), however, are limited. If the glutamine and asparagine residues at 4 and 5, respectively, are interchanged (Asn^{4},Gln^{5}-oxytocin) all activity is lost, whereas if the sole change is replacement of Gln^{4} by Asn^{4} (aspartocin) significant activity remains. Apparently, the net charge in this region of the molecule is important, since Glu^{4}-oxytocin (with a free carboxyl group) is almost completely inactive.

Other features of the oxytocin molecule which appear to be indispensable are the cyclic disulfide (Ala^{1,6}-oxytocin is devoid of activity), its size (4-isoglutamine, 5-isoasparagine, and 4β-alanine oxytocins are inactive), and the amide and carboxamide functions at residue 9 (Gly^{9} and 9-decarboxamide oxytocins). Only a trace (<5%) of activity survives replacement of the cysteine, tyrosine, isoleucine, proline, or leucine residues by their enantiomeric forms.

A basic side chain, with arginine, lysine, or ornithine at residue 8 appears to be a *sine-qua-non* for pressor or antidiuretic activity. Although oxytocin and mesotocin (Ile^{8}-oxytocin) possess moderate water balance activity on the bullfrog bladder, they possess little or no pressor or antidiuretic activity in mammals. The vasopressins, potent pressor and antidiuretic agents, have little effect on water balance in birds and amphibians; the latter property seems to be reserved for the vasotocins, compounds with the pentapeptide ring of oxytocin and the basic side chain characteristic of the vasopressins. With respect to water balance activity, the vasotocins are from five to eighty times as active as oxytocin; they also display an important measure of oxytocic and milk ejection activity, arginine vasotocin being from one-fourth to one-half as active as oxytocin.

Another interesting molecule is oxypressin, a hybrid with the pentapeptide ring of vasopressin and the oxytocin side chain (Phe^{3}-oxytocin or Leu^{8}-vasopressin). Unlike vasotocin, which retains potent pressor and water balance activity even in mammals, oxypressin displays only minimal activity in any of the assays listed.

Walter and Chen (1967) have prepared an interesting series of peptides–oxytocin analogs in which selenium has replaced sulfur (Table 12.3). If either cysteine residue is replaced by its selenium counterpart the resulting molecule retains nearly all the oxytocic and milk-ejecting activity of the parent molecule. In these compounds, as in oxytocin itself, removal of

TABLE 12.3 Biological Properties of Selenium Analogs of Oxytocin

	Activity, IU/mg				
Compound	Rat oxytocic	Avian depressor	Milk ejection	Rat pressor	Rat antidiuretic
Oxytocin	546	507	410	3.1	2.7
Desaminooxytocin	684	733	400	1.1	15.0
1-Se-Oxytocin[a]	362	361	351	3.1	5.7
Desamino-1-Se-oxytocin	560	613	248	1.7	24.0
6-Se-Oxytocin[a]	405	385	398	3.8	3.4
Desamino-6-Se-oxytocin	492	622	397	1.1	15.5

[a] *The numbers indicate the position of the cysteine residue in which Se replaces S.*

the terminal amino group markedly enhances oxytocic, avian-depressor, and milk-ejection activity, while diminishing pressor and antidiuretic activity.

IV. Neurophysin

In 1942, Van Dyke *et al.* reported the isolation, from bovine posterior pituitary lobes, of a protein which possessed oxytocic, pressor, and antidiuretic hormone activities in proportions similar to those found in the reference posterior pituitary standard. This material, which appeared to be homogeneous by several criteria then in general use, was described as having a molecular weight of 30,000. It was later discovered (Acher *et al.*, 1956; Chauvet *et al.*, 1960) that similar proteins could be isolated from the neurohypophyses of sheep, horses and pigs, and that oxytocin and vasopressin could be separated from the larger "carrier" molecule in acid solution. The name *neurophysin* was applied to the carrier protein by Acher, Chauvet, and Lenci (1958).

Recent studies of the chemical properties of neurophysin indicate that at least three well-defined proteins that bind the nonapeptide hormones stoichiometrically may be separated from extracts of bovine or porcine posterior pituitary glands (Rauch *et al.*, 1969; Cheng and Friesen, 1971). The bovine neurophysins (neurophysins-I, -II, and -C) are molecules of similar size, differing in amino acid composition and in electrophoretic mobility. Each appears to possess one binding site (for either oxytocin or vasopressin) per molecule. Crystalline complexes of arginine vasopressin with each of the bovine neurophysins have been isolated. Two of the porcine neurophysins are similar in size and amino acid composition to the corresponding bovine proteins; the third has a significantly higher molecular weight.

The complete amino acid sequences of bovine neurophysin-II and porcine neurophysin-I have been elucidated; each consists of a 97-amino acid peptide with 7 disulfide bridges (Schlesinger *et al.*, 1972; Wuu *et al.*, 1971). The amino terminal sequence of bovine neurophysin-I has also been reported (Capra *et al.*, 1972). Comparison of the known sequences indicates a high degree of homology, especially in the amino-terminal half of the molecule. Similarities of short sequences in some regions of the neurophysins to those found in oxytocin and vasopressin have suggested the possibility that ". . . the structural genes encoding the neurohypophyseal hormones may have been incorporated into the genes that eventually gave rise to their carriers, the neurohypophysins" (Capra *et al.*, 1972).

All of the neurophysins can bind either oxytocin or vasopressin *in vitro*.

In the gland itself, however, a selection process may occur. Dean *et al.* (1968) were able to sort out populations of neurosecretory granules, some of which were rich in oxytocin, others in vasopressin. Oxytocin was localized in granules containing predominantly neurophysin-I, whereas vasopressin-rich granules contained mostly neurophysin-II. Secretion of the posterior lobe hormones in association with different carriers may serve as a mechanism for independent release of oxytocin and vasopressin.

13

Hypothalamic-Releasing Hormones (RH)

The first attempt to directly demonstrate the existence of a pituitary regulating substance was the effort of Saffran and Schally (1955) to show the existence of a corticotropin-releasing hormone (CRH). Rat anterior pituitary lobes were incubated in the presence of fragments or extracts of other tissues for 1 hour. At the end of the incubation period, the medium and the recovered pituitary fragments were assayed separately for ACTH by the Saffran–Schally technique (see Chapter 10, Section II, A, 2). A positive response was recorded if the amount of ACTH released into the medium in the presence of the fragment or extract was greater than that released by the same weight of pituitary tissue in a control incubation.

Similar *in vitro* techniques have been used to show the existence of all releasing factors, as well as those substances which inhibit the release of prolactin and melanocyte-stimulating hormone, MSH. Rat anterior pituitary fragments cultured in a totally synthetic (199) medium have also been used (McCann and Brobek, 1954). Such explants, which remain functional for 2 weeks or longer, are especially useful for the study of release-inhibiting hormones.

The earliest *in vivo* assays of releasing hormones were also devised to detect CRH. Porter and Jones (1956) attempted to prove the existence of CRH in plasma obtained from hypothalamicohypophyseal vessels of hypophysectomized dogs by injecting the plasma into rats and measuring the fall in adrenal ascorbic acid. The rats were treated with hydrocortisone to suppress endogenous ACTH secretion, thus avoiding interference from stress occasioned by adrenalectomy. The same principle has been applied in the assay of TRH (release of ^{131}I from thyroids of ^{131}I-treated rats) and LH-RH (depletion of ovarian ascorbic acid). For the *in vivo* assay of FSH-RH and GH-RH, plasma concentrations of these hormones in recipient animals (also rats) were determined by suitable procedures, usually radioimmunoassays.

In 1965, David, Fraschini, and Martini, as well as Pecile *et al.* (1965) described experiments designed to establish the existence of FSH-RH and GH-RH; both were based upon the observation that the injection of a releasing hormone was quickly followed by a reduction in the pituitary stores of the corresponding tropic hormone. Subsequently, assays based upon the pituitary depletion principle were described for TRH, LH-RH and MRIH (MSH release-inhibiting hormone).

I. Thyrotropin-Releasing Hormone (TRH)

The existence of TRH was demonstrated about 10 years ago (Schreiber *et al.,* 1961; Guillemin *et al.,* 1963). Both bovine and porcine hypothalami

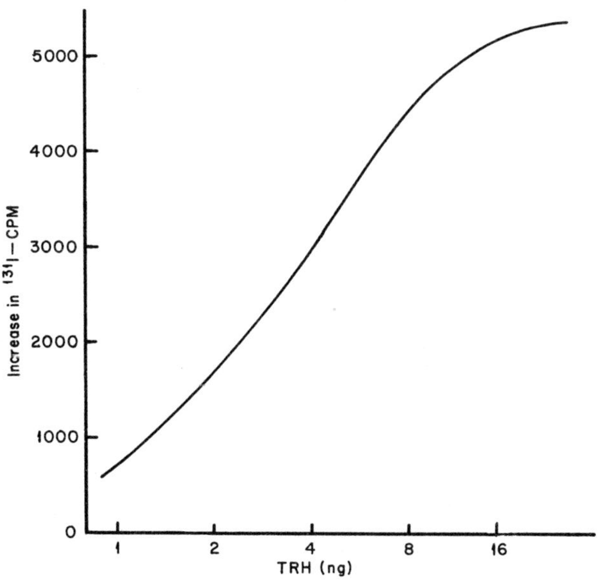

Fig. 13.1 *Assay of TRH in mice in vivo. Data of Boler et al. (1969).*

were used in these experiments. Because of the readier availability of porcine median eminences, TRH was first isolated from this source.

A. ASSAY

In vitro, TRH can be detected by incubating rat anterior pituitary sections with a hypothalamic extract, then assaying the TSH released into the medium by a standard TSH assay (e.g., discharge of labeled iodine into the circulation of rats previously given $Na^{131}I$). The *in vivo* assay essentially combines the separate steps into one; the experimental animals (mice) are first pretreated with labeled iodide, thyroxine, and codeine (to suppress endogenous TRH). After 48 hours, a solution containing TRH is injected and the radioactivity of the blood is determined 2 hours later (Redding *et al.*, 1966). A control blood sample is taken before TRH is injected. Figure 13.1 indicates the data obtained. Purified TRH is active in the codeine–thyroxine-blocked mouse at a dose of 15 ng or less, while 0.1 ng is sufficient for a response *in vitro.*

B. CHEMICAL PROPERTIES

Early work on the properties of TRH indicated that although part (but not all) of the compound could be accounted for by three amino acids (glutamic acid, histidine, and proline, present in approximately equimolar amounts) TRH was not a simple tripeptide. It lost activity when hydrolyzed with 6 *N* HCl, but it was resistant to a variety of proteolytic enzymes, including trypsin, chymotrypsin, pepsin, and aminopeptidase. Although the three amino acids accounted for only about 30% of the weight of the sample, the sequence Glu-His-Pro was always present. When TRH was chromatographed, activity invariably coincided with a Pauly-positive (i.e., imidazole) spot. Therefore attempts to identify the compound revolved around the properties of this tripeptide.

Folkers *et al.* (1969) tested eight synthetic peptides containing Glu (or Gln), Pro, and His, but none possessed significant TRH activity. This was not unexpected, since it was known that TRH possessed no free amino or carboxyl group. For this reason, further research centered about modifications of Glu-His-Pro. When this compound was esterified in methanolic HCl and the diester dissolved in methanolic ammonia, a highly active product resulted. Boler *et al.* (1969) subsequently identified TRH with pyroglutamylhistidylprolinamide (Fig. 13.2) by synthesizing the latter (which possessed high activity) and comparing its chromatographic and biological properties with those native TRH.

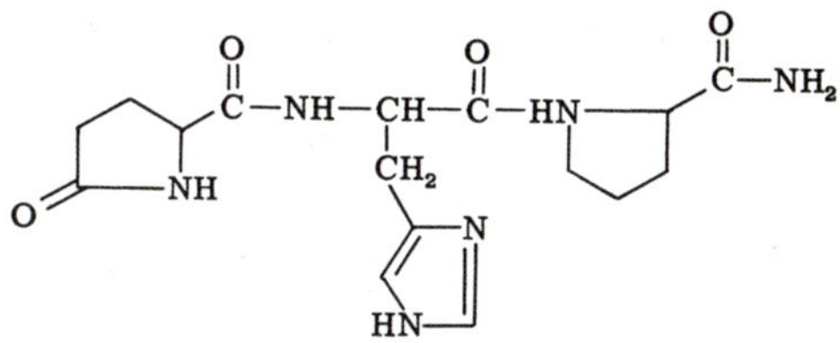

(I)

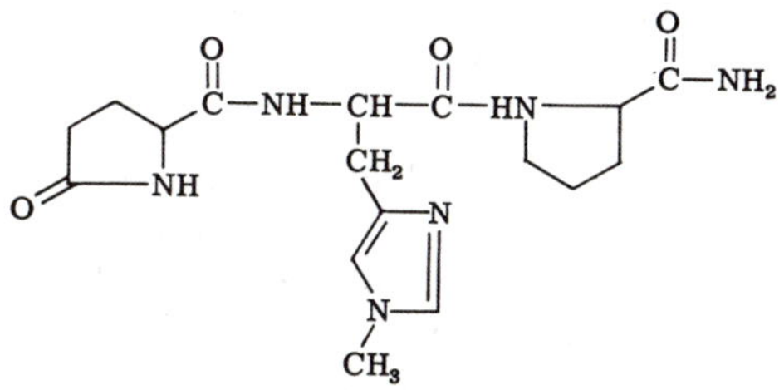

(II)

Fig. 13.2 *Structures of pyroglutamylhistidylprolinamide (TRH, I) and pyroglutamyl($N^{3\text{-Im}}$-methyl)histidylprolinamide (II).*

Bowers *et al.* (1970) have examined the properties of 15 synthetic tripeptides related to TRH. Most of the modifications involved changes in the imidazole or prolinamide parts of the molecule. Most were essentially inactive, but a few were 0.2–5.0% as active as native TRH. These included pyroGlu-His-Pro($NHCH_3$) (2%); pyroGlu-His-Val(NH_2) (0.2%); pyroGlu-His-Pro(OMe) (4%); pyroGlu-His-Ala(NH_2) (0.2%); and pyroGlu-β (3-pyrazolyl)-Ala-Pro(NH_2) (5%). Although the synthetic analogs were not as active as the native hormone, they were invariably more resistant than the latter to the TRH-inactivating action of serum.

Of the dozens of compounds which have been synthesized and tested for TRH activity only one has been found which approaches (indeed, exceeds) native TRH in biological activity (Vale *et al.*, 1971). This is pyroGlu-$N^{3\text{-Im}}$ Methyl-His-Pro(NH_2), the structure of which is also shown in Fig. 13.2.

This compound is approximately 8 times as active as native (or synthetic) TRH when tested on cultures of rat pituitary cells *in vitro*. If the methyl group is moved to N^5, activity is completely lost. The active methyl derivative was also more resistant than the native hormone to inactivation by serum.

II. Gonadotropin-Releasing Hormone (FSH- and LH-RH)

It was noted earlier (see Chapter 1, Section VII) that normal gonadal function in rats is critically dependent upon adequate vascular connections between the hypothalamus and the anterior pituitary. McCann, Taleisnik, and Friedman, in 1960, showed that acid extracts of stalk median eminence (SME) were able to deplete ovarian ascorbic acid and drew the conclusion that LH release was being stimulated. Later, Igarishi and McCann (1964) showed that similar extracts (including rat SME extracts) would elevate plasma FSH in estrogen- and progesterone-blocked rats; the existence of an FSH-releasing factor in median eminence extracts was confirmed by the pituitary depletion method (Kuroshima *et al.*, 1966) and by effects upon pituitary cells *in vitro* (Mittler and Meites, 1964; Kuroshima *et al.*, 1965).

During the fractionation of crude porcine hypothalamic extracts on Sephadex and carboxymethylcellulose, FSH- and LH-releasing activities were found to emerge in the same or overlapping fractions. Separation of the gonadotropin-releasing factors was reported when bovine SME extracts were chromatographed on Sephadex (Schally *et al.*, 1968a). Subsequently, Schally also claimed that porcine FSH-RH and LH-RH could be separated by column electrophoresis at pH 6.5 (at which pH LH-RH was essentially immobile). The FSH-RH preparation resulting from this experiment was active when tested *in vivo* in the range 4–10 ng, but 25–50 ng had no LH-RH activity. Later, however, it was found that a highly purified (10–25-ng effective dose) LH-RH preparation possessed intrinsic FSH-RH activity, and it was not possible to separate the two activities in any of 10 partition chromatography systems employed; furthermore, during the fractionation procedure the recovery of both activities approached 100%. Finally, a synthetic decapeptide identical in amino acid sequence with naturally occurring LH-RH proved to have FSH-releasing activity as well. At the present time, it appears that only one gonadotropic hormone-releasing factor (gon-RH) exists in mammalian hypothalami, and that both FSH and LH are subject to its control.*

Gon-RH has been isolated from bovine, ovine, and porcine hypothalami; in addition extracts containing FSH- and/or LH-releasing activity have been concentrated from rat, chicken, and human hypothalami. Bovine (or porcine) gon-RH will stimulate the release of LH from rat, hamster, rabbit, sheep, pig, monkey, cow, and human pituitaries and will cause premature ovulation in chickens (Schally, 1973). A concomitant release of

* Additional evidence for the existence of a separate FSH-releasing factor is based upon the observation that the maximum release of FSH from rat pituitaries which can be evoked by some side fractions is greater than that evoked by purified (or synthetic) gon-RH (Johansson *et al.*, 1973; Currie *et al.*, 1973; Bowers *et al.*, 1973).

FSH has also been shown in some of these animals. Usually, FSH release requires the injection of considerably higher concentrations of releasing hormone than does LH release.

A. ASSAY

1. *LH-RH*

The most commonly used procedure for the assay of LH-releasing hormone is essentially a modification of the Parlow assay for LH itself (see Chapter 10, Section III, A, 1). Rats are treated with chorionic gonadotropin and the ascorbic acid content of one ovary is determined. One hour after the injection of the sample, the ascorbic acid content of the other ovary is determined. A more or less linear relationship exists between the log dose of LH-RH and the depletion (expressed as percent decrease) of ovarian ascorbic acid (McCann and Taleisnik, 1962). Contamination by LH, which would obviously interfere, may be eliminated by heating or by ultrafiltration of the sample.

Measurement of plasma LH may also be used as an index of LH-RH activity. From the limited data available, it appears that peak LH concentrations are reached 10 minutes after injection of hypothalamic material. The test animal in this procedure is the ovariectomized, estrogen- and progesterone-blocked female, or the testosterone-treated castrated male rat. Assays for gonadotropin-releasing hormone which depend upon measurement of plasma LH are 20–40 times as sensitive as those which depend upon ovarian ascorbic acid depletion, but are not as amenable to quantitative application.

When rat hemipituitaries are incubated in a synthetic tissue culture (199) medium in the presence of LH-RH, a linear relationship exists between the amount of LH released into the medium and the logarithm of the amount of hypothalamic extract added. McCann (1970) has concluded that the *in vitro* assay for LH-RH is the best available.

2. *FSH-RH*

As with LH-RH, both *in vivo* and *in vitro* methods for FSH-RH assay are available. The optimal conditions for *in vivo* assays include the use of castrated female rats in which endogenous release of pituitary gonadotropins has been blocked by giving estrogen and progesterone a few days earlier. The animals are then injected with the sample and sacrificed within 25–60 minutes. Either the fall in pituitary FSH or the rise in plasma FSH may be measured; for pituitary FSH the Steelman–Pohley method (see Chapter 10,

Section III, A, 1) is most often used, while plasma FSH often requires the more sensitive mouse uterine weight augmentation method (Kuroshima *et al.*, 1966). Significant (50–60%) depletion of pituitary FSH can be brought about by the injection of no more than one-half to three-fourths of a rat hypothalamus (David *et al.*, 1965). Kuroshima and others have shown that the fall in pituitary FSH and the rise in plasma FSH following a single injection of bovine SME extract are mirror images of each other; minima and maxima, respectively, occur in about 20 minutes.

For the measurement of FSH-RH *in vitro,* two basic procedures have been used. Mittler and Meites (1964) cultured rat pituitary fragments for 3 days, and then added a hypothalamic extract; they found the medium contained considerably more FSH than if the extract had not been added. Rat pituitary fragments have also been exposed to median eminence extracts for shorter periods (Kuroshima *et al.*, 1965; Schally *et al.*, 1967). After a single hour of incubation with purified pig hypothalamic extract, pituitaries from ovariectomized, steroid-blocked rats released significant quantities of FSH.

Guinea pigs respond to the injection of adjuvant-treated gon-RH by developing a respectable antibody titer. Using guinea pig antiserum, a radioimmunoassay for gon-RH has been developed (Kerdelhue *et al.*, 1973). The useful range is 0.1–10 ng, and the curve obtained with median eminence extracts was superimposable over the standard curve obtained with the synthetic hormone.

B. CHEMICAL PROPERTIES

From 240,000 pig hypothalami, weighing 5.4 kg after lyophilization, Schally *et al.* (1971d) isolated 11.4 mg of purified gonadotropin-releasing hormone, shown to be homogeneous by chromatography and electrophoresis. This material increased the plasma LH of steroid-blocked ovariectomized rats by 60% when only 0.25 ng was given; it also released FSH from rat pituitaries *in vitro* when present at 0.5–2.0 ng/ml. The active compound proved to be a decapeptide with the sequence:

(pyro)-Glu-His-Trp-Ser-Tyr-Gly-Leu-Arg-Pro-Gly(NH_2)

(Schally *et al.*, 1971a; Matsuo *et al.*, 1971; Baba *et al.*, 1971). Final proof of the chemical identity of the decapeptide in gonadotropin-releasing hormone was achieved with its synthesis, in three laboratories, and with the demonstration of its biological identity with the native hormone (Schally *et al.*, 1971b; 1972). Ovine gon-RH, isolated by Amoss *et al.* (1971), has the same structure (Burgus *et al.*, 1972). The structures of gon-RH's from other kinds of animals are not known to be identical with the bovine hormone.

Jackson (1971b) compared the chromatographic properties of chicken and rat gon-RH. The two compounds could not be separated on a Sephadex G-25 column. This indicates that their molecular weights were similar, if not identical; however, on carboxymethyl Sephadex C-25, chicken gon-RH emerged first when a mixture of the two was chromatographed with an ammonium acetate gradient of increasing concentration and pH, pointing to a distinctly more basic character for rat gon-RH.

Since 1971, many laboratories have reported the synthesis of gon-RH by both classical and solid-phase methods. In addition, a considerable number of gon-RH analogs have been prepared and tested for FSH or LH releasing activity. Like TRH, gon-RH is less active when the pyroglutamyl ring is opened; the product (Glu^1-gon-RH) has only 6% of the activity of the native hormone. Removal of the N-terminal pyro-glu residue (des-pyro-glu-gon-RH) reduces activity more than a hundredfold. Ala^4-gon-RH (removing the OH group in residue 4) is only 6% as active as the parent decapeptide. Phe^5-gon-RH, in which phenylalanine replaces tyrosine, retains the full activity of the native hormone, but *p*-substitution of the benzene ring progressively reduces activity as the substituent becomes bulkier (*p*-amino-Phe^5-gon-RH, *p*-methoxy, Phe^5-gon-RH and *p*-nitro-Phe^5-gon-RH retain 37%, 24%, and 5%, respectively, of the original activity). Replacement of the leucine residue at position 7 by valine, isoleucine, or norleucine reduces activity by 50–85%, while Lys^8-gon-RH (in which lysine replaces arginine) is totally inactive. Although all activity is lost upon hydrolysis of the glycinamide terminus, some activity is restored upon the complete removal of the glycine residue. Thus $Gly(OH)^{10}$-gon-RH has less than 0.1%, but des-$Gly(NH_2)^{10}$-gon-RH retains about 10% of the activity of the native decapeptide. Further shortening of the chain at the C-terminal end, however, completely destroys activity (Sievertssen *et al.*, 1972; Chang *et al.*, 1972; Coy *et al.*, 1973; Yanaihara *et al.*, 1973; Rivier *et al.*, 1973).

Perhaps the most interesting series of gon-RH analogs were obtained by alkylation of the amide N of $Pro(NH_2)^9$,des-$Gly(NH_2)^{10}$-gon-RH; some of these compounds were distinctly more active than the parent hormone (Table 13.1).

Reversing the order of the Arg-Pro sequence at the C-terminal end (Pro^8,Arg^9 gon-RH) results in greatly diminished activity. Since such a change would result in a marked steric effect, it has been suggested that this region is probably involved when the molecule binds to its receptor site.

In general, changes in LH-RH activity are accompanied by corresponding changes in FSH-RH activity.

Des-His^2-gon-RH and Gly^2-gon-RH are both relatively inactive. When present in high concentration, however, either compound is capable of

TABLE 13.1 Activities of Gon-RH Analogs

Compound	LH-RH activity
pyroGlu · · · Pro-Gly(NH_2) (native FSH/LH-RH)	100
pyroGlu · · · Pro-GlyOH	0.1
pyroGlu · · · Pro(NH_2)	11
pyroGlu · · · ProNH(CH_3)	80–100
pyroGlu · · · ProNH(C_2H_5)	500
pyroGlu · · · ProNH(C_3H_7)	200–300
pyroGlu · · · ProNH(C_2H_4OH)	100–150

evoking a limited LH release. More interesting is the fact that they can act as LH-RH inhibitors. In the presence of 10^{-4}-10^{-5} *M* analog, the response of rat pituitary cultures to 10^{-8} *M* synthetic gon-RH was reduced by about 50%.

Grant and Vale (1972) have remarked upon some curious parallels between TRH and gon-RH. In both molecules, an N-terminal pyroglutamylhistidyl moiety is essential, as is a C-terminal amide (or substituted amide) feature. In both, a proline residue near the C-terminus is essential. As determined from molecular models, one of the stable configurations of gon-RH is one in which the C-terminal amide is juxtaposed to the N-terminal dipeptide, a configuration which is obligatory in TRH. The common features of the two releasing hormones are further emphasized by the fact that a highly potent TRH homolog, pyroGlu-His-Pro-Gly(NH_2) has some LH-RH activity. The juxtaposition of pyroglutamyl and prolineamide or glycineamide residues may constitute a "signal", recognized by various kinds of pituitary cells. Finally, it may be of some significance, not only that TSH, FSH, and LH are all glycoproteins, but also that their peptide chains bear more than a casual resemblance to each other.

III. Somatotropin-Releasing (GH-RH) and Release-Inhibiting Hormones (GH-RIH)

In 1960, Reichlin described the results of experiments which explored the effects of hypothalamic lesions upon the growth of young rats. He found that massive lesions, especially those involving the anterior half of the median eminence, reduced growth rates significantly. Atrophy or dysfunction of the thyroid, gonad, or adrenal glands were excluded as possible causes, and he concluded that growth hormone secretion was deficient in lesioned animals. Electrical stimulation of the median eminence, on the other hand, was followed by an increase in the concentration of circulating growth hormone (Frohman and Bernardis, 1968). Some hypothalamic extracts, added to rat pituitaries *in vitro* or injected into monkeys, sheep, or properly prepared rats, will increase the amount of growth hormone released into the medium or into the circulation (Deuben and Meites, 1964; Pecile *et al.,* 1965). Other hypothalamic preparations, added to growth hormone-secreting pituitary cells in monolayer cultures, will significantly depress the release of growth hormone (Brazeau *et al.,* 1973). These facts, as well as others, point to the existence of both growth hormone releasing (GH-RH) and growth hormone release-inhibiting (GH-RIH) factors in the hypothalamus.

A. GH-RH

Growth hormone releasing activity has been demonstrated in hypothalamic extracts prepared from cattle, pigs, dogs, rabbits, and pigeons (Ishida *et al.,* 1965; Mueller *et al.,* 1967). Less significant effects were obtained with extracts of frog, mouse, and kitten hypothalami. Human hypothalamus has also been found to contain GH-RH.

1. *Assay*

Assays for GH-RH utilize both *in vitro* and *in vivo* (pituitary depletion) methods. Schally *et al.* (1968b) preincubated rat pituitary fragments for 30–60 minutes, discarded the medium, and continued the incubation for 6–7 hours in the presence of the sample being assayed. Growth hormone in the medium was determined by means of the tibia test (see Chapter 10, Section I, A). The addition of 0.03–10 μg of purified GH-RH to 5 ml of incubation medium resulted in the release (during 6–7 hours) of 180–300 μg of GH (NIH-GH-S7 equivalents) into the medium; however the data did not provide a useful dose–response curve. Later, however, Schally showed that a graded response to 0.1–10 pg of purified porcine GH-RH could be achieved. When the incubation period was extended to 24 hours the amount of GH-RH released also increased, but irregularly. The release of growth hormone into the medium was not accompanied by a significant decrease in the growth hormone content of the tissue, except during prolonged (24 hours) incubation. This implied that GH-RH stimulated synthesis, as well as release of growth hormone; it was not surprising, therefore, to find that, unlike the results of similar experiments with gonadotropin-releasing hormone, the addition of actinomycin D completely inhibited the response.

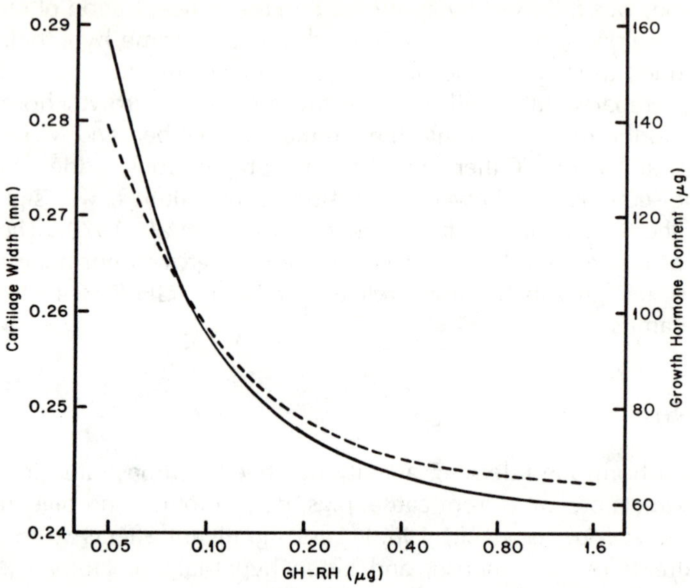

Fig. 13.3 *Effect of GH-RH upon the growth hormone content of rat pituitaries in vivo. The solid line represents the growth hormone content of 1.2 mg of rat pituitary (right ordinate); the broken line indicates the corresponding effect upon tibial epiphyseal width (left ordinate). Data of Schally et al. (1969).*

Somewhat more satisfactory estimates of GH-RH concentration are provided by an *in vivo* assay taking advantage of its ability to deplete pituitary STH in rats. One-tenth of a microgram of purified GH-RH reduced the growth hormone content of rat pituitary from 133 μg/mg to 80 μg/mg (NIH-GH-S7 equivalents) within a few minutes of its injection, and a reasonable log dose–response curve was obtained within the range 0.05–0.5 μg (Fig. 13.3).

2. *Chemistry*

Schally *et al.* (1969) purified the GH-RH extracted from a total of 200,000 pork hypothalami by 2 *N* acetic acid and obtained a product which appeared to be homogeneous on the basis of thin-layer chromatography in two solvent systems and thin-layer electrophoresis at 3 pH's. About 50 mg of product was obtained; the lyophilized starting material weighed something over 3 kg. In pituitary depletion assays the product was active at a total dose of 1.0 ng; *in vitro,* only 0.1–1.0 pg was needed to release STH from pituitary fragments.

The usual techniques of peptide analysis revealed that porcine GH-RH is a decapeptide with the amino acid sequence:

Val-His-Leu-Ser-Ala-Glu-Glu-Lys-Glu-Ala

(Schally *et al.*, 1971c). A synthetic preparation with this composition possessed GH-releasing activity both *in vivo* and *in vitro*.

When crude hypothalamic extracts are tested for growth hormone releasing activity by the pituitary depletion test *in vivo*, either bioassay (tibia test) or radioimmunoassay can be used to monitor the reduction in pituitary GH or the increase in plasma GH. Both methods give substantially the same answer. This is not true, however, with tests of the releasing activity of purified GH-RH preparations or of the pure decapeptide (natural or synthetic). With both of these materials, the amount of bioassayable GH released from rat pituitaries is much greater than that detectable by radioimmunoassay, despite the greater sensitivity of the latter method.

Other discrepancies also exist. Synthetic "GH-RH" does not release growth hormone in humans, nor does it stimulate growth in intact nongrowing rats or hypophysectomized rats with pituitary grafts (Schally *et al.*, 1973). These facts make it unlikely that the decapeptide isolated by Schally is the physiological growth hormone-releasing substance. In the same paper, Schally *et al.* reported the detection, in hypothalamic extracts, of a substance which releases immunoreactive GH from rat pituitaries. From its behavior on Sephadex columns, this substance appears to be a smaller molecule than the decapeptide described above.

B. GH-RIH

Brazeau *et al.* (1973) studied the effects of hypothalamic extracts upon growth hormone release by monolayer cultures of dispersed rat pituitary cells. From 350 to 400 ng GH/hour, as determined by radioimmunoassay, are produced by such cultures. An extract equivalent to 0.001 hypothalamus (porcine) reduced this by about 50%, and the inhibition increased with the amount of extract added. Purification of the inhibitory material resulted in the isolation of a small amount (8.5 mg) of a tetradecapeptide, identified as:

Ala-Gly-Cys-Lys-Asn-Phe-Phe-Trp-Lys-Thr-Phe-Thr-Ser-CysOH

The structure has been confirmed by synthesis (Burgus *et al.*, 1973). As little as 0.2 n*M* of either native or synthetic GH-RIH is sufficient to reduce GH release in monolayer cultures by about 50%, and the effect is dose dependent. Plasma GH in pentobarbital-treated rats was also reduced (from 66 to 32 ng/ml) by synthetic GH-RIH. Brazeau *et al.* have proposed the name "somatostatin" for this regulatory hormone.

IV. Corticotropin-Releasing Hormone (CRH)

Studies of the release of ACTH from rat anterior pituitary fragments *in vitro* provided the first direct evidence for the humoral control of anterior pituitary function. ACTH-releasing factors have been isolated from both the neurohypophysis and the hypothalamus; furthermore, the existence of two kinds of CRH, separable by countercurrent distribution, has been reported.

Despite this early and promising beginning, progress toward the identification and characterization of CRH has been negligible during the past 8 years, possibly because of its instability. While there is an imposing amount of literature, inconsistent and contradictory reports are frequently encountered.

A. ASSAY

Reference has already been made to the Saffran–Schally *in vitro* assay for CRH. In their early work, the addition of arterenol (or other catecholamines) to incubation mixtures significantly potentiated the ACTH-releasing effects of either neurohypophyseal fragments or extracts. Subsequently, however, Guillemin *et al.* (1957) could find no potentiating (or permissive) effect of catecholamines in the *in vitro* assay, and the addition of arterenol to the incubation medium has generally been abandoned. Unsupplemented extracts containing the equivalent of 10 μg of either hypothalamic or neurohypophyseal tissue are capable of increasing the amount of ACTH released by pituitary fragments 1.5- to threefold.

In order to assay CRH *in vivo,* the endogenous secretion of ACTH induced by the stresses of the experiment must be avoided, and both surgically- and pharmacologically-lesioned rats have been used to achieve this end. Manual destruction of the hypothalamus involves the risk of interfering with blood circulation to the pituitary. A number of drugs (Nembutal, morphine, various steroids) have been used to block stress-induced responses; it has not always been recognized that some of these compounds also suppress the response of the adrenal gland to ACTH. Small doses of hydrocortisone (2.5–7.5 mg/100 gm body weight) have been shown to be effective inhibitors of the stress response with no discernable effect upon the response to ACTH; although dexamethasone is frequently used as a blocking agent, its possible limitations are unknown (Vernikos-Danellis and Marks, 1970). Arimura *et al.* (1967) have shown that dexamethasone suppresses the rise in plasma corticosterone which normally follows the injection of stalk median eminence extracts (rat) into rats treated with monase and Nembutal.

Vernikos–Danellis (1964) described an *in vivo* assay for CRH which employed hydrocortisone-blocked rats. CRH samples were injected into the carotid artery and 1.25 minutes was allowed for a maximal response. Blood was collected by decapitation and assayed for ACTH by the ascorbic acid depletion method in hypophysectomized rats. The log dose–response curve to median eminence extracts paralleled the response to ACTH. As little as one-half the median eminence from a single rat was sufficient to cause a measurable increase in circulating ACTH.

Arimura *et al.* (1967) have described an assay for CRH which depends upon the increase in plasma corticosterone following the injection of a test sample into suitably prepared, i.e., monase- and Nembutal-blocked, rats. Just one-half of a rat superior median eminence increased plasma corticosterone from 16 to 38 μg/100 ml.

B. CHEMISTRY

Corticotropin-releasing factors have been isolated from both porcine and bovine neurohypophyses, as well as from porcine, bovine, ovine, and canine hypothalami. Although lysine vasopressin is a frequent contaminant of neurohypophyseal CRH preparations, amounts of lysine vasopressin which are equivalent in pressor activity to active CRH preparations are without significant CRH activity.

Neurohypophyseal extracts which are rich in CRH activity can be separated, by countercurrent distribution, into two active fractions. α-CRH is active *in vivo* when 1.0 μg is injected; it also possesses intrinsic MSH activity (equivalent to that of α-MSH). Its amino acid composition is also similar to that of α-MSH, but the latter possesses no CRH activity. Schally *et al.* (1962) have suggested that the two molecules differ in structure at the amino terminus (serine in MSH), since α-CRH is more basic than α-MSH.

β-CRH has been reported to be a smaller molecule, containing, in addition to the amino acids of lysine vasopressin, serine and histidine, as well. β-CRH is active (*in vivo*) in amounts considerably smaller than effective doses of α-CRH (0.01–0.3 μg). Hypothalamic CRH can also be separated into two active fractions.

In order to avoid the inevitable loss of hypothalamic CRH which occurs during the slaughter of domestic animals, Chan *et al.* (1970) turned to the isolation of CRH from rat median eminences collected under carefully controlled conditions. The active fraction was similar to lysine vasopressin in its chromatographic properties, but again had little pressor activity. Treatment of rat median eminence CRH with pepsin, with thioglycolate, or with dilute acid at 100° removed about one-third the initial activity. The rest of the activity may be due to a different compound.

V. The Control of Prolactin Secretion

In mammals, control of prolactin secretion appears to differ in a major way from the manner in which the other pituitary hormones are controlled, since any procedure which removes the pituitary from hypothalamic influence (transplantation, stalk section, or hypothalamic lesions) leads to *increased* prolactin synthesis. Indices of prolactin secretion which have been used in such studies include mammary growth and lactation in rats, mice, and rabbits, as well as prolongation of the life of functional corpora lutea in rats (Meites, 1966). When cultured *in vitro,* rat anterior pituitary fragments continue to synthesize (and secrete) prolactin for at least 6 days; by this time, the amount of prolactin cumulatively secreted into the medium was 2–14 times greater than that present in the gland initially. When extracts of rat hypothalamus were added to the incubation fluid, its prolactin content was reduced by 40–70%; the decrease was reflected both in the amount in the medium as well as that left in the gland.

Schally *et al.* (1965a) found that extracts made from bovine, ovine, or porcine hypothalami would also inhibit prolactin release *in vitro.* The equivalent of half a median eminence from any one of these animals reduced prolactin secretion by 70–80%; the effect was not duplicated by vasopressin, oxytocin, FSH- or LH-RH, nor any of a large number of simpler compounds, among them epinephrine, norepinephrine, acetyl choline, histamine, or serotonin. Both rat and human hypothalamic extracts inhibited prolactin secretion by human anterior pituitary explants.

In birds, the hypothalamus exerts a positive, rather than a negative control on prolactin secretion. Interference with the vascular connections between the hypothalamus and the pituitary in pigeons did not lead to an increase in prolactin secretion; in ducks, stalk section results in apparent atrophy of the "prolactin cells" of the anterior pituitary.

In vitro the addition of extracts containing the equivalent of one pigeon hypothalamus increased the secretion of prolactin by explants of homologous pituitaries two- to fourfold within 4 hours. Rat hypothalamic extracts had no apparent effect on prolactin release by pigeon pituitaries, but chicken hypothalamus was an effective stimulant.

In other species both inhibitory and stimulatory patterns are seen. Teleost fishes and amphibians follow the mammalian pattern (inhibition) while some reptiles (turtles) display the stimulatory pattern characteristic of birds. It appears that a dual mechanism for the control of this important hormone has evolved, with different roles having been defined for the hypothalamus in birds and mammals. This functional difference may be related in some fashion to the different functions of prolactin in the two kinds of animals.

The chemical natures of the hypothalamic factors that modify prolactin secretion are, as yet, unknown. TRH stimulates prolactin release in some mammals, but Schally and others have reported that it is possible to separate TRH and an active placental lactogen-RH fraction. From their behavior during gel filtration, it seems likely that both hormones are of low molecular weight and probably polypeptide in nature. Studies are under way to evaluate the usefulness of TRH in increasing milk production in cattle.

VI. MSH Control in Mammals and Amphibians

Although claims have been made for the existence of both stimulatory and inhibitory hypothalamic factors controlling the secretion of melanocyte-stimulating hormone (MSH), it appears that control of MSH secretion is normally effected by an inhibitory hormone (Schally *et al.*, 1968a; Burgus and Guillemin, 1970). Evidence for the existence of MIF (MSH-release inhibiting factor) has been documented for seven mammalian (rat, cat, rabbit, pig, sheep, cow, human) and one amphibian (frog) species. In all instances, the inhibitory activity was tested in rats. An extract corresponding to one-tenth of a vertebrate SME was required to increase the pituitary MSH content by approximately 100%.

A. ASSAY

Both *in vitro* and *in vivo* assays have been used. The earliest work which led to the conclusion that MIF existed was based upon the ability of hypothalamic extracts to reduce the amount of MSH released into the medium when rat pituitaries were cultured for 4 days. MIF may also be detected by injecting a sample into an ether-anesthetized rat and determining the MSH content of the pituitary after 20 minutes. Many modifications of the basic rat pituitary-accumulating assay have been suggested (Kastin *et al.*, 1970). Amphibians may also be used in a direct test for MIF. After removal of the hypothalamus from frogs, the animals darken, since release of MSH is no longer inhibited. Injection of MIF causes the skin to lighten; the degree of paling can be compared to that induced by a standard dose of melatonin (5-methoxy-N-acetyltryptamine).

B. CHEMISTRY

Schally and Kastin (1966) purified bovine MIF, recovering 39 mg of active material from 2.5 kg of hypothalamic tissue. This material was active *in vivo* (rats) when as little as 60 ng were injected, reducing the MSH con-

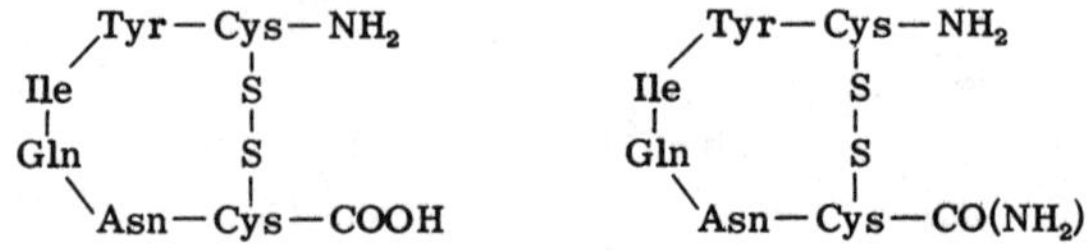

Tocinoic acid Tocinamide

Fig. 13.4 *Structures of tocinoic acid and tocinamide.*

tent of the rat's pituitary by 75%. After further purification (by thin-layer chromatography on cellulose) an apparently homogeneous preparation was obtained, which was identified as Pro-Leu-Gly(NH_2) (Nair *et al.*, 1971). Synthetic Pro-Leu-Gly(NH_2), tested in median eminence-treated rats, inhibited MSH release when as little as 10 ng were injected (Celis *et al.*, 1972).

Celis *et al.* (1971a) reported that while oxytocin and some of its open-chain analogs had no intrinsic MIF activity, several of these compounds (including oxytocin itself) were converted to products with MIF activity by a microsomal enzyme present in rat median eminence. The product was active both *in vivo* and *in vitro.* They concluded that in the rat, at least, MIF arose by enzymatic digestion of oxytocin to the tripeptide Pro-Leu-Gly(NH_2).

The identification of MIF as Pro-Leu-Gly(NH_2) has been challenged by Bower *et al.* (1971; Bower and Hadley, 1972). She and her colleagues have reported that in their experiments the tripeptide was unable to inhibit MSH release in either amphibian or rat pituitaries *in vitro;* on the other hand, tocinoic acid, the cyclic hexapeptide representing the rest of the oxytocin molecule (Fig. 13.4) effectively inhibited the release of MSH from rat pituitaries *in vitro* when present at a concentration of 10^{-9} gm/ml (Hruby *et al.*, 1972). Tocinamide was active at even lower concentrations. Neither of these substances affected the MSH content of amphibian pituitaries except at much higher concentrations. Bower and Hadley (1972) concluded that the exact nature of mammalian MIF is still unsettled, and she left open the possibility that some as yet unidentified compound serves as a vertebrate MIF, active in both amphibians and mammals.

Celis *et al.* (1971b) found that some rat median eminence extracts evoked the release of MSH when injected into other rats. Extracts of paraventricular nuclei had similar properties. Because the latter organ is also the site of oxytocin synthesis, it was considered possible (indeed probable) that a metabolite of oxytocin was involved. A synthetic peptide corresponding to the opened ring of oxytocin, but lacking one cysteine residue:

Cys-Tyr-Ile-Gln-AsnOH

was found to be active at a dose of 20 ng/animal. Oxytocin itself had no effect.

14

The Gastrointestinal Hormones

I. Gastrin

A. ASSAY

Gastrin is generally estimated by its ability to stimulate acid secretion by the stomach. Dog and cats have been used as test animals; with both species, conscious animals prepared with denervated fundic pouches offer the most consistent results. Sometimes the volume, but more frequently the number of milliequivalents of acid produced during a 15-minute interval after subcutaneous or intravenous injection of the hormone is determined. Until synthetic gastrin, or smaller polypeptides with gastrin activity, became available, there was no general agreement on a standard preparation, although in some instances the effects of gastrin-containing extracts were compared to a standard dose of histamine. Even with chemically defined preparations, however, there is a curious lack of information concerning the effectiveness of gastrin in dogs or cats.

Using human gastrin dispersed in adjuvant as an antigen, Odell *et al.* (1968) were able to induce antibody formation in rabbits. A double antibody radioimmunoassay was developed, which permitted the estimation of gastrin at concentrations of 1–50 ng/ml.

B. CHEMISTRY

All the known gastrins are single-chain heptadecapeptides; their sequences are shown in Fig. 14.1. Two forms of gastrin have been isolated from both porcine and human intestinal mucosa; porcine gastrin II and human gastrin II are phenolic sulfates of the compounds shown. Activity is undiminished if the methionine in residue 15 is replaced by leucine (Wuensch *et al.*, 1972).

The pentaglutamyl sequence (residues 6–11) of gastrin is an unusual structural feature among polypeptide hormones, as is the complete absence of basic amino acids. The first feature is not an absolute requirement, however, since a tetradecapeptide with three of the glutamic acid residues eliminated was fully active. One of the fragments produced when gastrin is submitted to digestion by papain is the C-terminal tetrapeptide, Trp-Met-Asp-Phe(NH_2), a compound which elicits the full range of physiological actions characteristic of gastrin. On a weight basis, the tetrapeptide is only about one-fifth as active as the native hormone (one-twentieth on a molar basis). As the peptide is lengthened by the addition of amino acids to this N-terminus, activity progressively increases. However, the N-terminal tridecapeptide (gastrin$^{1-13}$) is completely inactive.

The observation that a relatively simple tetrapeptide possesses gastrin activity has stimulated an intensive study of essential structural features of simple molecules with gastrin activity. Allowable changes include some modifications of the free amino group, modifications of the indolyl side chain, replacement of methionine by leucine or norleucine, and substitution into or reduction of the phenylalanyl residue. A limited number of alterations of the C-terminal amide, such as its methylation, or replacement by an azide, were permissible, but conversion to the free acid or ester destroyed activity.

Almost any change in the aspartic acid residue resulted in inactivation. The only modification which permitted retention of activity was replacement of the carboxymethyl side chain by the equally bulky tetrazolymethyl

	1	2	3	4	5	6	7	8	9	10	11	12	13	14	15	16	17
Porcine	(pyro)Glu-	Gly-	Pro-	Trp-	Met-	Glu-	Glu-	Glu-	Glu-	Glu-	Ala-	Tyr-	Gly-	Trp-	Met-	Asp-	Phe(NH_2)
Bovine, ovine					-Val-					-Ala-							
Canine								-Ala-									
Feline					-Leu-					-Ala-							
Human					-Leu-												

Fig. 14.1 *Amino acid sequences of several gastrins. In most species a sulfated (at Tyr^{12}) form is also found.*

group. Insertion of another amino acid between any of the four existing ones diminished or abolished gastrin activity. It has been suggested that the three dispensable amino acids function as "affinity" determinants, i.e., are concerned with binding at the site of action, while the aspartic acid residue serves a functional role (*see also* Morley, 1968).

An important incentive for the study of structure–function relationships in the gastrin series has been the lure of a compound with "anti-gastrin" properties, with its obvious application to the control of stomach acid secretion. To date, however, none of the many synthetic peptides tested has displayed significant ability to inhibit histamine- or gastrin-induced HCl secretion.* An apparently unrelated peptide with anti-gastrin activity, urogastrone, has been isolated from human urine. Purified urogastrone is an effective anti-gastrin in dogs when injected at a dose of 2 μg/kg. It is a single-chain polypeptide with a molecular weight near 4000 (Gregory, 1970).

The molecular weight of human gastrin is 2100. Yalow and Berson (1972) filtered extracts of human jejunum through Sephadex G-50 and examined the effluent for substances which would react with anti-gastrin antibody. In addition to gastrin itself, two other immunoreactive peaks were found with molecular weights of 7000 ("big" gastrin) and at least 65,000 ("big-big" gastrin), respectively. When the extracts were digested with trypsin, "big-big" gastrin disappeared, with the formation of an immunoreactive heptadecapeptide. Similar experimental results were obtained using plasmas of patients with Zollinger–Ellison syndrome. It was suggested that the larger molecules represented two forms of pro-gastrin.

II. Secretin

A. ASSAY

The earliest assays for secretin depended upon measurement of the flow of pancreatic juice from a cannulated pancreatic duct in response to the injection of a test sample. In 1928 Hammersten introduced the technique of titrating the alkali in the pancreatic juice collected during a 15-minute interval following the intravenous injection of secretin into an anesthetized cat. One cat unit (HCU = Hammersten cat unit) was defined as the amount of secretin required to stimulate the secretin of 0.01 MEq of bicarbonate. Purified secretin contains 80,000–400,000 HCU/mg; thus as little as 0.002–0.01 μg of secretin will provoke a measurable response.

* However, burimamide, a thiourea derivative, is a potent inhibitor of both histamine- and gastrin-stimulated acid secretion (Black *et al.*, 1972).

Porcine secretin is antigenic in rabbits if it is first conjugated with rabbit serum albumin. A radioimmunoassay specific for secretin has been described by Young *et al.* (1968) using rabbit anti-secretin antibody and radioiodinated secretin. Sensitivity to 0.1 ng of the hormone was claimed.

B. CHEMISTRY

Although the discovery of secretin antedated the discoveries of all the other hormones, its chemistry was not resolved until 1966, when Mutt and Jorpes (1967) characterized porcine secretin as a 27-amino acid peptide:

His-Ser-Asp-Gly-Thr-Phe-Thr-Ser-Glu-Leu-Ser-Arg-Leu-Arg-
Asp-Ser-Ala-Arg-Leu-Gln-Arg-Leu-Leu-Gln-Gly-Leu-Val(NH_2)

The synthesis of secretin has been reported by Bodanszky *et al.* (1966). Pure secretin contains about 400,000 HCU/mg, and both it and the synthetic product display all the activities shown by less active preparations, including stimulation of the flow of water and bicarbonate from the pancreas and of bile from the liver. The activity of secretin is very sensitive to modifications at the amino terminal end of the molecule. Brief exposure to alkali reduces its activity by 70–80%; this has been attributed to the formation of a cyclic amide involving Asp^3 and His^1. Removal of the N-terminal histidine leads to almost complete inactivation, and smaller C-terminal fragments are also inactive. While it is known that the N-terminal tetradecapeptide His- . . . -Arg(NH_2) possesses very slight activity, the minimal sequence for a useful secretin analog is apparently not yet known.

Said and Mutt (1972) have isolated a compound from the upper intestinal wall of pigs which appears to be a 28-amino acid peptide, also with His at its N-terminus, but of substantially different amino acid composition than secretin. Its principal physiological effect seems to be exerted upon peripheral and splanchnic blood flow, but it also has modest secretin activity (about 5–10% that of native secretin).

A high degree of homology is found when the amino acid sequence of secretin is compared with that of another hormone originating in the gastrointestinal tract, pancreatic glucagon (*see* Chapter 7, Section II, C). Both molecules begin with an N-terminal histidine, and 13 of the next 26 residues are identical. Furthermore, of the remaining 13 positions common to both molecules, six are occupied by amino acids of similar polarities: Asp^3 vs Gln^3, Glu^9 vs Asp^9, Arg^{12} vs Lys^{12}, Leu^{22} vs Phe^{22}, Leu^{23} vs Val^{23}, and Val^{27} vs Met^{27}. Track (1973) has noted that of the 13 nonmatching amino acids in the two molecules, the trinucleotide codons of six require only a single base change, and four required only two base changes to complete a glucagon-secretin transition. Track also compared hypothetical mRNA sequences for the gastrointestinal peptides proinsulin and gastrin as well as secretin; a single (forward) frameshift mutation in the mRNA sequence, corresponding to the last 25 amino acids of proinsulin, followed by a single nucleotide change in 13 codons, generated an mRNA sequence with 75% homology to secretin mRNA; a similar, but different set of nucleotide changes resulted in a gastrin-like sequence. Track suggested that a primordial proinsulin-like protein served as the evolutionary progenitor of gastrin, glucagon, and secretin, as well as of proinsulin itself. This hypothesis suggests that a search for gastrin- and secretin-like molecules among the gastrointestinal secretions of animals of lower phyla might be rewarding.

III. Cholecystokinin (CCK) and Pancreozymin (PZ)

A. ASSAY

In 1928, Ivy and Oldberg discovered that extracts of intestinal mucosa would stimulate gallbladder contractions. From the same source, Harper and Raper in 1943 extracted a material which would stimulate the secretion of various enzymes (amylase, lipase, and trypsinogen) from a pancreas which was already secreting alkali in response to secretin. When efforts were made to isolate the agents responsible for these phenomena, they were found to parallel each other very closely, and there is now little doubt that a single hormone (abbreviated CCK-PZ) accounts for both activities.

Ivy's original assay consisted of measuring the pressure changes occurring in dog gallbladders when intestinal extracts were given to the intact animal. One Ivy dog unit (IDU) was the amount required to produce maximum contraction of the gallbladder in an anesthetized dog. A more convenient assay uses a guinea pig gallbladder exposed *in situ*. Strips of guinea pig gallbladder suspended in physiological salt solution will also respond to cholecystokinin-containing preparations. This has been made the basis for a relatively simple *in vitro* assay.

Pancreozymic activity is assayed in anesthetized cats prepared in the same manner as for secretin assay. The pancreas is first stimulated by secretin, then PZ is injected. Under these conditions, no proteins other than the three enzymes are secreted, hence a simple determination of the protein content of the pancreatic juice provides a measure of the pancreozymic effect. Crick *et al.* (1950) defined a unit of PZ activity as that contained in 1 mg of a partly purified preparation from hog intestinal mucosa. This amount of PZ was sufficient to increase the amylase output sixfold.

B. CHEMISTRY

Both cholecystokinin and pancreozymin activities are contained in a side fraction left over from the purification of secretin from hog intestinal extracts. The two activities follow each other when purified (Mutt and Jorpes, 1967); the final product was a seemingly homogeneous peptide which contained 3000 IDU of CCK and 12,000 Crick units of PZ per milligram.

Porcine CCK–PZ is a sulfated, 33-amino acid peptide, with the structure:

Lys-Ala-Pro-Ser-Gly-Arg-Val-Ser-Met-Ile-Lys-Asn-Leu-Gln-Ser-Leu-Asp-
Pro-Ser-His-Arg-Ile-Ser-Asp-Arg-Asp-Tyr-Met-Gly-Trp-Met-Asp-Phe(NH_2)
SO_3H

The C-terminal pentapeptide sequence in CCK–PZ is identical with that found in gastrin; the neighboring tyrosine residue is also sulfated. However, while unsulfated gastrin is as active as its O-sulfate, removal of the sulfate moiety from some active CCK–PZ analogs reduces activity more than 90%.

The biological activity of CCK–PZ, like that of gastrin, is severely dependent upon the proper configuration of amino acids at the C-terminal end. The C-terminal hexapeptide of CCK–PZ (Met . . . . . Phe(NH_2)) is completely inactive, but extension of the sequence toward the N-terminal end gives rise to compounds which may be ten or more times as active (2.5 times as active on a molar basis) as native CCK–PZ (Table 14.1). Elimination of the sulfate group or moving it to the 3′ position in the C-terminal octapeptide reduces activity by more than 90%.* Other modifications of the C-terminal octapeptide which result in significant (50–95%) diminution of activity are: (1) replacement of the penultimate Asp residue by Ala; (2) replacement of the N-terminal Asp residue by Ala; (3) transposition of Asp^1 and $Tyr(SO_3H)^2$; (4) transposition of $Tyr(SO_3H)^2$ and Met^3; and (5) replacement of Met^6 by leucine.

The most active analog described by Ondetti *et al.* (1970) was the β-Asp^1 derivative corresponding to the C-terminal octapeptide, which was found to be 40 times as active as native CCK–PZ *in vitro.* While the data in Table 14.1 include assays of gallbladder activity only, the octapeptide possesses the full range of CCK–PZ activities, including evocation of pancreatic enzyme secretion and stimulation of duodenal contractility.

CCK–PZ activity has been found in extracts of the intestines of *Chimaera,* lampreys, and other eels (Barrington and Dockray, 1972).

Of the other gastrointestinal hormones which have been described from

* However, the unsulfated octapeptide with its free amino group blocked by a *tert*-butyl carbonyl residue is nearly as active as the sulfated octapeptide. It may be that the net charge (or lack of one) at this end of the molecule is an important determinant of function.

TABLE 14.1 Activities of C-Terminal Peptides Related to CCK-PZ[a]

Peptide	Activity, IDU/mg	
	In vitro	*In vivo*
Asp-Tyr(SO_3H)-Met-Gly(OH)	3	3
Asp-Tyr(SO_3H)-Met-Gly(NH_2)	8	1
Met-Gly-Trp-Met-Asp-Phe(NH_2)	1	1
Tyr(SO_3H)-Met-Gly-Trp-Met-Asp-Phe(NH_2)	—	22,000
Asp-Tyr——Met-Gly-Trp-Met-Asp-Phe(NH_2)	200	200
Asp-Tyr(SO_3H)-Met-Gly-Trp-Met-Asp-Phe(NH_2)	26,000	30,000
Asp-Arg-Asp-Tyr(SO_3H)-Met-Gly-Trp-Met-Asp-Phe(NH_2)	48,000	56,000
Ile-Ser-Asp-Arg-Asp-Tyr(SO_3H)-Met-Gly-Trp-Met-Asp-Phe(NH_2)	56,000	11,900

[a] *From Ondetti et al. (1970).*

time to time (including enterocrinin, villicrinin, and duocrinin) only enterogastrone has received more than cursory attention. Enterogastrone inhibits secretin- (but not histamine-) induced gastric acid production. Like the other hormones described in this chapter, it is secreted by the small intestine. Brown *et al.* (1970) obtained a potent enterogastrone preparation from impure CCK–PZ; it was effective (in dogs) at a total dose of 0.50 μg. Although some data on amino acid composition were reported, no estimate of molecular size or covalent structure was obtained.

15

Erythropoietin

I. Assay

As mentioned earlier, the definition of erythropoietin as a physiological and humoral entity was based upon its ability to increase the total red cell mass of various experimental animals. Early efforts to measure erythropoietin depended upon an increase in the percentage of reticulocytes in the blood of treated rabbits, or upon increases in hemoglobin, hematocrit, or reticulocytes in the blood of rats injected with erythropoietin-rich preparations. These procedures have now been replaced by methods which depend upon the incorporation of radioactive iron (^{59}Fe) into red blood cells. Other improvements in the assay include suppression of endogenous erythropoietin production and red cell formation by starvation or hypophysectomy (rats) or by inducing polycythemia (mice). A variety of methods are employed to obtain plethoric mice; the most convenient is to expose animals of an appropriate strain to reduced atmospheric pressure (0.5 atm) for 14 days. Erythropoietin is injected subcutaneously on the fifteenth and sixteenth day, followed by the intravenous injection of radioactive iron citrate. Two to three days later, the faction of ^{59}Fe originally injected which has been incorporated into erythrocytes is determined (Camiscoli *et al.*, 1968).

Very early in the history of erythropoietin research it was discovered that the injection of a small amount of cobalt chloride into a fasted rat produced an erythropoietic response, and that the responses to graded amounts of cobalt paralleled those induced by erythropoietin concentrates. Accordingly, a "unit" of erythropoietin activity was defined as that equivalent, physiologically, to 5 μmoles of cobalt chloride. While this represented a convenient standardization procedure, the cobalt standard is limited in application, since not all strains of rats are responsive. More recently, erythropoietin concentrates prepared from plasma of anemic sheep or from human urine have accepted as International Reference Standards. The current erythropoietin "unit" (1.48 mg of International Reference Standard B) is approximately equivalent to 1 cobalt unit when assayed in rats. In hypobaric-polycythemic mice the fraction of administered radioactive iron incorporated is linear with the logarithm of the dose between 0.05–1.0 U (Fig. 15.1).

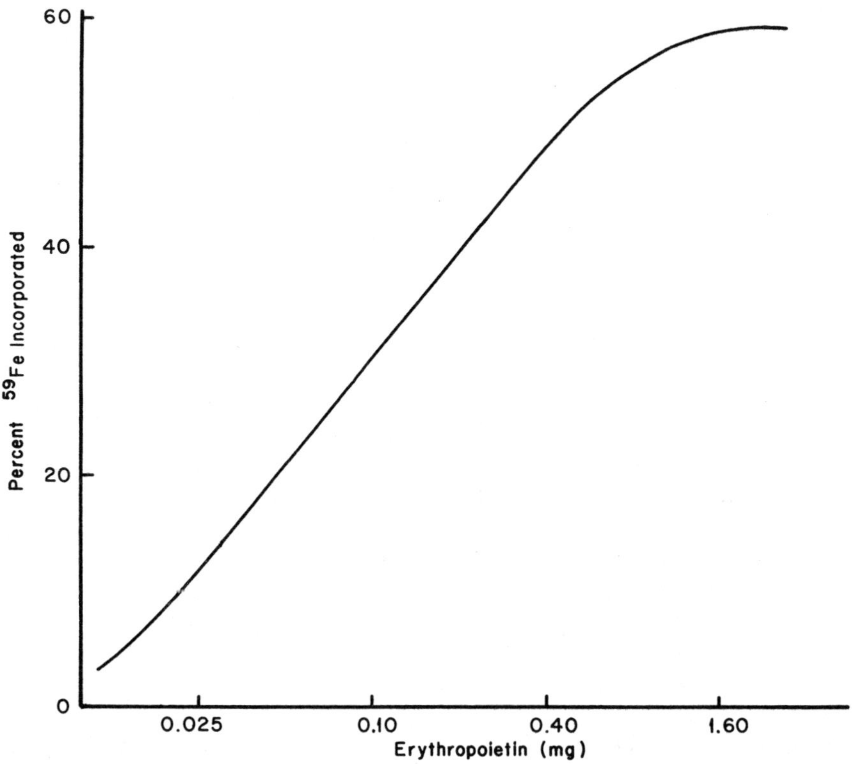

Fig. 15.1 *Effect of human urinary erythropoietin upon incorporation of radioactive Fe into the erythrocytes of hypobaric-polycythemic mice. Data of Keighley (1968).*

Krantz *et al.* (1963) incubated rat bone marrow cells with $^{59}FeCl_3$ and later isolated radioactive heme from a lysate of the cell suspension. If erythropoietin was added to the incubation medium, the amount of label in heme was increased two to twentyfold, with a linear log C-response curve spanning the range 0.01–1.5 U/ml of erythropoietin. Similar results were obtained with bone marrow cells from dogs (Ward, 1967). More recently, Stephenson and Axelrod (1971) were able to assay erythropoietin by relying on the ability of fetal mouse liver cells, maintained in tissue culture, to synthesize heme. These cells were about ten times as sensitive as rat bone marrow cells; graded responses were obtained with 0.005–0.16 U/ml.

II. Occurrence

Evidence for the existence of erythropoietin, or of erythropoietin-like activity has been claimed for the plasmas of at least a dozen species of mammals, birds, and fish. Mammalian erythropoietin is inactive in birds and virtually inactive in fish; correspondingly, avian erythropoietin is inactive in polycythemic mice. The role played by erythropoietin in erythrocyte formation in amphibians and reptiles is unknown. The various mammalian erythropoietins (sheep, rabbit, monkey, and human) gave identical regression lines when assayed in polycythemic mice, while antisera to human urinary erythropoietin, raised in rabbits, neutralized mouse, rat, rabbit, and sheep, as well as human, erythropoietin.

III. Isolation and Chemical Properties

Highly purified erythropoietin has been obtained from plasma of sheep made anemic by bleeding, and from the urine of anemic humans. Goldwasser and Kung (1968, 1971, 1972) concentrated sheep plasma erythropoietin more than one millionfold to obtain a product which had a single major peak on acrylamide gel electrophoresis and assayed 9200 U/mg. The molecular weight of radioiodinated ovine erythropoietin was determined by electrophoresis in SDS*-containing gels to be 46,000 daltons. Comparable activity (8000 U/mg) was displayed by purified human urinary erythropoietin (Espada *et al.*, 1972). Human erythropoietin contained about 30% carbohydrate (13% hexose, 9% hexoseamine, and 7.5% sialic acid). Its amino acid analysis was unremarkable.

Erythropoietin-containing plasma may be boiled 15 minutes without loss

* Sodium dodecyl sulfate.

of activity, while more potent preparations readily lose activity unless another protein (serum albumin, orosomucoid, gelatin) is added (Goldwasser and Kung, 1968). Erythropoietin is inactivated by trypsin, and experiments with a variety of reagents suggest that activity is dependent upon intact carboxyl, indole, amino, and phenolic hydroxyl groups; —SH groups and aliphatic hydroxyls are either unimportant for biological activity, or inaccessible.

Erythropoietin which has had part of its sialic acid removed by neuraminidase is inactive in mice and rats, but retains its activity *in vitro* (marrow cell cultures); concomitantly, its isoelectric point (as determined by isoelectric focusing) is raised from about 4 to about 6 (Lubowsky and Painter, 1972). Oxidation of desialized erythropoietin by galactose oxidase or horseradish peroxidase has been reported to restore activity *in vivo.*

The exact role of the kidney in the biogenesis of erythropoietin is uncertain. Burlington *et al.* (1972) reported that prolonged culture of goat kidney glomeruli resulted in the appearance of erythropoietic activity in the culture medium. Contreras *et al.* (1966) found that after all the residual plasma was removed from kidneys of hypoxic male mice, there remained a particulate-bound erythropoietic material. This substance appeared to be concentrated in the "light" mitochondrial fraction (sedimenting between 6800 and 20,200 *g*) and possessed little intrinsic erythropoietic activity in hypobaric-polycythemic mice; however, when it was incubated for short periods with normal rat serum at 37°, potent erythropoietic activity was generated. This material has been designated the "renal erythropoietic factor" (REF) by its discoverers. REF differs significantly from erythropoietin of plasma in its stability to weak acid solutions (pH 5.0) and to heat. It has been suggested that REF represents either (1) a molecule which has to be complexed or combined with a factor present in serum to give rise to erythropoietin activity, or (2) an enzyme which acts upon serum to produce erythropoietin (much as renin acts on plasma substrate to form angiotensin). The latter possibility seems more in keeping with the relative heat- and acid-labilities of the various entities concerned.

The existence of extra-renal sites for the production of erythropoietin has been suggested (Peschle *et al.*, 1973).

References

Abraham, G. E., Odell, W. D., Edwards, R., and Purdy, J. M. (1970). *Acta Endocrinol. (Copenhagen), Suppl.* **147,** 332.

Abramowitz, A. A., Money, W. L., Zarrow, M. X., Talmage, R. V., Kleinholz, L. H., and Hisaw, F. L. (1944). *Endocrinology* **34,** 103.

Abramson, D., Hurwit, E., and Lesnick, G. (1937). *Surg., Gynecol. Obstet.* **65,** 335.

Acher, R., Chauvet, J., and Olivry, G. (1956). *Biochim. Biophys. Acta* **22,** 421.

Acher, R., Chauvet, J., and Lenci, M. T. (1958). *Bull. Soc. Chim. Biol.* **40,** 2005.

Acher, R., Chauvet, J., and Chauvet, M. T. (1972). *Eur. J. Biochem.* **29,** 12.

Adams, D. D., and Purves, H. D. (1955). *Endocrinology* **57,** 17.

Adams, D. D., and Purves, H. D. (1957). *Can. J. Biochem. Physiol.* **35,** 993.

Adamson, J. W., and Stamatoyannopoulous, G. (1973). *Science* **180,** 310.

Allen, E., and Doisy, E. A. (1923). *J. Amer. Med. Ass.* **81,** 819.

Amir, S. M. (1972). *Acta Endocrinol. (Copenhagen)* **70,** 21.

Amoss, M., Burgus, R., Blackwell, R., Vale, W., Fellows, R., and Guillemin, R. (1971). *Biochem. Biophys. Res. Commun.* **44,** 205.

Anderson, E., and Long, J. A. (1948). *Recent Progr. Horm. Res.* **2,** 209.

Andrews, P. (1966). *Nature (London)* **209,** 155.

Andrews, P., and Folley, S. J. (1963). *Biochem. J.* **87,** 3P.

Arimura, A., Saito, T., and Schally, A. V. (1967). *Endocrinology* **81,** 235.

Arquila, E. R., and Stavisky, A. B. (1956). *J. Clin. Invest.* **35,** 458.

Aschheim, S., and Zondek, B. (1927). *Klin. Wochenschr.* **6,** 1322.

Ashitaka, Y., Tohura, Y., Tane, M., Mochizuki, M., and Tojo, S. (1970). *Endocrinology* **87,** 233.

Astwood, E. B. (1938). *Endocrinology* **23,** 25.

Aurbach, G. D. (1959). *Endocrinology* **64,** 296.

Baba, Y., Matsuo, H., and Schally, A. V. (1971). *Biochem. Biophys. Res. Commun.* **44,** 459.

Bahl, O. P. (1969). *J. Biol. Chem.* **244,** 567.

Baldratti, G., Barbieri, W., Consonni, A., Sciaky, R., Scrasia, E., and Suchowsky, G. K. (1969). *Experientia* **25,** 1018.

Banting, F., and Best, C. H. (1922). *J. Lab. Clin. Med.* **7,** 251.

Barker, J. A., Last, J. A., Adams, S. L., Nienhuis, A. W., and Anderson, W. F. (1973). *Proc. Nat. Acad. Sci. U.S.* **70,** 1739.

Barker, S. B. (1956). *Endocrinology* **59,** 548.

Barrington, E. J. W., and Dockray, G. J. (1972). *Gen. Comp. Endocrinol.* **19,** 80.

Bell, E. T., Mukerji, S., and Loraine, J. A. (1964). *J. Endocrinol.* **28,** 321.

Bell, J., Canfield, R. E., and Sciarra, J. J. (1969). *Endocrinology* **84,** 298.

Bell. P. H. (1954). *J. Amer. Chem. Soc.* **76,** 5565.

Bell, P. H., Howard, K. S., Shepherd, R. G., Finn, B. M., and Meisenhelder, J. H. (1956). *J. Amer. Chem. Soc.* **78,** 5059.

Bellisario, R., Carlson, R. B., and Bahl, O. P. (1973). *J. Biol. Chem.* **248,** 6796.

Berson, S. A., Yalow, R. S., Aurbach, G. D., and Potts, J. T. (1963). *Proc. Nat. Acad. Sci. U.S.* **49,** 613.

Bethune, J. E., Inoue, H., and Turpin, R. A. (1967). *Endocrinology* **81,** 67.

Black, J. W., Duncan, W. A. M., Durant, C. J., Ganellin, C. R., and Parsons, E. M. (1972). *Nature (London)* **236,** 385.

Bodanszky, M., Ondetti, M. A., Levine, S. D., Narayanan, V. L., von Saltza, M., Sheehan, J. T., Williams, N. J., and Sabo, E. F. (1966). *Chem. Ind. (London)* p. 1757.

Boissonas, R. A., Guttman, S., Waller, J. P., and Jacquenoud, P. A. (1956). *Experientia* **12,** 446.

Boissonas, R. A., Guttman, S., and Pless, J. (1966). *Experientia* **22,** 526.

Boler, J., Enzmann, F., Folkers, K., Bowers, C. Y., and Schally, A. V. (1969). *Biochem. Biophys. Res. Commun.* **37,** 705.

Borell, U., and Holmgren, H. (1949). *Acta Endocrinol. (Copenhagen)* **3,** 331.

Boright, H. A., Engel, F. L., Lebovitz, H. E., Kostyo, J. L., and White, J. E., Jr. (1962). *Biochem. J.* **83,** 95.

Bottari, P. M., Donovan, B. T., and El Kabir, D. J. (1963). *J. Physiol. (London)* **169,** 278.

Botticelli, C. R., Hisaw, F. L., Jr., and Wotiz, H. H. (1961). *Proc. Soc. Exp. Biol. Med.* **106,** 887.

Bourke, J. R., Hawker, R. W., and Manley, S. W. (1969). *Endocrinology* **84,** 1292.

Bower, A., and Hadley, M. E. (1972). *Science* **176,** 1331.

Bower, A., Hadley, M. E., and Hruby, V. J. (1971). *Biochem. Biophys. Res. Commun.* **45,** 1185.

Bowers, C. Y., Weil, A., Chang, J. K., Sievertsson, H., Enzmann, F., and Folkers, K. (1970). *Biochem. Biophys. Res. Commun.* **40,** 683.

Bowers, C. Y., Currie, B. L., Johansson, K. N. G., and Folkers, K. (1973). *Biochem. Biophys. Res. Commun.* **50,** 20.

Brazeau, P., Vale, R., Ling, N., Butcher, M., Rivier, J., and Guillemin, R. (1973). *Science* **179,** 77.

Brewer, H. B. (1969). *Fed. Proc., Fed. Amer. Soc. Exp. Biol.* **28,** 383.

Brewer, H. B., Fairwell, T., Ronan, R., Sizemore, G. W., and Arnaud, C. D. (1972). *Proc. Nat. Acad. Sci. U.S.* **69,** 3585.

Briggs, M. H., and Brotherton, J. (1970). "Steroid Biochemistry and Pharmacology," p. 106. Academic Press, New York.

Brink, N. G., Kuehll, F. A., Jr., Richter, J. W., Bazemore, A. W., Meisinger, M. A. P., Ayer, D. D., and Folkers, K. (1952). *J. Amer. Chem. Soc.* **74,** 2120.

Bromer, W. W. (1964). *Abstr., Int. Congr. Biochem., 6th, 1964* Vol. II, p. 24.
Bromer, W. W., and Behrens, O. K. (1962). *Methods Horm. Res.* **2,** 163.
Bromer, W. W., Sinn, L. G., and Behrens, O. K. (1957). *J. Amer. Chem. Soc.* **79,** 2807.
Brown, J. C., Mutt, V., and Pederson, R. A. (1970). *J. Physiol. (London)* **209,** 57.
Brown, P. S. (1955). *J. Endocrinol.* **13,** 59.
Brown, P. S., and Billewicz, W. Z. (1962). *J. Endocrinol.* **24,** 65.
Bruice, T. C., Winzler, R. J., and Kharasch, N. (1954). *J. Biol. Chem.* **210,** 1.
Bruice, T. C., Kharasch, N., and Winzler, R. J. (1956). *Arch. Biochem. Biophys.* **62,** 305.
Bryant, G. D. (1972). *Endocrinology* **91,** 1113.
Burgus, R., and Guillemin, R. (1970). *Annu. Rev. Biochem.* **39,** 499.
Burgus, R., Butcher, M., Amoss, M., Ling, N., Monahan, M., Rivier, J., Fellows, R., Blackwell, R., Vale, W., and Guillemin, R. (1972). *Proc. Nat. Acad. Sci. U.S.* **69,** 278.
Burgus, R., Ling, N., Butcher, M. and Guillemin, R. (1973). *Proc. Nat. Acad. Sci. U.S.* **70,** 684.
Burlington, H., Cronkite, E. P., Reineke, U., and Zanjani, E. D. (1972). *Proc. Nat. Acad. Sci. U.S.* **69,** 3547.
Burzawa-Gerard, E., and Fontaine, Y. A. (1972). *Gen. Comp. Endocrinol., Suppl.* **3,** 715.
Byfield, P. G. H., Clark, M. B., Turner, K., Foster, G. V., and MacIntyre, I. (1972). *Biochem. J.* **127,** 199.
Cahill, C. L., and Hart, K. M. (1969). *Biochim. Biophys. Acta* **194,** 227.
Cahill, C. L., Shetlar, M. R., Payne, R. W., Endicott, B., and Li, Y. T. (1968). *Biochim. Biophys. Acta* **154,** 40.
Callingham, B. A. (1967). *In* "Hormones in Blood" (C. H. Gray and A. L. Bacharach, eds.), 2nd rev. ed., Vol. 2, p. 519. Academic Press, New York.
Camiscoli, J. F., Weintraub, A. H., and Gordon, A. S. (1968). *Ann. N.Y. Acad. Sci.* **149,** 40.
Canterbury, J. M., and Reiss, E. (1972). *Proc. Soc. Exp. Biol. Med.* **140,** 1393.
Capra, J. D., Kehoe, J. M., Kotelchuck, D., Walter, R., and Breslow, E. (1972). *Proc. Nat. Acad. Sci. U.S.* **69,** 431.
Carlsen, R. B., Bahl, O. P., and Swaminathan, N. (1973). *J. Biol. Chem.* **248,** 6810.
Carnot, P., and DeFlandre, C. (1906). *C. R. Acad. Sci.* **143,** 384.
Celis, M. E., Taleisnik, S., and Walter, R. (1971a). *Proc. Nat. Acad. Sci. U.S.* **68,** 1428.
Celis, M. E., Taleisnik, S., and Walter, R. (1971b). *Biochem. Biophys. Res. Commun.* **45,** 564.
Celis, M. E., Hase, S. and Walter, R. (1972). *FEBS (Fed. Eur. Biochem. Soc.) Lett.* **27,** 327.
Chan, L. T., Schaal, S. M., and Saffran, M. (1970). *In* "Hypophysiotropic Hormones of the Hypothalamus" (J. Meites, ed.), p. 253. Williams & Wilkins, Baltimore, Maryland.
Chang, J. K., Sievertsson, H., Currie, B. L., Bogentoft, C., and Folkers, K. (1972). *J. Med. Chem.* **15,** 623.
Chard, T. (1973). *J. Endocrinol.* **58,** 143.
Chauvet, J., Lenci, M. T., and Acher, R. (1960). *Biochim. Biophys. Acta* **38,** 266.
Cheng, K. W., and Friesen, H. G. (1972). *J. Biol. Chem.* **246,** 7656.
Chillemi, F., and Pecile, A. (1971). *Experientia* **27,** 385.
Chu, L. H., McGregor, R. R., Hamilton, J. W., and Cohn, D. V. (1971). *Endocrinology* **89,** 1425.
Churchill, W. H., and Tapley, D. F. (1964). *Nature (London)* **202,** 29.
Claesson, L., Hogberg, B., Rosenberg, T., and Westman, A. (1948). *Acta Endocrinol. (Copenhagen)* **1,** 1.
Clark, I., Bowers, W., and Geoffroy, R. (1960). *Endocrinology* **66,** 527.
Clauberg, C. (1930). *Zentralbl. Gynaekol.* **54,** 2757.
Clossett, J., Hennen, G., and Lequin, R. M. (1972). *FEBS (Fed. Eur. Biochem. Soc.) Lett.* **21,** 325.
Cohen, A. I., and Frieden, E. H. (1961). *J. Biol. Chem.* **236,** 765.
Cohen, A. I., and Frieden, E. H. (1963). *Acta Endocrinol. (Copenhagen)* **42,** 209.

Cohen, A. I., and Furth, J. (1959). *Cancer Res.* **19,** 72.

Cohen, A. I., Bloch, E., and Celozzi, E. (1957). *Proc. Soc. Exp. Biol. Med.* **95,** 304.

Cohen, H. (1963). *Endocrinology* **72,** 164.

Cohen, H., and Steinetz, B. G. (1966). *Proc. Soc. Exp. Biol. Med.* **122,** 268.

Cohn, D. V., MacGregor, R. R., Chu, L. H., Kimmel, J. R., and Hamilton, J. W. (1972). *Proc. Nat. Acad. Sci. U.S.* **69,** 1521.

Cole, R. D., and Li, C. H. (1955). *J. Biol. Chem.* **213,** 197.

Collip, J. B. (1925). *J. Biol. Chem.* **63,** 395.

Collip, J. B., Anderson, E. B., and Thomson, D. L. (1933). *Lancet* **2,** 347.

Condliffe, P., and Jakoby, W. B. (1967). *Endocrinology* **80,** 203.

Contreras, J. F., Gordon, A. S., and Weintraub, A. H. (1966). *Blood* **28,** 330.

Cooper, C. W., Hirsch, P. P., Toverud, S. U., and Munson, P. L. (1967). *Endocrinology* **81,** 610.

Copp, D. H. (1970). *Annu. Rev. Physiol.* **32,** 61.

Copp, D. H., and Kuczerpa, A. V. (1968). *In* "Calcitonin: Symposium on Thyrocalcitonin and the C Cells" (S. F. Taylor, ed.), Conference 1967, p. 18 Heinemann, London.

Corker, C. S., Exley, D., and Naftolin, F. (1970). *Acta Endocrinol. (Copenhagen), Suppl.* **147,** 305.

Corner, G., and Allen, E. (1929). *Amer. J. Physiol.* **88,** 326.

Courte, C., Hurault, M., Clary, C., De la Llosa, P., and Jutisz, M. (1972). *Gen. Comp. Endocrinol.* **18,** 284.

Coy, D. H., Coy, E. J., and Schally, A. V. (1973). *J. Med. Chem.* **16,** 83.

Crick, J., Harper, A. A., and Raper, H. S. (1950). *J. Physiol. (London)* **110,** 367.

Cunningham, N. F., and Hebert, C. N. (1973). *J. Endocrinol.* **58,** 239.

Currie, B. L., Johansson, K. N. G., Folkers, K., and Bowers, C. Y. (1973). *Biochem. Biophys. Res. Commun.* **50,** 14.

Dacke, C. G., and Kenny, C. D. (1973). *Endocrinology* **92,** 463.

Dallenbach, F. D., and Dallenbach-Hellweg, G. (1964). *Virchows Arch. Pathol. Anat. Physiol.* **331,** 301.

David, M. A., Fraschini, F., and Martini, L. (1965). *Experientia* **21,** 483.

Davies, B. M. A., Gordon, A. H., and Mussett, M. V. (1954). *J. Physiol. (London)* **125,** 383.

Davies, B. M. A., Gordon, A. H., and Mussett, M. V. (1955). *J. Physiol. (London)* **130,** 79.

Dayhoff, M. O. (1972). "Atlas of Protein Sequences." Nat. Biomed. Res. Found., Washington, D.C.

Dean, C. R., Hope, D. B., and Kazic, T. (1968). *Brit. J. Pharmacol.* **34,** 192P.

Deftos, L. H. (1971). *Metab., Clin. Exp.* **20,** 1122.

De la Llosa, P., and Jutisz, M. (1969). *In* "Protein and Polypeptide Hormones" (M. Margoulies, ed.), Int. Congr. Ser. No. 161, p. 229. Excerpta Med. Found., Amsterdam.

Delfs, E. (1941). *Endocrinology* **28,** 196.

Dellacha, J. M., Santome, J. A., and Paladini, A. C. (1968). *Ann. N.Y. Acad. Sci.* **148,** 313.

De Martinez, N. R., Garcia, M. C., Salas, M., and Candela, J. L. R. (1973). *Gen. Comp. Endocrinol.* **20,** 305.

Deuben, R. R., and Meites, J. (1964). *Endocrinology* **74,** 408.

Dietrich, F. M., and Rittel, W. (1970). *Nature (London)* **225,** 75.

Dixon, H. B. F. (1962). *Biochem. J.* **83,** 91.

Dixon, H. B. F., and Stack-Dunne, M. P. (1955). *Biochem. J.* **61,** 483.

Dodds, E. C., Goldberg, L., Lawson, W., and Robinson, R. (1938). *Nature (London)* **141,** 247.

Donini, P., Puzzuoli, D., D'Alessio, I., Bergisi, G., and Donini, S. (1968). *In* "Gonadotropins, 1968" (E. Rosemberg, ed.), p. 204. Geron-X, Los Altos, California.

Donini, S., Olivieri, V., Ricci, G., and Donini, P. (1973). *Acta Endocrinol.* (*Copenhagen*) **73,** 133.

Dorfman, R. I. (1948a). *In* "The Hormones" (G. Pincus, and K. V. Thimann, eds.), Vol. 1, p. 484. Academic Press, New York.
Dorfman, R. I. (1948b). *Endocrinology* **42,** 1.
Dorfman, R. I. (1962). *Methods Horm. Res.* **2,** 340.
Dorfman, R. I., and Kincl, F. A. (1963). *Endocrinology* **72,** 259.
Dorfman, R. I., and Kincl, F. A. (1964). *Steroids* **3,** 109.
Dorfman, R. I., Potts, A. M., and Feil, M. (1947). *Endocrinology* **41,** 464.
Drill, V. A. (1959). *Fed. Proc., Fed. Amer. Soc. Exp. Biol.* **18,** 1040.
Drill, V. A., and Riegel, B. (1958). *Recent Progr. Horm. Res.* **14,** 29.
Dufau, M. L., Dulmanis, A., Catt, K. J., and Hudson, B. (1970). *J. Clin. Endocrinol. Metab.* **30,** 351.
du Vigneaud, V., Ressler, C., and Trippett, S. (1953). *J. Biol. Chem.* **205,** 949.
Dyer, F. J., Kidd, D. A. A., and Walker, J. (1952). *J. Chem. Soc. London* p. 4778.
Eisenberg, E., and Gordan, G. S. (1950). *J. Pharmacol. Exp. Ther.* **99,** 38.
Elliott, F. H., Birmingham, M. K., Schally, A. V., and Schonbaum, E. (1954). *Endocrinology* **55,** 721.
Ellis, S. (1961). *Endocrinology* **68,** 334.
Emmens, C. W. (1962a). *Methods Horm. Res.* **2,** 80.
Emmens, C. W. (1962b). *Methods Horm. Res.* **2,** 94.
Erslev, A. (1953). *Blood* **8,** 349.
Espada, J., Langton, A. A., and Dorado, M. (1972). *Biochim. Biophys. Acta* **285,** 427.
Falkmer, S. (1972). *Gen. Comp. Endocrinol., Suppl.* **3,** 184.
Fellows, R. E., Rogel, A. D., and Mudge, A. (1972). *In* "Growth and Growth Hormone" (A. Pecile and E. E. Müller, eds.), Int. Congr. Ser. No. 244, p. 166. Excerpta Med. Found., Amsterdam.
Felton, L., Frieden, E. H., and Bryant, H. H. (1953). *J. Pharmacol. Exp. Ther.* **107,** 160.
Fernandez, H. N., Pena, C., Poskus, E., Biscoglio, M. J., Paladini, A. C., Dellacha, J. M., and Santome, J. A. (1972). *FEBS (Fed. Eur. Biochem. Soc.) Lett.* **25,** 265.
Fieser, L. F., and Fieser, M. (1959). "Steroids," p. 519. Van Nostrand-Reinhold, Princeton, New Jersey.
Fisher, J. D. (1962). *Methods Horm. Res.* **2,** 655.
Florini, J. R., Tonelli, G., Breuer, C. B., Coppola, J., Ringler, I., and Bell, P. H. (1966). *Endocrinology* **79,** 692.
Florsheim, W. H., Moskowitz, N., Schwartz, J. R., and Morton, M. E. (1957). *Endocrinology* **60,** 683.
Folkers, K., Enzmann, F., Boler, J., Bowers, C. Y., and Schally, A. V. (1969). *Biochem. Biophys. Res. Commun.* **37,** 123.
Forsyth, I. (1969). *In* "Lactogenesis" (S. M. Reynolds and S. J. Folley, eds.), p. 197. Univ. of Pennsylvania Press, Philadelphia.
Fried, J., and Borman, A. (1958). *Vitam. Horm. (New York)* **16,** 303.
Fried, W., Plzak, L. F., Jacobson, L. O., and Goldwasser, E. (1957). *Proc. Soc. Exp. Biol. Med.* **94,** 237.
Frieden, E. (1968). *In* "Metamorphosis" (W. Etkin and L. I. Gilbert, eds.), p. 349. Appleton, New York.
Frieden, E., and Lipner, H. (1971). "Biochemical Endocrinology of the Vertebrates," Chapter 3. Prentice-Hall, Englewood, New Jersey.
Frieden, E., and Westmark, G. W. (1961). *Science* **133,** 1487.
Frieden, E., and Winzler, R. (1948). *J. Biol. Chem.* **176,** 155.
Frieden, E. H. (1964). *In* "Actions of Hormones on Molecular Processes" (G. Litwak and D. Krichevsky, eds.), p. 509. Wiley, New York.
Frieden, E. H., and Hisaw, F. L. (1950). *Arch. Biochem.* **29,** 166.

Frieden, E. H., and Hisaw, F. L. (1953). *Recent Progr. Horm. Res.* **8,** 333.
Frieden, E. H., Fischbein, J., and Hisaw, F. L. (1948). *Arch. Biochem.* **17,** 183.
Frieden, E. H., Chen, S. W., and Rawitch, A. B. (1974). *Fed. Proc., Fed. Amer. Soc. Exp. Biol.* **33,** 1358.
Friesen, H. G. (1965). *Endocrinology* **76,** 369.
Friesen, H. G. (1968). *Acta Endocrinol. (Copenhagen)* **58,** 157.
Frohman, L. A., and Bernardis, L. L. (1968). *Endocrinology* **82,** 1125.
Frohman, L. A., Burek, L., and Stachura, M. E. (1972). *Endocrinology* **91,** 262.
Fujino, M., Hatanaka, C., and Nishimura, O. (1970a). *Chem. Pharm. Bull.* **18,** 1288.
Fujino, M., Nishimura, O., and Hatanaka, C. (1970b). *Chem. Pharm. Bull.* **18,** 1291.
Gabe, M., Karlson, P., and Roche, J. (1964). *Comp. Biochem.* **6,** 294.
Gabuzda, T. G., Schumann, M. A., Silver, R. K., and Lewis, H. B. (1968). *J. Clin. Endocrinol. Metab.* **47,** 1895.
Gaddum, J. H. (1927). *J. Physiol. (London)* **64,** 246.
Geiger, V. R., Sturm, K., Vogel, G., and Seidel, W. (1964). *Z. Naturforsch. B* **19,** 858.
Gemmill, C. L. (1940). *Bull. Johns Hopkins Hosp.* **66,** 232.
Gemzell, C., and Roos, P. (1966). *In* "The Pituitary Gland" (G. W. Harris and B. T. Donovan, eds.), Vol. 1, p. 492. Univ. of California Press, Berkeley.
Glick, S. M., Roth, J., Yalow, R. S., and Berson, S. A. (1963). *Nature (London)* **199,** 784.
Givol, D., de Lorenzo, F., Goldberger, R. F., and Anfinsen, C. B. (1965). *Proc. Nat. Acad. Sci. U.S.* **53,** 676.
Goldwasser, E., and Kung, C. K. H. (1968). *Ann. N.Y. Acad. Sci.* **149,** 49.
Goldwasser, E., and Kung, C. K. H. (1971). *Proc. Nat. Acad. Sci. U.S.* **68,** 697.
Goldwasser, E., and Kung, C. K. H. (1972). *J. Biol. Chem.* **247,** 5159.
Goldwasser, E., Jacobson, L. O., Fried, W., and Plzak, L. F. (1958). *Blood* **13,** 55.
Goodfriend, L., and Sehon, A. H. (1960). *Nature (London)* **185,** 764.
Got, R., and Bourrillon, R. (1960). *Biochim. Biophys. Acta* **42,** 505.
Graesslin, D., Weise, H. C., and Braendle, W. (1972). *FEBS (Fed. Eur. Biochem. Soc.) Lett.* **20,** 87.
Grant, G., and Vale, W. (1972). *Nature (London), New Biol.* **237,** 182.
Grant, P. T., and Reid, K. B. M. (1968). *Biochem. J.* **110,** 281.
Greep, R. O., Van Dyke, H. B., and Chow, B. F. (1941). *Proc. Soc. Exp. Biol. Med.* **46,** 644.
Gregory, H. (1970). *Amer. J. Dig. Dis.* **15,** 141.
Gross, J., and Pitt–Rivers, R. (1952). *Lancet* **i,** 439.
Grosvenor, C. E., and Turner, C. W. (1958). *Endocrinology* **63,** 530.
Gudernatsch, J. F. (1912). *Arch. Entwicklungsmech. Organismen* **35,** 457.
Guillemin, R., Hearn, W. R., Cheek, W. R., and Householder, D. E. (1957). *Endocrinology* **60,** 488.
Guillemin, R., Yamazaki, E., Gard, D. A., Jutisz, M., and Sakiz, E. (1963). *Endocrinology* **73,** 564.
Gurin, S., Bachman, C., and Wilson, D. W. (1939). *J. Biol. Chem.* **128,** 525.
Gurin, S., Bachman, C., and Wilson, D. W. (1940). *J. Biol. Chem.* **133,** 467.
Guyda, H. J., and Friesen, H. G. (1971). *Biochem. Biophys. Res. Commun.* **42,** 1068.
Habener, J. F., Segré, G. V., Powell, D., Murray, T. M., and Potts, J. T. (1972). *Nature (London), New Biol.* **238,** 152.
Haggendal, J. (1966). *Pharmacol. Rev.* **18,** 325.
Hales, C. N., and Randle, P. J. (1963). *Biochem. J.* **88,** 137.
Halkes, S. J., Hartog, J., Morsink, L., and de Wachter, A. M. (1972). *J. Med. Chem.* **15,** 1288.
Hall, K., and Newton, W. H. (1947). *J. Physiol. (London)* **106,** 18.
Hano, K., Koida, M., Kubo, K., and Yajima, H. (1964). *Biochim. Biophys. Acta* **90,** 201.
Harper, A. A., and Raper, H. S. (1943). *J. Physiol. (London)* **102,** 115.

Harris, G. W., and Jacobsohn, D. (1952). *Proc. Roy. Soc. Ser. B* **139,** 263.
Hartree, A. S., and Cunningham, F. J. (1969). *J. Endocrinol.* **43,** 609.
Hartung, W. H. (1945). *Ind. Eng. Chem.* **37,** 126.
Haugaard, N., and Marsh, J. B. (1952). *J. Biol. Chem.* **194,** 33.
Hayashida, T. (1969). *Nature (London)* **222,** 294.
Heard, R. D. H., Bligh, E. G., Cann, M. C., Jellinck, P. H., O'Donnell, V. J., Rao, B. G., and Webb, J. L. (1956). *Recent Progr. Horm. Res.* **12,** 45.
Heller, H. (1941). *J. Physiol. (London)* **100,** 125.
Hench, P. S., Kendall, E. C., Slocumb, C. H., and Polley, H. F. (1949). *Proc. Staff Meet. Mayo Clin.* **24,** 181.
Herrick, R. B., McGibbon, W. H., and McShan, W. H. (1962). *Endocrinology* **71,** 487.
Hershberger, L. G., Shipley, E. G., and Meyer, R. K. (1953). *Proc. Soc. Exp. Biol. Med.* **83,** 175.
Hirsch, P. F., Gauthier, G. F., and Munson, P. (1963). *Endocrinology* **73,** 244.
Hirsch, P. F., Voelkel, E. F., and Munson, P. L. (1964). *Science* **146,** 412.
Hodgen, G. D., Nixon, W. E., Vaitukaitis, J. L., Tullner, W. W., and Ross, G. T. (1973). *Endocrinology* **92,** 705.
Hofmann, K. (1962). *Annu. Rev. Biochem.* **31,** 213.
Hofmann, K., and Yajima, H. (1962). *Recent Progr. Horm. Res.* **18,** 41.
Hofmann, K., Yajima, H., Yamaihara, N., Liu, T., and Lande, S. (1961). *J. Amer. Chem. Soc.* **83,** 487.
Hofmann, K., Yajima, H., Liu, T. Y., Yanaihara, N., Yanaihara, C., and Humes, J. L. (1962). *J. Amer. Chem. Soc.* **84,** 4481.
Hofmann, K., Andreatta, R., Bohn, H., and Morode., L. (1970). *J. Med. Chem.* **13,** 339.
Hogg, J. A., and Korman, J. (1956). *Med. Chem. (New York)* **2,** 34.
Holtkamp, D. E., Ochs, S., Pfeiffer, C. C., and Heming, A. E. (1955). *Endocrinology* **56,** 93.
Hooker, C. W., and Forbes, T. R. (1947). *Endocrinology* **41,** 158.
Howard, S. M., and Pierce, J. G. (1969). *J. Biol. Chem.* **244,** 6468.
Hruby, V. J., Smith, C. W., Bower, A., and Hadley, M. E. (1972). *Science* **176,** 1331.
Hsu, T. H., and Bledsoe, T. (1970). *J. Clin. Endocrinol. Metab.* **30,** 443.
Huisman, T. H. J., Adams, H. R., Dimmock, M. O., Edwards, W. E., and Wilson, J. B. (1967). *J. Biol. Chem.* **242,** 2534.
Humbel, R. E. (1963). *Biochim. Biophys. Acta* **74,** 96.
Humbel, R. E. (1965). *Proc. Nat. Acad. Sci. U.S.* **53,** 853.
Hunter, W. M., and Greenwood, F. C. (1964). *Biochem. J.* **91,** 43.
Igarishi, M., and McCann, S. M. (1964). *Endocrinology* **74,** 446.
Ishida, Y., Kuroshima, A., Bowers, C. Y., and Schally, A. V. (1965). *Endocrinology* **77,** 759.
Ivy, A. C., and Oldberg, E. (1928). *Amer. J. Physiol.* **86,** 599.
Jackson, G. L. (1971a). *Endocrinology* **89,** 1454.
Jackson, G. L. (1971b). *Endocrinology* **89,** 1460.
Jensen, E. V., and De Sombre, E. R. (1973). *Science* **182,** 126.
Johansson, K. N. G., Currie, B. L., Folkers, K., and Bowers, C. Y. (1973). *Biochem. Biophys. Res. Commun.* **50,** 8.
Jorgensen, E. C., and Block, P. (1973). *J. Med. Chem.* **16,** 307.
Josimovich, J. B., and MacLaren, J. A. (1962). *Endocrinology* **71,** 209.
Jost, K., and Rudinger, J. (1969). *Colloq. Int. Cent. Nat. Rech. Sci.* **117,** 13.
Kakiuchi, S., and Tomizawa, H. H. (1964). *J. Biol. Chem.* **239,** 2160.
Kastin, A. J., Schally, A. V., Yajima, H., and Kubo, K. (1965). *Nature (London)* **207,** 978.
Kastin, A. J., Viosca, S., and Schally, A. V. (1970). *In* "Hypophysiotropic Hormones of the Hypothalamus" (J. Meites, ed.), p. 171. Williams & Wilkins, Baltimore, Maryland.
Katsoyannis, P. G., and du Vigneaud, V. (1958). *J. Biol. Chem.* **233,** 1352.

Katsoyannis, P. G., Trakatellis, A. C., Zalut, C., Johnson, S., Tometsko, A., Schwartz, G., and Ginos, T. (1967). *Biochemistry* **6,** 2656.
Keighley, G. (1968). *Ann. N.Y. Acad. Sci.* **149,** 18.
Kemper, B., Habener, J. F., Potts, J. T., and Rich, A. (1972). *Proc. Nat. Acad. Sci. U.S.* **69,** 643.
Kenny, A. D., and Munson, P. L. (1959). *Endocrinology* **64,** 513.
Kerdelhue, B., Jutisz, M., Gillessen, D., and Studer, R. O. (1973). *Biochim. Biophys. Acta* **297,** 540.
Keutmann, H. T., Parsons, J. A., Potts, J. T., and Schleuter, R. J. (1970). *J. Biol. Chem.* **245,** 1491.
Keutmann, H. T., Dawson, B. F., Aurbach, G. D., and Potts, J. T. (1972). *Biochemistry* **11,** 1973.
Kimball, C. P., and Murlin, J. R. (1923). *J. Biol. Chem.* **58,** 337.
Kirkham, K. E. (1962). *J. Endocrinol.* **25,** 259.
Kliman, B., and Greep, R. O. (1958). *Endocrinology* **63,** 586.
Knobil, E., and Greep, R. O. (1959). *Recent Progr. Horm. Res.* **15,** 3.
Kochakian, C. D., and Murlin, J. D. (1935). *J. Nutr.* **10,** 437.
Koida, M., Hano, K., and Iso, T. (1966). *Jap. J. Pharmacol.* **16,** 243.
Korenman, S. G., Tulchinsky, D., and William, E. L. (1970). *Acta Endocrinol. (Copenhagen), Suppl.* **147,** 291.
Krantz, S. B., Gallien-Lartigue, O., and Goldwasser, E. (1963). *J. Biol. Chem.* **238,** 4085.
Kroc, R. L., Steinetz, B. G., and Beach, V. L. (1959). *Ann. N.Y. Acad. Sci.* **75,** 942.
Kumar, S., Seelig, S., and Sayers, G. (1972). *Biochem. Biophys. Res. Commun.* **49,** 1316.
Kuroshima, A., Ishida, Y., Bowers, C. Y., and Schally, A. V. (1965). *Endocrinology* **76,** 614.
Kuroshima, A., Arimura, A., Saito, T., Ishida, Y., Bowers, C. Y., and Schally, A. V. (1966). *Endocrinology* **78,** 1105.
Kwa, H. G., and Verhofstad, F. (1967). *Biochim. Biophys. Acta* **133,** 186.
Kwa, H. G., Van der Bent, E. M., and Prop, F. J. A. (1967). *Biochim. Biophys. Acta* **133,** 301.
Laljec, H. C. R., Smith, R. N., and Dorrington, K. J. (1967). *J. Endocrinol.* **39,** 507.
Lande, S., and Lerner, A. B. (1967). *Pharmacol. Rev.* **19,** 1.
Landgrebe, F. W., and Waring, H. (1944). *Quart. J. Exp. Physiol. Cog. Med. Sci.* **33,** 1.
Landgrebe, F. W., and Waring, H. (1962). *Methods Horm. Res.* **2,** 549.
Lauson, H. D., Heller, C. G., Golden, J. B., and Severinghaus, E. L. (1939). *Endocrinology* **24,** 35.
Lee, T. H., and Buettner-Janusch, V. (1963). *J. Biol. Chem.* **238,** 2012.
Leidenberger, F., and Reichert, L. E. (1973). *Endocrinology* **92,** 646.
Lequin, R. M., Hackeng, W. H. L., and Schopman, W. (1969). *J. Endocrinol.* **44,** 283.
Lerner, A. B. (1965). *Proc. Int. Congr. Endocrinol., 2nd, 1964* Int. Congr. Ser. No. 83, p. 392.
Levy, R. P., McGuire, W. L., and Heideman, M. L., Jr. (1962). *Proc. Soc. Exp. Biol. Med.* **110,** 598.
Lewis, U. J., Singh, R. N. P., and Seavey, B. K. (1971). *Biochem. Biophys. Res. Commun.* **44,** 1169.
Li, C. H. (1945). *J. Biol. Chem.* **155,** 45.
Li, C. H. (1956) *Advan. Protein Chem.* **11,** 101.
Li, C. H. (1957). *Advan. Protein Chem.* **12,** 269.
Li, C. H. (1959). *Science* **129,** 969.
Li, C. H. (1972). *Biochem. Biophys. Res. Commun.* **49,** 835.
Li, C. H., and Dixon, J. S. (1956). *Science* **124,** 934.
Li, C. H., and Evans, H. M. (1948). *In* "The Hormones" (G. Pincus and K. V. Thimann, eds.), Vol. I, p. 674. Academic Press, New York.
Li, C. H., and Oelofson, W. (1967). *In* "The Adrenal Cortex" (A. B. Eisenstein, ed.), p. 185. Little, Brown, Boston, Massachusetts.

Li, C. H., and Pedersen, K. O. (1953). *J. Biol. Chem.* **201,** 595.

Li, C. H., and Yamashiro, D. (1970). *J. Amer. Chem. Soc.* **92,** 7608.

Li, C. H., Evans, H. M., and Simpson, M. (1943). *J. Biol. Chem.* **149,** 413.

Li, C. H., Evans, H. M., and Simpson, M. (1945). *J. Biol. Chem.* **159,** 353.

Li, C. H., Fonns-Bech, P., Geschwind, I. I., Hayashida, G. F., Lostroh, A. J., Lyons, W. R., Moon, H. D., Reinhardt, W. O., and Sideman, M. (1957). *J. Exp. Med.* **105,** 335.

Li, C. H., Papkoff, H., and Jordan, C. W. (1959). *Proc. Soc. Exp. Biol. Med.* **100,** 44.

Li, C. H., Dixon, J. S., and Liu, W. K. (1969). *Arch. Biochem. Biophys.* **133,** 70.

Li, C. H., Dixon, J. S., Lo, T. B., Schmidt, K. D., and Pankov, Y. A. (1970). *Arch. Biochem. Biophys.* **141,** 705.

Li, C. H., Dixon, J. S., and Chung, D. (1971). *Science* **173,** 56.

Li, C. H., Gordon, D., and Knorr, J. (1973). *Arch. Biochem. Biophys.* **156,** 493.

Liao, T. H., and Pierce, J. G. (1970). *J. Biol. Chem.* **245,** 3275.

Liao, T. H., and Pierce, J. G. (1971). *J. Biol. Chem.* **246,** 850.

Liao, T. H., Hennen, G., Howard, S. M., Shome, B., and Pierce, J. G. (1969). *J. Biol. Chem.* **244,** 6458.

Licht, P. (1972). *Gen. Comp. Endocrinol.* **19,** 273.

Liddle, G. W., Island, D., and Meador, C. K. (1962). *Recent Progr. Horm. Res.* **18,** 125.

Lieberman, S., Erlanger, B. F., Beiser, S. M., and Agate, F. J., Jr. (1959). *Recent Progr. Horm. Res.* **15,** 165.

Linman, J. W., and Bethell, F. H. (1956). *Blood* **11,** 310.

Linnel, W. H., Mathieson, D. W., and Williams, G. (1951). *Nature (London)* **167,** 237.

Lipscomb, H. S., and Nelson, D. H. (1962). *Endocrinology* **71,** 13.

Loraine, J. A., and Gaddum, J. H. (1950). *J. Endocrinol.* **6,** 319.

Lubowsky, W. A., and Painter, R. H. (1972). *Can. J. Biochem.* **50,** 509.

Lyons, W. R. (1969). *In* "Lactogenesis" (M. Reynolds and S. J. Folley, eds.), p. 223. Univ. of Pennsylvania Press, Philadelphia.

McCann, S. M. (1970). *In* "Hypophysiotropic Hormones of the Hypothalamus" (J. Meites, ed.), p. 90. Williams & Wilkins, Baltimore, Maryland.

McCann, S. M., and Brobek, J. R. (1954). *Proc. Soc. Exp. Biol. Med.* **87,** 318.

McCann, S. M., and Taleisnik, S. (1962). *Amer. J. Physiol.* **202,** 395.

McCann, S. M., Taleisnik, S., and Friedman, H. M. (1960). *Proc. Soc. Exp. Biol. Med.* **104,** 432.

McGinty, D. A., Anderson, C. P., and McCullough, N. B. (1939). *Endocrinology* **24,** 839.

MacGregor, R. R., Chu, L. L. H., Hamilton, J. W., and Cohn, D. V. (1972). *Endocrinology* **92,** 1312.

McKenzie, J. M. (1958). *Endocrinology* **63,** 372.

Maclagen, N. F., and Sheahan, M. M. (1950). *J. Endocrinol.* **6,** 456.

Maghuin-Register, G., and Dockier, A. (1971). *FEBS (Fed. Eur. Biochem. Soc.) Lett.* **19,** 209.

Maghuin-Register, G., and Hennen, G. (1972). *FEBS (Fed. Eur. Biochem. Soc.) Lett.* **23,** 225.

Maghuin-Register, G., Combarnous, Y., and Hennen, G. (1972). *FEBS (Fed. Eur. Biochem. Soc.) Lett.* **25,** 57.

Makman, M. H., and Sutherland, E. W. (1964). *Endocrinology* **75,** 127.

Manley, S. W., Bourke, J. R., and Hawker, R. W. (1969). *Endocrinology* **84,** 1286.

Manning, M., Coy, E. J., Sawyer, W. H., and Acosta, M. (1973). *J. Med. Chem.* **16,** 463.

Marcus, R., and Aurbach, G. D. (1969). *Endocrinology* **85,** 801.

Matsuo, H., Baba, Y., Nair, R. M. G., Arimura, A., and Schally, A. V. (1971). *Biochem. Biophys. Res. Commun.* **43,** 1334.

Mayes, D., and Nugent, C. A. (1970). *Steroids* **15,** 389.

Meites, J. (1966). *In* "Neuroendocrinology" (L. Martini and W. F. Ganong, eds.), Vol. 1, p. 690. Academic Press, New York.

Midgley, A. R. (1966). *Endocrinology* **79,** 10.
Midgley, A. R. (1967). *J. Clin. Endocrinol. Metab.* **27,** 295.
Midgley, A. R., and Niswender, G. D. (1970). *Acta Endocrinol. (Copenhagen), Suppl.* **147,** 320.
Mikhail, G., Wu, C. H., Ferin, M., and Vande Wiele, R. L. (1970). *Steroids* **15,** 333.
Mittler, J. C., and Meites, J. (1964). *Proc. Soc. Exp. Biol. Med.* **117,** 309.
Miyake, T. (1962). *Methods Horm. Res.* **2,** 136.
Miyake, T., and Rooks, W. H. (1966). *Methods Horm. Res.* **5,** 59.
Moffezoli, R. D., Kaplan, G. N., and Chrambach, A. (1972). *J. Clin. Endocrinol. Metab.* **34,** 375.
Money, W. L., Meltzer, R. I., Young, J., and Rawson, R. W. (1958). *Endocrinology* **63,** 20.
Money, W. L., Meltzer, R. I., Feldman, D., and Rawson, R. W. (1959). *Endocrinology* **64,** 123.
Mori, K. F., and Hollands, T. R. (1971). *J. Biol. Chem.* **246,** 7223.
Morley, J. S. (1968). *Proc. Roy. Soc., Ser. B.* **170,** 97.
Motta, M., Piva, F., and Martini, L. (1970). *In* "The Hypothalamus" (L. Martini, M. Motta, and F. Fraschini, eds.), p. 463. Academic Press, New York.
Mueller, E. E., Sawano, S., and Schally, A. V. (1967). *Gen. Comp. Endocrinol.* **9,** 349.
Munsick, R. A., Sawyer, W. H., and Van Dyke, H. B. (1960). *Endocrinology* **66,** 860.
Munson, P. L. (1955). *Ann. N.Y. Acad. Sci.* **60,** 776.
Munson, P. L., and Sheps, M. C. (1958). *Endocrinology* **62,** 173.
Munson, P. L., and Toepel, W. (1958). *Endocrinology* **63,** 785.
Murphy, B. P. (1965). *J. Lab. Clin. Med.* **66,** 161.
Murphy, B. P. (1967). *J. Clin. Endocrinol. Metab.* **27,** 973.
Murphy, B. P. (1969). *Recent Progr. Horm. Res.* **25,** 563.
Murphy, B. P., Engelberg, W., and Pattee, C. J. (1963). *J. Clin. Endocrinol. Metab.* **23,** 293.
Mutt, V., and Jorpes, J. E. (1967). *Recent Progr. Horm. Res.* **23,** 483.
Nagai, S. (1966). *Tohoku J. Exp. Med.* **90,** 219.
Nair, R. M. G., Kastin, A. J., and Schally, A. V. (1971). *Biochem. Biophys. Res. Commun.* **43,** 1376.
Nandi, J. (1967). *Amer. Zool.* **7,** 115.
Newcomer, W. S., and Barrett, R. A. (1960). *Endocrinology* **66,** 409.
Niall, H. D. (1971). *Nature (London), New Biol.* **230,** 90.
Niall, H. D., Hogen, M. L., Tregear, G. W., Segré, G. V., Hwang, P., and Friesen, H. (1973). *Recent Progr. Horm. Res.* **29,** 387.
Nicoll, C. S., and Bern, H. A. (1968). *Gen. Comp. Endocrinol.* **11,** 5.
Nicoll, C. S., and Nichols, C. W., Jr. (1971). *Gen. Comp. Endocrinol.* **17,** 300.
Nuti, L. C., Grimek, H. J., Braselton, W. E., and McShan, W. H. (1972). *Endocrinology* **91,** 1418.
Odell, W. D., Ross, G. T., and Rayford, P. L. (1967a). *J. Clin. Invest.* **46,** 248.
Odell, W. D., Wilber, J. F., and Utiger, R. D. (1967b). *Recent Progr. Horm. Res.* **23,** 47.
Odell, W. D., Charters, A. C., Davidson, W. D., and Thompson, J. C. (1968). *J. Clin. Endocrinol. Metab.* **28,** 1840.
Ondetti, M. A., Rubin, B., Engel, S. L., Pluscec, J., and Sheehan, J. T. (1970). *Amer. J. Dig. Dis.* **15,** 149.
O'Riordan, J. L. H., Potts, J. T., Jr., and Aurbach, G. D. (1971). *Endocrinology* **89,** 234
Östlund, E., Bloom, G., Adams-Ray, J., Ritzen, M., Siegman, M., Nordenstam, H., Lishajko, F., and von Euler, U. S. (1960). *Nature (London)* **188,** 324.
Pabst, M. L., Sheppard, R., and Kuizenga, M. H. (1947). *Endocrinology* **41,** 55.
Pala, A., Meirinho, M., and Benagiano, G. (1973). *J. Endocrinol.* **56,** 441.
Pang, P. K. T. (1971). *J. Exp. Zool.* **178,** 89.
Papkoff, H. (1972). *Gen. Comp. Endocrinol., Suppl.* **3,** 609.

Papkoff, H., and Ekblad, M. (1970). *Biochem. Biophys. Res. Commun.* **40,** 614.
Papkoff, H., and Samy, T. S. A. (1967). *Biochim. Biophys. Acta* **147,** 175.
Papkoff, H., Gospodarowicz, D., and Li, C. H. (1967). *Arch. Biochem. Biophys.* **120,** 434.
Papkoff, H., Solis-Wallckermann, J., Martin, M., and Li, C. H. (1971). *Arch. Biochem. Biophys.* **143,** 226.
Papkoff, H., Sairam, M. R., Farmer, S. W., and Li, C. H. (1973). *Recent Progr. Horm. Res.* **29,** 533.
Parlow, A. F. (1961). *In* "Human Pituitary Gonadotropins" (A. Albert, ed.), p. 300. Thomas, Springfield, Illinois.
Parlow, A. F., and Shome, B. (1974). *J. Clin. Endocrinol. Metab.* **39,** 195.
Parlow, A. F., Kovacic, N., and Bhalla, R. C. (1972). *J. Clin. Endocrinol. Metab.* **35,** 319.
Parsons, J. A., and Reynolds, J. J. (1968). *Lancet* **1,** 1067.
Parsons, J. A., Reit, B., and Robinson, C. J. (1973). *Endocrinology* **92,** 454.
Payne, R. W., Raben, M. S., and Astwood, E. B. (1950). *J. Biol. Chem.* **187,** 719.
Pecile, A., Müller, E., Falconi, G., and Martini, L. (1965). *Endocrinology* **77,** 241.
Peckham, W. D., and Parlow, A. F. (1969). *Endocrinology* **85,** 618.
Peschle, C., D'Avanzo, A., Rappaport, I. A., Russolillo, S., Marone, G., and Condorelli, M. (1973). *Nature (London), New Biol.* **243,** 539.
Pierce, J. G. (1971). *Endocrinology* **89,** 1331.
Pierce, J. G., and Nyc, J. F. (1956). *J. Biol. Chem.* **222,** 777.
Pierce, J. G., Bahl, O. P., Cornell, J. S., and Swaminathan, N. (1971a). *J. Biol. Chem.* **246,** 2321.
Pierce, J. G., Liao, T., Howard, S. M., Shome, B., and Cornell, J. S. (1971b). *Recent. Progr. Horm. Res.* **27,** 165.
Pincus, G. (1948). *In* "The Hormones" (G. Pincus and K. V. Thimann, eds.), Vol. 1, p. 333. Academic Press, New York.
Pless, J., Bauer, W., Bossert, H., Zehnder, K., and Guttman, S. (1972). *Nature (London), New Biol.* **240,** 62.
Pommerenke, W. T. (1934). *Amer. J. Obstet. Gynecol.* **27,** 708.
Porter, J. C., and Jones, J. C. (1956). *Endocrinology* **58,** 62.
Postel, S. (1956). *Endocrinology* **58,** 557.
Potts, J. T., Jr., Keutmann, H. T., Niall, H. D., and Tregear, G. W. (1971). *Vitam. Horm. (New York)* **29,** 41.
Pruss, T. P., Maengwyn-Davies, G. D., and Wurzel, M. (1965). *J. Pharmacol.* **147,** 76.
Psychoyos, S., Ma, D. S., Czernik, A. J., Bowers, H. S., Atkins, C. D., and Cash, W. D. (1973). *Endocrinology* **92,** 243.
Randle, P. J. (1956). *J. Endocrinol.* **14,** 82.
Rasmussen, H., and Westall, R. G. (1957). *Biochem. J.* **67,** 658.
Rauch, R., Hollenberg, M. D., and Hope, D. B. (1969). *Biochem. J.,* **115,** 473.
Rayford, P. L., Vaitukaitis, J. L., Ross, G. T., Morgan, F. J., and Canfield, R. E. (1972). *Endocrinology* **91,** 144.
Redding, T. W., Bowers, C. Y., and Schally, A. V. (1966). *Endocrinology* **79,** 229.
Reed, C. H., and Bryan, G. T. (1960). *Recent Progr. Horm. Res.* **16,** 187.
Reichert, L. E. (1971). *Endocrinology* **89,** 925.
Reichert, L. E., and Lawson, G. M. (1973). *Endocrinology* **93,** 1034.
Reichert, L. E., Leidenberger, F., and Trowbridge, C. G. (1973). *Rec. Progr. Horm. Res.* **29,** 497.
Reichlin, S. (1960). *Endocrinology* **67,** 760.
Reisfield, R. A., and Hertz, R. (1960). *Biochim. Biophys. Acta* **43,** 540.
Renold, A. E., Martin, D. B., Dagenais, Y. M., Steinke, J., Nickerson, R. J., and Sheps, M. C. (1960). *J. Clin. Invest.* **39,** 1487.

Ringold, I. (1961). *In* "Mechanism of Action of Steroid Hormones" (C. A. Villee and L. L. Engel, eds.) p. 200. Pergamon, Oxford.
Riniker, B., Neher, R., Maier, R., Kahnt, F. W., Byfield, P. G. H., Gudmunsson, T. V., Galante, L., and MacIntyre, I. (1968). *Helv. Chim. Acta* **51,** 1738.
Rivier, J., Vale, W., Burgus, R., Ling, N., Amoss, M., Blackwell, R., and Guillemin, R. (1973). *J. Med. Chem.* **16,** 545.
Robinson, R. G., and Fanestil, D. D. (1970). *Acta Endocrinol. (Copenhagen), Suppl.* **147,** 275.
Roche, J., Fontaine, M., and Leloup, J. (1963). *Comp. Biochem.* **5,** 493.
Roos, P., and Gemzell, C. A. (1964). *Biochim. Biophys. Acta* **82,** 218.
Roos, P., and Gemzell, C. A. (1965). "Gonadotropins," *Ciba Found. Symp.* p. 11.
Ryan, R. J., Jiang, N. S., and Hanlon, S. (1970). *Recent Progr. Horm. Res.* **26,** 105.
Ryle, A. P., Sanger, F., Smith, L. F., and Kitai, R. (1955). *Biochem. J.* **60,** 541.
Saffran, M., and Bayliss, M. J. (1953). *Endocrinology* **52,** 140.
Saffran, M., and Schally, A. V. (1955). *Can. J. Biochem. Physiol.* **33,** 408.
Said, S. I., and Mutt, V. (1972). *Eur. J. Biochem.* **28,** 199.
Sairam, M. R., and Li, C. H. (1973a). *Biochem. Biophys. Res. Commun.* **51,** 336.
Sairam, M. R., and Li, C. H. (1973b). *Biochem. Biophys. Res. Commun.* **54,** 426.
Sairam, M. R., Papkoff, H., and Li, C. H. (1972). *Biochem. Biophys. Res. Commun.* **48,** 530.
Sand, T., and Torjesen, P. A. (1973). *Acta Endocrinol. (Copenhagen)* **73,** 444.
Sawyer, W. H. (1966a). *Res. Publ. Ass. Rev. Nerv. Ment. Dis.* **46,** 132.
Sawyer, W. H. (1966b). *In* "The Pituitary Gland" (G. W. Harris and B. T. Donovan, eds.), Vol. 3, p. 288. Univ. of California Press, Berkeley.
Sawyer, W. H., Martin, A. S., and Frieden, E. H. (1953). *Amer. J. Physiol.* **172,** 547.
Saxena, B. B., and Rathnam, P. (1971). *J. Biol. Chem.* **246,** 3549.
Sayers, G., White, A., and Long, C. N. H. (1943). *J. Biol. Chem.* **149,** 425.
Sayers, M. A., Sayers, G., and Woodbury, L. A. (1948). *Endocrinology* **42,** 379.
Schally, A. V. (1973). *Science* **179,** 341.
Schally, A. V., and Kastin, A. J. (1966). *Endocrinology* **79,** 768.
Schally, A. V., Lipscomb, H. S., and Guillemin, R. (1962). *Endocrinology* **71,** 164.
Schally, A. V., Kuroshima, A., Ishidi, Y., Redding, T. W., and Bowers, C. Y. (1965). *Proc. Soc. Exp. Biol. Med.* **118,** 350.
Schally, A. V., Saito, T., Arimura, A., Sawano, S., Bowers, C. Y., White, W. H., and Cohen, A. I. (1967). *Endocrinology* **81,** 882.
Schally, A. V., Arimura, A., Bowers, C. Y., Kastin, A. J., Sawano, S., and Redding, T. W. (1968a). *Recent. Progr. Horm. Res.* **24,** 497.
Schally, A. V., Muller, E. E., and Sawano, S. (1968b). *Endocrinology* **82,** 271.
Schally, A. V., Sawano, S., Arimura, A., Barrett, J. F., Wakayabayashi, I., and Bowers, C. Y. (1969). *Endocrinology* **84,** 1493.
Schally, A. V., Arimura, A., Baba, Y., Nair, R. M. G., Matsuo, H., Redding, T. W., Debeljuk, L., and White, W. F. (1971a). *Biochem. Biophys. Res. Commun.* **43,** 393.
Schally, A. V., Arimura, A., Kastin, A. J., Matsuo, H., Baba, Y., Redding, T. W., Nair, R. M. G., and Debeljuk, L. (1971b). *Science* **173,** 1036.
Schally, A. V., Baba, Y., Nair, R. M. G., and Bennett, C. D. (1971c). *J. Biol. Chem.* **246,** 6647.
Schally, A V., Nair, R. M. G., Redding, T. W., and Arimura, A. (1971d). *J. Biol. Chem.* **246,** 7230.
Schally, A. V., Redding, T. W., Matsuo, H., and Arimura, A. (1972). *Endocrinology* **90,** 1561.
Schally, A. V., Arimura, A., and Kastin, A. J. (1973). *Science* **179,** 341.
Schellabarger, C. J., and Godwin, J. T. (1954). *Endocrinology,* **54,** 230.
Schlesinger, D. H., Frangione, B., and Walter, R. (1972). *Proc. Nat. Acad. Sci. U.S.* **69,** 3350.
Schlumberger, H. D. (1968). *Z. Naturforsch. B* **23,** 1412.
Schmidt-Elmendorff, H., Loraine, J. A., and Bell, E. T. (1962). *J. Endocrinol.* **24,** 349.

Schreiber, V., Eckertova, A., Franc, Z., Koci, J., Rybak, J., and Kmentova, V. (1961). *Experientia* **17,** 264.
Schwartz, I. L., and Livingston, L. M. (1964). *Vitam. Horm. (New York)* **22,** 261.
Schwyzer, R., and Kappeler, H. (1963). *Helv. Chim. Acta* **46,** 1550.
Schwyzer, R., Schiller, P., Seelig, S., and Sayers, G. (1971). *FEBS (Fed. Eur. Biochem. Soc.) Lett.* **19,** 229.
Seavey, B. K., and Lewis, U. J. (1971). *Biochem. Biophys. Res. Commun.* **42,** 905.
Seelig, S., and Sayers, G. (1973). *Arch. Biochem. Biophys.* **154,** 230.
Seelig, S., Sayers, G., Schwyzer, R., and Schiller, P. (1971). *FEBS (Fed. Eur. Biochem. Soc.) Lett.* **19,** 232.
Selenkow, H. A., and Asper, S. P. (1955). *Physiol. Rev.* **35,** 426.
Shaw, W. N., and Chance, R. E. (1968). *Diabetes* **17,** 737.
Shepherd, R. G., Willson, S. D., Howard, K. S., Bell, P. H., Davies, D. S., Davis, S. B., Eigner, E. A., and Shakespeare, N. E. (1956). *J. Amer. Chem. Soc.* **78,** 5067.
Sherwood, C. D., and O'Byrne, E. M. (1974). *Arch. Biochem. Biophys.* **160,** 185.
Sherwood, O. D., Grimek, H. J., and McShan, W. H. (1970). *J. Biol. Chem.* **245,** 2328.
Sherwood, O. D., Rosentreter, K. R., and Birkhimer, M. L. (1975). *Endocrinology,* **96,** 1106.
Shiu, R. P. C., Kelley, P. A., and Friesen, H. G. (1973). *Science* **180,** 968.
Shizume, K., Lerner, A. B., and Fitzpatrick, T. B. (1954). *Endocrinology* **54,** 553.
Shome, B., and Parlow, A. F. (1973). *J. Clin. Endocrinol. Metab.* **36,** 618.
Shome, B., and Parlow, A. F. (1974a). *J. Clin. Endocrinol. Metab.* **39,** 199.
Shome, B., and Parlow, A. F. (1974b). *J. Clin. Endocrinol. Metab.* **39,** 203.
Shome, B., Brown, D. M., Howard, S. M., and Pierce, J. G. (1968). *Arch. Biochem. Biophys.* **126,** 456.
Shoppee, C. W. (1964). "Chemistry of the Steroids," 2nd ed. p. 151. Butterworth, Washington, D.C.
Sievertssen, H., Chang, J. K., von Klandy, A., Bogentoft, C., Currie, B., and Folkers, K. (1972). *J. Med. Chem.* **15,** 222.
Simpson, S. A., and Tait, J. F. (1952). *Endocrinology* **50,** 150.
Skosey, J. L., and Goldstein, D. P. (1966). *Endocrinology* **78,** 218.
Sluyser, M., and Li, C. H. (1964). *Biochim. Biophys. Acta* **82,** 595.
Smith, A. U., Emmens, C. H., and Parkes, A. S. (1947). *J. Endocrinol.* **5,** 186.
Smith, P. E. (1930). *Amer. J. Anat.* **45,** 205.
Sonnenberg, M., Kikutani, M., Free, C. A., Nadler, A. C., and Dellacha, J. M. (1968). *Ann. N.Y. Acad. Sci.* **148,** 532.
Sonnenberg, M., Dellacha, J. M., Free, C. A., and Nadler, A. C. (1969). *J. Endocrinol.* **44,** 255.
Spiegel, A. M., and Bitensky, M. W. (1969). *Endocrinology* **85,** 638.
Stachura, M. E., and Frohman, L. A. (1973). *Endocrinology* **92,** 1708.
Staehlin, M. (1972). *J. Mol. Evol.* **1,** 258.
Stasilli, N. R., Kroc, R. L., and Meltzer, R. I. (1963). *Endocrinology* **64,** 62.
Staub, A., Sinn, L., and Behrens, O. K. (1955). *J. Biol. Chem.* **214,** 619.
Steelman, S. L., and Guillemin, R. (1959). *Proc. Soc. Exp. Biol. Med.* **101,** 600.
Steelman, S. L., and Hirschmann, R. (1967). *In* "The Adrenal Cortex" (A. B. Eisenstein, ed.), p. 345. Little, Brown, Boston, Massachusetts.
Steelman, S. L., and Pohley, F. M. (1953). *Endocrinology* **53,** 604.
Stehle, R. L. (1938). *Ergeb. Vitamin-Hormonforsch.* **1,** 115.
Steiner, D. F., Cunningham, D., Spiegelman, L., and Aten, B. (1967). *Science* **157,** 697.
Steiner, D. F., Clark, J. L., Nolan, C., Rubenstein, A. H., Margoliash, E., Aten, B., and Oyer, P. E. (1969). *Recent Progr. Horm. Res.* **25,** 207.
Steinetz, B. G. (1959). *In* "Recent Progress in the Endocrinology of Reproduction" (C. W. Lloyd, ed.), p. 389. Academic, New York.
Steinetz, B. G., Beach, V. L., and Kroc, R. L. (1962). *Methods Horm. Res.* **2,** 565.

Stephenson, J. R., and Axelrod, A. A. (1971). *Endocrinology* **88,** 1519.
Stetten, D., Jr. (1956). *Science* **124,** 365.
Struck, H. (1967). *Z. Vitam.-, Hormon-Fermentforsch.* **14,** 370.
Swaminathan, N., and Bahl, O. P. (1970). *Biochem. Biophys. Res. Commun.* **40,** 422.
Tashjian, A., Levine, L., and Munson, P. L. (1964). *Endocrinology* **74,** 244.
Tashjian, A., Levine, L., and Wilhelmi, A. E. (1965). *Endocrinology* **77,** 563.
Thomas, K., and Ferin, J. (1968). *J. Clin. Endocrinol. Metab.* **28,** 1667.
Thompson, R. E., and Fisher, J. D. (1953). *Methods Horm. Res.* **2,** 655.
Thomsen, J., Kristiansen, K., Brunfeldt, K., and Sundby, F. (1972). *FEBS (Fed. Eur. Biochem. Soc.) Lett.* **21,** 315.
Thurmon, T. F., Boyer, S. H., Crosby, E. F., Shepard, M. K., Noyes, A. N., and Stohlman, F., Jr. (1970). *Blood* **36,** 598.
Tolksdorf, S., Battin, M. L., Cassidy, J. W., MacLeod, R. M., Warren, F. M., and Perlman, P. L. (1956). *Proc. Soc. Exp. Biol. Med.* **92,** 207.
Tomich, E. G., and Woolett, E. A. (1954). *J. Endocrinol.* **11,** 134.
Track, N. S. (1973). *Comp. Biochem. Physiol. B* **45,** 291.
Tregear, G. W., van Rietshoten, J., Greene, E., Keutmann, H. T., Niall, H. D., Reit, B., Parsons, J. A., and Potts, J. T. (1973). *Endocrinology* **93,** 1349.
Tsuruhara, T., Dufau, M. L., Hickman, J., and Catt, K. J. (1972). *Endocrinology* **91,** 296.
Tuppy, H., and Michl, H. (1953). *Monatsh. Chem.* **84,** 1011.
Unger, R. H., Eisentraut, A. M., McCall, M. S., Keller, S., Lanz, H. C., and Madison, L. L. (1959). *Proc. Soc. Exp. Biol. Med.* **102,** 621.
Unger, R. H., Eisentraut, A. M., McCall, M. S., and Madison, L. I. (1961). *J. Clin. Invest.* **40,** 1280.
Utiger, R. D., Parker, M. L., and Daughaday, W. H. (1962). *J. Clin. Invest.* **41,** 254.
Utiger, R. D., Odell, W. D., and Condliffe, P. G. (1963). *Endocrinology* **73,** 359.
Vaitukaitis, J. L., Ross, G. T., and Reichert, L. E. (1972). *Endocrinology* **92,** 411.
Vale, W., Rivier, J., and Burgus, R. (1971). *Endocrinology* **89,** 1485.
Van Dyke, H. B., Chow, B. F., Greep, R. O., and Rothen, A. (1942). *J. Pharmacol. Exp. Ther.* **74,** 190.
Vane, J. R. (1964). *Brit. J. Pharmacol. Chemother.* **23,** 360.
Vane, J. R. (1966). *Pharmacol. Rev.* **18,** 317.
Van Hell, H., Goverde, B. C., Schuurs, A. H. W. M., De Jager, E., Matthijsen, R., and Homan, J. D. H. (1966). *Nature (London)* **212,** 261.
Van Vliet, G., and Huisman, T. H. J. (1964). *Biochem. J.* **93,** 401.
Vermuelen, A., and Verdonck, L. (1970). *Acta Endocrinol. (Copenhagen), Suppl.* **147,** 204 and 239.
Vernikos-Danellis, J. (1964). *Endocrinology* **75,** 514.
Vernikos-Danellis, J., and Marks, B. H. (1970). *In* "Hypophysiotropic Hormones of the Hypothalamus" (J. Meites, ed.), p. 60. Williams & Wilkins, Baltimore, Maryland.
Vida, J. A. (1969). "Androgens and Anabolic Agents." Academic Press, New York.
Vinik, A. I., Kaplan, S. L., and Grumbach, M. M. (1973). *Endocrinology* **92,** 1051.
von Euler, U. S. (1961). *Nature (London)* **190,** 170.
Von Mering, J., and Minkowski, O. (1889). *Arch. Exp. Pathol. Pharmakol.* **26,** 371.
Walter, R., and Chen, W. Y. (1967). *J. Amer. Chem. Soc.* **89,** 3892.
Wang, S. S., and Carpenter, F. H. (1965). *J. Biol. Chem.* **240,** 1619.
Ward, D. N., Reichert, L. E., Jr., Liu, W. K., Nahm, H. S., Hsia, J., Lamkin, W. M., and Jones, N. S. (1973). *Rec. Progr. Horm. Res.* **29,** 533.
Ward, H. P. (1967). *Proc. Soc. Exp. Biol. Med.* **125,** 370.
Weber, v.W., Hornle, S., Grieser, G., Herzog, K. H., and Weitzel, G. (1967). *Hoppe-Seyler's Z. Physiol. Chem.* **348,** 1715.
Weil-Malherbe, H. (1968). *Methods Biochem. Anal.* **16,** 293.

Wherry, F. E., Pennington, L. L., Bates, R. W., Garrison, M. M., Ehle, A. L., and Mason, J. W. (1970). *Endocrinology* **86,** 769.
White, A., Bosnes, R. W., and Long, C. N. H. (1942). *J. Biol. Chem.* **143,** 447.
White, A., Handler, P., and Smith, E. L. (1973). "Principles of Biochemistry," p. 1084. McGraw-Hill, New York.
White, W. F. (1953). *J. Amer. Chem. Soc.* **75,** 503.
Whittlestone, W. G. (1969). *Chem. N. Z.* **33,** 69.
Wide, L., Nillius, S. J., Gemzell, C., and Roos, P. (1973). *Acta Endocrinol. (Copenhagen), Suppl.* **174,** 7.
Wilde, C. E., and Bagshawe, K. D. (1965). *Gonadotropins, Ciba Found. Symp.* p. 46.
Wilde, C. E., Orr, A. H., and Bagshawe, K. D. (1967). *J. Endocrinol.* **37,** 23.
Wilhelmi, A. E. (1955). *Hypophyseal Growth Horm., Nature Actions, Henry Ford Hosp. Int. Symp., 1954* p. 59.
Wilhelmi, A. E. (1968). *Yale J. Biol. Med.* **41,** 199.
Wilhelmi, A. E., and Mills, J. B. (1968). *Colloq. Int. Cent. Nat. Rech. Sci.* **177,** 165.
Winegrad, A. I., and Renold, A. E. (1958). *J. Biol. Chem.* **233,** 273.
Wiqvist, N., and Paul, K. G. (1958). *Acta Endocrinol. (Copenhagen)* **29,** 135.
Woodhead, J. S., O'Riordan, J. L. H., Keutmann, H. T., Stoltz, M. L., Dawson, B. F., Niall, H. D., Robinson, C. J., and Potts, J. T. (1971). *Biochemistry* **10,** 2787.
Wright, A. D., and Taylor, K. W. (1967). *In* "Hormones in Blood" (C. H. Gray and A. L. Bacharach, eds.) 2nd rev. ed., Vol. 1, p. 40. Academic Press, New York.
Wright, P. A. (1948). *J. Cell. Comp. Physiol.* **31,** 111.
Wuensch, E. (1967). *Z. Naturforsch. B* **22,** 1269.
Wuensch, E., and Wendelberger, G. (1968). *Chem. Ber.* **101,** 341.
Wuensch, E., Jaeger, E., Deffner, M., and Scharf, R. (1972). *Hoppe-Seyler's Z. Physiol. Chem.* **353,** 1716.
Wurtman, R. J. (1970). *In* "Hypophysiotropic Hormones of the Hypothalamus" (J. Meites, ed.), p. 184. Williams & Wilkins, Baltimore, Maryland.
Wuu, T. C., Crumm, S., and Saffran, M. (1971). *J. Biol. Chem.* **246,** 6043.
Yajima, H., Kubo, K., Kinomura, Y., and Lande, S. (1966). *Biochim. Biophys. Acta* **127,** 545.
Yalow, R. S., and Berson, S. A. (1960). *J. Clin. Invest.* **39,** 1157.
Yalow, R. S., and Berson, S. A. (1961). *Diabetes* **10,** 339.
Yalow, R. S., and Berson, S. A. (1972). *Biochem. Biophys. Res. Commun.* **48,** 391.
Yamasaki, N., Kikutani, M., and Sonenberg, M. (1970). *Biochemistry* **9,** 1107.
Yamasaki, N., Kangawa, K., Kobayashi, S., Kikutani, M., and Sonenberg, M. (1972). *J. Biol. Chem.* **247,** 3874.
Yanaihara, N., Yanaihara, C., Sakagami, M., Tsuji, K., Hashimoto, T., Kaneko, T., Oka, H., Schally, A. V., Arimura, A., and Redding, T. (1973). *J. Med. Chem.* **16,** 373.
Yoshimi, T., and Lipsett, M. B. (1968). *Steroids* **11,** 527.
Young, J. D., Lazarus, L., Chisholm, D. J., and Atkinson, F. F. V. (1968). *J. Nucl. Med.* **9,** 641.
Zanati, G., and Wolff, M. E. (1973). *J. Exp. Med.* **16,** 90.
Zanelli, J. M., Lea, D. J., and Nisber, J. A. (1969). *J. Endocrinol.* **43,** 33.
Zander, J., Forbes, T. R., Von Munstermann, A. M., and Naher, R. (1958). *J. Clin. Endocrinol. Metab.* **18,** 337.
Zilliacus, H., and Roos, B. E. (1951). *Acta Endocrinol. (Copenhagen)* **6,** 147.

Index

Tabular material is indicated by (T) next to the page number.

U

V

6
7
8
9
0
1
2
3
4
5